How to access the supplemental web resource

We are pleased to provide access to a web resource that supplements *Guidelines for Cardiac Rehabilitation and Secondary Prevention Programs, Fifth Edition.* This resource offers reproducible questionnaires, charts, consent forms, protocols, records, checkl

Access
Follow   w book:

1. Visit **w**
   Guideli   ograms.

2. Click th   ition
   book cover.

3. Click the Sign In link on the left or top of the page. If you do not have an account with Human Kinetics, you will be prompted to create one.

4. If the online product you purchased does not appear in the Ancillary Items box on the left of the page, click the Enter Key Code option in that box. Enter the key code that is printed at the right, including all hyphens. Click the Submit button to unlock your online product.

5. After you have entered your key code the first time, you will never have to enter it again to access this product. Once unlocked, a link to your product will permanently appear in the menu on the left. For future visits, all you need to do is sign in to the textbook's website and follow the link that appears in the left menu!

→ Click the Need Help? button on the textbook's website if you need assistance along the way.

How to access the web resource if you purchased a used book:

You may purchase access to the web resource by visiting the text's website, **www.HumanKinetics.com/ GuidelinesForCardiacRehabilitationAndSecondaryPreventionPrograms,** or by calling the following:

800-747-4457 . . . . U.S. customers
800-465-7301 . . . . .Canadian customers
+44 (0) 113 255 5665 . . . . European customers
08 8372 0999 . . . . Australian customers
0800 222 062 . . . . .New Zealand customers
217-351-5076 . . . . .International customers

`D1342577`

For technical support, send an e-mail to:
support@hkusa.com . . . . U.S. and international customers
info@hkcanada.com . . . . Canadian customers
academic@hkeurope.com . . . . European customers
keycodesupport@hkaustralia.com . . . . . Australian and New Zealand customers

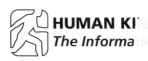

HUMAN KINETICS
The Informa   *ity & Health*

WG
219
AME
07-2013

Product: Guidelines for Cardiac Rehabilitation and Secondary Prevention Programs, Fifth Edition, web resource

Key code: AACVPR-VJPSKB-OSG

This unique code allows you access to the web resource.

Access is provided if you have purchased a new book. Once submitted, the code may not be entered for any other user.

Guidelines for Cardiac Rehabilitation and Secondary Prevention Programs

Fifth Edition

American Association of Cardiovascular
and Pulmonary Rehabilitation

This book has been reviewed and endorsed
by the American Heart Association

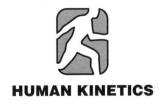

HUMAN KINETICS

Library of Congress Cataloging-in-Publication Data

American Association of Cardiovascular & Pulmonary Rehabilitation, author.
  Guidelines for cardiac rehabilitation and secondary prevention programs / American Association of Cardiovascular and Pulmonary Rehabilitation. -- Fifth edition.
      p. ; cm.
  Preceded by: Guidelines for cardiac rehabilitation and secondary prevention programs / American Association of Cardiovascular and Pulmonary Rehabilitation. 4th ed. c2004.
  Includes bibliographical references and index.
  I. Title.
  [DNLM: 1. Heart Diseases--rehabilitation--Guideline. 2. Heart Diseases--prevention & control--Guideline.WG 210]
  RC682
  616.1'203--dc23
                    2013022228

ISBN-13: 978-1-4504-5963-1

This book is a revised edition of *Guidelines for Cardiac Rehabilitation Programs,* published in 1991, 1995, and 1999 by American Association of Cardiovascular and Pulmonary Rehabilitation, Inc.

The web addresses cited in this text were current as of May 16, 2013, unless otherwise noted.

Acquisitions Editor: Amy Tocco; **Developmental Editor:** Kevin Matz; **Assistant Editors:** Susi Huls and Melissa Zavala; **Copyeditor:** Joyce Sexton; **Indexer:** Nancy Ball; **Permissions Manager:** Dalene Reeder; **Graphic Designer:** Joe Buck; **Graphic Artists:** Nancy Rasmus and Yvonne Griffith; **Cover Designer:** Keith Blomberg; **Photographs (interior):** Steve Kowalski: A Better Exposure/© Human Kinetics, unless otherwise noted, photo on page 32 courtesy of Mark Williams; **Visual Production Assistant:** Joyce Brumfield; **Photo Production Manager:** Jason Allen; **Art Manager:** Kelly Hendren; **Associate Art Manager:** Alan L. Wilborn; **Illustrations:** © Human Kinetics; **Printer:** Sheridan Books

We thank the Cardiac Center of Creighton University in Omaha, Nebraska, for assistance in providing the location for the photo shoot for this book.

Printed in the United States of America

10 9 8 7 6 5 4 3 2

The paper in this book is certified under a sustainable forestry program.

Human Kinetics
Website: www.HumanKinetics.com

United States: Human Kinetics
P.O. Box 5076
Champaign, IL 61825-5076
800-747-4457
e-mail: humank@hkusa.com

Canada: Human Kinetics
475 Devonshire Road Unit 100
Windsor, ON N8Y 2L5
800-465-7301 (in Canada only)
e-mail: info@hkcanada.com

Europe: Human Kinetics
107 Bradford Road
Stanningley
Leeds LS28 6AT, United Kingdom
+44 (0) 113 255 5665
e-mail: hk@hkeurope.com

Australia: Human Kinetics
57A Price Avenue
Lower Mitcham, South Australia 5062
08 8372 0999
e-mail: info@hkaustralia.com

New Zealand: Human Kinetics
P.O. Box 80
Torrens Park, South Australia 5062
0800 222 062
e-mail: info@hknewzealand.com

E5992

Contents

Contributors vii

Preface xi

Chapter 1 Cardiac Rehabilitation, Secondary Prevention Programs, and the Evolution of Health Care: Providing Optimal Care for All Patients 1

Cardiac Rehabilitation: Finding Its Place in the Evolving Health Care Arena . . . 2

Cardiac Rehabilitation Programs as Secondary Prevention Centers 3

Summary 4

Chapter 2 The Continuum of Care: From Inpatient and Outpatient Cardiac Rehabilitation to Long-Term Secondary Prevention . . . 5

Cardiovascular Continuum of Care 6

Efforts to Reduce Gaps in the Continuum of Care 13

The Role of CR/SP in the Continuum of Care 17

Putting It All Together 17

Summary 18

Chapter 3 Behavior Modification and Risk Factor Reduction: Guiding Principles and Practices 19

Overview of Patient Education and Health Behavior Change 20

Summary 28

Chapter 4 Nutrition Guidelines 31

Dietary Patterns 32

Obesity and Weight Control 32

Fat Versus Sugar Intake 34

Anti-Inflammatory Diet 35

Dietary Supplements 36

Relevant Guideline Updates 37

Summary 38

Chapter 5 Cardiac Rehabilitation in the Inpatient and
Transitional Settings 41

Assessment, Mobilization, and Risk-Factor Management 42
Discharge Planning 47
Clinical Pathways 49
Staffing 50
Space and Equipment 52
Transitional Programming 52
Summary 54

Chapter 6 Medical Evaluation and Exercise Testing 57

Physical Examination 59
Risk Stratification and Identification of Contraindications for
    Exercise Training 60
Summary 70

Chapter 7 Outpatient Cardiovascular Rehabilitation and
Secondary Prevention 71

Structure of Secondary Prevention. 76
Coaching and Case Management 77
Assessment and Management of Risk Factors for Disease Progression 77
Innovation in CR/SP 85
Maintenance CR/SP 85
Implementation of Secondary Prevention 88
Summary 88

Chapter 8 Modifiable Cardiovascular Disease Risk Factors 89

Tobacco Use 90
Abnormal Lipids 95
Hypertension. 106
Physical Inactivity 109
Diabetes. 122
Psychosocial Considerations. 130
Overweight and Obesity 137
Emerging Risk Factors 141
Summary 142

Chapter 9   Special Populations. 143

     Older and Younger Adults 144

     Women 150

     Racial and Cultural Diversity. 154

     Revascularization and Valve Surgery. 162

     Dysrhythmias. 166

     Heart Failure and Left Ventricular Assist Devices. 170

     Cardiac Transplantation 179

     Peripheral Arterial Disease. 185

     Chronic Lung Disease 189

     Summary. 191

Chapter 10   Program Administration. 193

     Program Priorities 194

     Facilities and Equipment 200

     Organizational Policies and Procedures. 202

     Insurance and Reimbursement 203

     Documentation 205

     Personnel 207

     Continuum of Care and Services 210

     Summary. 210

Chapter 11   Outcomes Assessment and Utilization 211

     Outcomes Matrix 212

     Outcomes in Contrast to Performance Measures 218

     Resources 223

     Summary 223

Chapter 12   Management of Medical Problems and Emergencies 225

     Potential Risks in Outpatient CR/SP 226

     Intervention Summary 228

     Nontraditional Programs. 232

     Summary 234

     Appendices. 235

     References 273

     Index 313

     About the AACVPR 323

Contributors

Mark A. Williams, PhD, MAACVPR, FACSM, Editor
Jeffrey L. Roitman, EdD, FACSM, Editor

CONTRIBUTORS

Philip A. Ades, MD, FAACVPR

Professor of Medicine, Division of Cardiology

University of Vermont College of Medicine

Burlington, VT

Chapter 9—Special Populations: Older and Younger Adults

Gary J. Balady, MD, FAHA, FACC

Director, Non-Invasive Cardiovascular Labs and Preventive Cardiology, Boston Medical Center

Professor of Medicine, Boston University School of Medicine

Boston, MA

Chapter 6—Medical Evaluation and Exercise Testing

Theresa M. Beckie, PhD, FAHA

Professor, College of Nursing

University of South Florida

Tampa, FL

Chapter 9—Special Populations: Women

Kathy Berra, MSN, NP-C, FAHA, FAACVPR, FPCNA, FAAN

Cardiovascular Nurse Practitioner

Stanford Prevention Research Center

Stanford University School of Medicine

Stanford, CA

Chapter 1—Cardiac Rehabilitation, Secondary Prevention Programs, and the Evolution of Health Care: Providing Optimal Care for All Patients

Jenna B. Brinks, MS

Clinical Exercise Physiologist

Beaumont Health System

Royal Oak, MI

Chapter 7—Outpatient Cardiovascular Rehabilitation and Secondary Prevention

Jennifer J. Cameron, PhD

Staff Psychologist

Hunter Holmes McGuire VA Medical Center

Richmond, VA

Chapter 8—Modifiable Cardiovascular Disease Risk Factors: Psychosocial Considerations

Brian W. Carlin, MD, MAACVPR

Assistant Professor of Medicine

Drexel University School of Medicine

Sleep Medicine and Lung Health Consultants

Pittsburgh, PA

Chapter 9—Special Populations: Chronic Lung Disease

Rita A. Frickel, MS, RD, LMNT

Clinical Dietitian, Division of Cardiology

Creighton University School of Medicine

Omaha, NE

Chapter 8—Modifiable Cardiovascular Disease Risk Factors: Hypertension

Christopher D. Gardner, PhD

Associate Professor of Medicine, Stanford Prevention Research Center

Stanford University

Stanford, CA

Chapter 4—Nutrition Guidelines

Helen L. Graham, PhD, MSN, RN-BC

Manager, Cardiac Rehabilitation Program, Cardiology Quality Programs

Nurse Manager Cardiovascular Services

Centura Health, Penrose-St. Francis Health Services

Colorado Springs, CO

Chapter 11—Outcomes Assessment and Utilization

Larry F. Hamm, PhD, MAACVPR, FACSM

Professor of Exercise Science

School of Public Health and Health Services

The George Washington University

Washington, DC

Chapter 9—Special Populations: Revascularization and Valve Surgery

Karen K. Hardy, RN, BSN

Coordinator, Cardiovascular Disease Prevention and Rehabilitation

Cardiac Center of Creighton University

Omaha, NE

Chapter 12—Management of Medical Problems and Emergencies

Tom T. Hee, MD, FACC

Professor of Medicine and Director, Cardiac Electrophysiology Laboratory and Arrhythmia Device Clinic

Creighton University School of Medicine, Division of Cardiology

Omaha, NE

Chapter 9—Special Populations: Dysrhythmias

Leonard A. Kaminsky, PhD, FACSM

Professor of Exercise Science

Director, Clinical Exercise Physiology Program

Ball State University

Muncie, IN

Chapter 8—Modifiable Cardiovascular Disease Risk Factors: Physical Inactivity

Dennis Kerrigan, PhD

Senior Exercise Physiologist

Division of Cardiovascular Medicine

Henry Ford Hospital

Detroit, MI

Chapter 9—Special Populations: Heart Failure and Left Ventricular Assist Devices

Steven J. Keteyian, PhD, FAACVPR, FACSM

Director, Preventive Cardiology

Division of Cardiovascular Medicine

Henry Ford Hospital

Detroit, MI

Chapter 9—Special Populations: Heart Failure and Left Ventricular Assist Devices

Tom LaFontaine, PhD, ACSM RCEP, FAACVPR

Clinical Exercise Physiologist, Independent Contractor

Optimus: The Center for Health

Columbia, MO

Chapter 8—Modifiable Cardiovascular Disease Risk Factors: Emerging Risk Factors

Cindy Lamendola, MSN, NP, FAACVPR, FAHA

Clinical Research Nurse Coordinator

Stanford University School of Medicine

Stanford, CA

Chapter 8—Modifiable Cardiovascular Disease Risk Factors: Abnormal Lipids

Steven W. Lichtman, EdD, FAACVPR

Director, Cardiopulmonary Outpatient Services

Helen Hayes Hospital

West Haverstraw, NY

Chapter 5—Cardiac Rehabilitation in the Inpatient and Transitional Settings

Karen Lui, RN, MS, MAACVPR

GRQ, LLC

Vienna, VA

Chapter 10—Program Administration

Tom Mahady, MS, CSCS

Senior Exercise Physiologist, Cardiac Prevention and Rehabilitation

Hackensack University Medical Center

Hackensack, NJ

Chapter 8—Modifiable Cardiovascular Disease Risk Factors: Diabetes

Patrick McBride, MD, MPH, FACC, FAHA

Professor of Medicine and Family Medicine and Associate Director, Preventive Cardiology

University of Wisconsin School of Medicine and Public Health

Madison, WI

Chapter 1—Cardiac Rehabilitation, Secondary Prevention Programs, and the Evolution of Health Care: Providing Optimal Care for All Patients

Nancy Houston Miller, RN, BSN, FAHA, FAACVPR

Associate Director of the Stanford Cardiac Rehabilitation Program

Stanford University, Stanford, CA

Adjunct Clinical Assistant Professor

University of California, San Francisco School of Nursing

San Francisco, CA

Chapter 8—Modifiable Cardiovascular Disease Risk Factors: Tobacco Use

Ana Mola, MA, RN, ANP-BC, CTTS, FAACVPR

Program Director, Joan and Joel Smilow Cardiopulmonary Rehabilitation and Prevention Center, Rusk Institute of Rehabilitation Medicine

New York University Langone Medical Center

New York, NY

Chapter 9—Special Populations: Racial and Cultural Diversity

Jeffrey L. Roitman, EdD, FACSM

Chair, Associate Professor

Department of Exercise and Sport Science

Rockhurst University

Kansas City, MO

Chapter 7—Outpatient Cardiovascular Rehabilitation and Secondary Prevention

Patrick D. Savage, MS, FAACVPR

Senior Exercise Physiologist, Cardiac Rehabilitation

Fletcher Allen Health Care

Burlington, VT

Chapter 8—Modifiable Cardiovascular Disease Risk Factors: Overweight and Obesity

Lisa A. Benz Scott, PhD

Director, Program in Public Health

Stony Brook University Health Sciences Center

Associate Professor, Schools of Health Technology and Management, and Medicine

Stony Brook University

Stony Brook, NY

Chapter 3— Behavior Modification and Risk Factor Reduction: Guiding Principles and Practices

Paul Sorace, MS, ACSM RCEP, CSCS

Clinical Exercise Physiologist, Cardiac Prevention and Rehabilitation

Hackensack University Medical Center

Hackensack, NJ

Chapter 8—Modifiable Cardiovascular Disease Risk Factors: Diabetes

Douglas R. Southard, PhD, MPH, PA-C, FAACVPR

Dean, College of Graduate and Professional Studies

Franklin Pierce University

Manchester, NH

Chapter 8—Modifiable Cardiovascular Disease Risk Factors: Psychosocial Considerations

Ray W. Squires, PhD, FACSM, FAACVPR, FAHA

Professor of Medicine, Division of Cardiovascular Diseases and Internal Medicine

Mayo Clinic

Rochester, MN

Chapter 9—Special Populations: Cardiac Transplantation

Kerry J. Stewart, EdD, FAHA, MAACVPR, FACSM

Professor of Medicine and Director Clinical and Research Exercise Physiology

Johns Hopkins University School of Medicine

Baltimore, MD

Chapter 9—Special Populations: Dysrhythmias

Chapter 9—Special Populations: Peripheral Arterial Disease

Randal J. Thomas, MD, MS, FAACVPR, FACC, FACP, FAHA

Director, Cardiovascular Health Clinic, Cardiovascular Division

Mayo Clinic and Foundation

Rochester, MN

Chapter 2—The Continuum of Care: From Inpatient and Outpatient Cardiac Rehabilitation to Long-Term Secondary Prevention

Carmen M. Terzic, MD, PhD

Department of Internal Medicine, Division of Cardiovascular Diseases and Department of Physical Medicine and Rehabilitation

Mayo Clinic

Rochester, MN

Chapter 9—Special Populations: Racial and Cultural Diversity

Mitchell H. Whaley, PhD, FACSM

Professor of Exercise Science

Dean, College of Applied Sciences and Technology

Ball State University

Muncie, IN

Chapter 8—Modifiable Cardiovascular Disease Risk Factors: Physical Inactivity

Michael D. White, MD, FACC

Associate Dean for Medical Education and Assistant Professor of Medicine, Division of Cardiology

Creighton University School of Medicine

Omaha, NE

Chapter 8—Modifiable Cardiovascular Disease Risk Factors: Hypertension

REVIEWERS

Ross Arena, PhD, PT, FAACVPR, FAHA, FACSM

Professor and Head, Department of Physical Therapy, College of Applied Health Sciences

University of Illinois at Chicago

Chicago, IL

Gerene S. Bauldoff, PhD, RN, FAACVPR, FAAN

Professor of Clinical Nursing

Ohio State University College of Nursing

Columbus, OH

Todd M. Brown, MD, MSPH, FACC

Assistant Professor of Medicine, Division of Cardiovascular Diseases

University of Alabama at Birmingham

Birmingham, AL

Eileen G. Collins, PhD, RN, FAACVPR, FAAN

Research Career Scientist, Edward Hines Jr., VA Hospital

Professor, College of Nursing, University of Illinois at Chicago

Chicago, IL

Barb Fagan, MS, RCEP, FAACVPR

Director of Employer Services and Cardiopulmonary Rehabilitation Services

Froedtert Health

Milwaukee, WI

Rita A. Frickel, MS, RD, LMNT

Clinical Dietitian, Division of Cardiology

Creighton University School of Medicine

Omaha, NE

Chris Garvey FNP, MSN, MPA, FAACVPR

Manager, Seton Pulmonary and Cardiac Rehabilitation

Daly City, CA

Nurse Practitioner, UCSF Sleep Disorders

San Francisco, CA

Anne M. Gavic, MPA, FAACVPR

Manager, Cardiopulmonary Rehabilitation

Northwest Community Hospital

Arlington Heights, IL

Karen K. Hardy, RN, BSN

Coordinator, Cardiovascular Disease Prevention and Rehabilitation

Cardiac Center of Creighton University

Omaha, NE

Tom T. Hee, MD, FACC

Professor of Medicine and Director, Cardiac Electrophysiology Laboratory

Division of Cardiology, Creighton University School of Medicine

Omaha, NE

Reed Humphrey, PT, PhD, MAACVPR

Professor and Chair, School of Physical Therapy and Rehabilitation Science

College of Health Professions and Biomedical Sciences

University of Montana

Missoula, MT

Marjorie King, MD, FACC, MAACVPR

Director, Cardiac Services, Helen Hayes Hospital

West Haverstraw, NY

Assistant Clinical Professor of Medicine, Columbia University

New York, NY

Carl "Chip" J. Lavie, MD, FACC, FACP, FCCP

Professor of Medicine, Ochsner Heart and Vascular Institute

Ochsner Clinical School, The University of Queensland School of Medicine

New Orleans, LA

Department of Preventive Medicine

Pennington Biomedical Research Center, Louisiana State University System

Baton Rouge, LA

Murray Low, EdD, MAACVPR, FACSM

Director, Cardiac Rehabilitation

Stamford Hospital

Stamford, CT

Karen Lui, RN, MS, MAACVPR

GRQ, LLC

Vienna, VA

Timothy R. McConnell, PhD, FAACVPR, FACSM

Chair and Professor, Department of Exercise Science

Bloomsburg University

Bloomsburg, PA

Michael McNamara, MS, FAACVPR

Cardiovascular Health Program

Montana Department of Public Health and Human Services

Helena, MT

Joseph F. Norman, PhD, PT, CCS, FAACVPR

Professor, Physical Therapy Education

University of Nebraska Medical Center

Omaha, NE

Gayla Oakley, RN, FAACVPR

Director, Cardiology Services and Prevention

Boone County Health Center

Albion, NE

Bonnie K. Sanderson, PhD, RN, FAACVPR

Associate Professor, School of Nursing

Auburn University

Auburn, AL

Patrick D. Savage, MS, FAACVPR

Senior Exercise Physiologist, Cardiac Rehabilitation

Fletcher Allen Health Care

Burlington, VT

Randal J. Thomas, MD, MS, FAACVPR, FACC, FACP, FAHA

Director, Cardiovascular Health Clinic, Cardiovascular Division

Mayo Clinic and Foundation

Rochester, MN

Preface

The time between the publication of the previous edition and this Fifth Edition of the American Association of Cardiovascular and Pulmonary Rehabilitation (AACVPR) *Guidelines for Cardiac Rehabilitation and Secondary Prevention Programs* has provided additional, stronger evidence of two significant facts:

- Participation in outpatient cardiac rehabilitation and secondary prevention (CR/SP) decreases mortality and recurrent morbidity after a cardiac event.
- Despite this conclusive evidence, medical referral to and participation in CR/SP has not increased significantly, remaining at a level that belies its safety, efficacy, and cost-effectiveness.

The literature clearly supports the efficacy of participating in CR/SP, as well as the efficacy of risk factor intervention and lifestyle change for prevention of primary and recurrent cardiovascular events. These components must be the essential focus of all CR/SP programs. However, changes in (and interpretation of) federal regulations affecting reimbursement and program design continue to influence CR/SP programs and professionals. For CR/SP professionals, this has been affirming (reimbursement coverage for six diagnoses) but at the same time challenging (as yet, no specific coverage for heart failure). Consequently, it is likely that CR/SP will remain a rehabilitative and a secondary preventive service that functions both within and outside traditional health care institutions. Nonetheless, programs that are not current with ongoing research, regulatory developments, and practice guidelines and are not responsive to changes in the practice environment may become stagnant and limited in their effectiveness.

Cardiac rehabilitation and secondary prevention programs must remain connected to the larger continuum of care both in and out of the hospital. New program models (see chapter 10) are developing in accordance with evolving regulatory guidelines. Older, more established models also have the opportunity to become more creative with programming, which may in turn enhance participation and efficacy. Cooperative and creative partnerships with other health care providers, as well as with individuals and institutions involved in community health and fitness programming, will become more the norm than the exception. CR/SP professionals and their programs must maintain diligence in helping people make lifestyle changes that reduce the risk of onset and progression of chronic disease and vascular events. And all of this must be tempered by the economic realities of our time. The editors of these *Guidelines* believe that CR/SP is well positioned because our programs are lifesaving and cost-effective. Participation in CR/SP reduces the incidence and progression of heart disease and directly addresses lifestyle and health behaviors known to be associated with and causative of atherosclerosis and a wide range of chronic diseases that threaten so many individuals and families.

We must discern how to provide patients with low-cost, high-quality programming that moves patients toward taking personal responsibility for disease management and secondary prevention over a lifetime. A major challenge for all CR programs is to increase opportunities to provide risk intervention and promote positive health behavior patterns within the finite limit of available resources. Disease management involves using efficacious approaches for risk factor intervention, implementing more effective education and coaching techniques, increasing physical activity and discouraging sedentary behavior, and urging symptom recognition before acute episodes occur to decrease cardiovascular disease morbidity and mortality.

Importantly, this secondary prevention model also allows for program transition into the management of other chronic diseases that have similar underlying pathophysiology. Many chronic diseases, including coronary heart disease, hypertension, obesity, diabetes, and peripheral vascular disease, have a common underlying pathophysiology. Thus, the preventive and rehabilitative aspects of CR programs can (and should) be adapted to address six

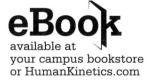

eBook
available at
your campus bookstore
or HumanKinetics.com

lifestyle-related risk factors—smoking, hypertension, obesity, type 2 diabetes, inappropriate diet, and sedentary lifestyle. The key to effective chronic disease management is adherence to a healthy lifestyle, including high levels of physical activity, no tobacco use, and a healthy dietary pattern. Adherence to existing medical therapy underpins the healthy lifestyle choices. Thus, CR/SP programs can be models for other disease management programs.

In this Fifth Edition of the *Guidelines,* we have provided complete chapter revisions along with several new sections. Chapter 3, "Behavior Modification and Risk Factor Reduction: Guiding Principles and Practices," has been moved closer to the beginning of the book as an indication of our belief in the critical importance of effectively addressing behavior change in secondary prevention programs. This chapter contains new and updated information and is one that the professional practitioner should read and refer to constantly. There is perhaps no more important or "fluid" topic in lifestyle behavior than nutrition, discussed in chapter 4. Chapter 7, "Outpatient Cardiovascular Rehabilitation and Secondary Prevention," includes suggestions for models that comply with the new regulatory guidelines. Each of chapters 8 and 9, "Modifiable Cardiovascular Disease Risk Factors" and "Special Populations," has been completely rewritten with the most recent information. Finally, chapter 10, "Program Administration," has also been completely rewritten to include new regulations and reimbursement standards, as well as additional suggestions for new models for CR/SP. In addition, the most recently published "Core Competencies for Cardiac Rehabilitation and Secondary Prevention Professionals" has been included in its entirety.

The information in the Fifth Edition covers the entire scope of practice for CR/SP programs and professionals. Keeping up with change is a professional necessity, while keeping up with the science is a professional responsibility. The Fifth Edition of the *Guidelines* is an essential tool to help CR/SP professionals meet future program structure and delivery challenges. By participating in writing these *Guidelines,* more than 50 leaders in the field of cardiac rehabilitation and secondary prevention, cardiovascular risk reduction, reimbursement, and public policy have provided CR professionals with the latest tools and information to successfully start new programs or update and enhance existing ones.

As with the previous edition, it is acknowledged that all programs may not have the personnel or resources to provide specific expertise in each area, but the core components should be some part of every program. Changes in program delivery and professional expertise of CR practitioners, as identified in the core competencies and core components documents, may be necessary to make this happen. The Fifth Edition of the *Guidelines* provides the basis to address the essential components in a manner that is in keeping with the delivery of a comprehensive CR program. The challenge to CR professionals is to select, develop, and deliver appropriate, state-of-the-art rehabilitative and secondary preventive services to patients and to tailor the method of delivery of these services to individual needs of each patient. Determination of the best approach in each case should involve both health care provider recommendations and patient preferences. The strategy for success should reflect a desire for progressive patient independence in cardiac rehabilitation and continued compliance with the appropriate lifestyle change.

The AACVPR and these guidelines are critical links to keeping our profession and the services that we provide recognized and valued by the scientific community; federal agencies; third-party payers; and, most importantly, the patients, families, and communities whose lives we touch. The Fifth Edition of the AACVPR *Guidelines* provides significant support to help us achieve our goals of continuing professional development and program excellence.

Web Resource

To complement the text, *Guidelines for Cardiac Rehabilitation and Secondary Prevention Programs, Fifth Edition,* has a companion web resource. This resource includes 21 reproducible questionnaires, charts, consent forms, protocols, records, checklists, and logs for use in creating or assessing programs. These are also found within the book, providing users with practical information to support their work. The web resource will also serve as a location for AACVPR to post biannual updates to book content, as necessary, keeping the guidelines up to date between editions of the text. The web resource can be accessed at **www.HumanKinetics.com/GuidelinesFor CardiacRehabilitationAndSecondary PreventionPrograms**.

Cardiac Rehabilitation, Secondary Prevention Programs, and the Evolution of Health Care

Providing Optimal Care for All Patients

Guidelines for Cardiac Rehabilitation and Secondary Prevention, Fifth Edition, fully embraces the increasing incidence of coronary heart disease (CHD), the changing demographics of the patient populations we serve, and the growing importance of the services we provide in the 21st century. Cardiac rehabilitation and secondary prevention (CR/SP) has evolved substantially over the past 50 years. The patient population using these program services has progressed from a predominantly white male population, physically and emotionally debilitated from an acute myocardial infarction (MI) followed by prolonged bed rest, to an ethnically diverse population of men and women receiving individualized programs of intensive secondary prevention for CHD and other cardiac illness or procedures, with or without a precedent hospitalization.[1-3] Significant challenges continue with the underreferral of cardiac patients to CR/SP, particularly women, the elderly, and the medically underserved.[4] In spite of the knowledge that patients referred to CR/SP are more likely to receive guideline-based care, to improve all lifestyle habits, and to report improved quality of life and physical and psychological function, referral to CR/SP occurs in less than 30% of eligible patients.[5]

OBJECTIVES

This chapter identifies

- the current status and future directions of CR/SP and
- the challenges and opportunities that face those who work within the CR/SP discipline.

In 2013, hospitalization following an acute coronary syndrome (ACS) seldom lasted longer than 5 to 7 days. Advances in cardiovascular (CV) preventive care over the past 20 years have resulted in fewer acute MIs and bypass surgeries, with the number of percutaneous interventions (PCI) remaining relatively unchanged.[6] Patients are discharged and eligible for CR/SP earlier in the course of their disease and are quickly transitioning back to work and to usual activities. This rapid transition from hospital to home and to normal life routines requires the immediate services of CR/SP to implement secondary prevention efforts much sooner than in previous decades, as well as to be more flexible in the provision of these services, including home-based programs. These efforts have been shown to reduce hospitalization, depression, recurrent ACS, disability, and stroke and to improve medication adherence and quality of life.[1,5,7] The recent MI FREEE trial (Post-Myocardial Infarction Free Rx and Economic Evaluation) demonstrated that even when recommended medical therapies were provided at no cost to persons following acute MI, the overall adherence rate improved but remained less than ideal at around 50%.[8] The role of CR/SP is to improve overall adherence to these lifesaving medical therapies by addressing barriers to adherence through behavioral strategies and support. Poor adherence to lifesaving medications remains a major challenge to patients and providers and is significantly enhanced by participation in CR/SP.[7]

Intensive secondary prevention in persons with CHD has been widely studied. A seminal study, published in 1994, demonstrated the benefits of intensive secondary prevention. Haskell and colleagues[9] randomized 300 men and women with documented CHD to a program of intensive risk reduction versus usual care and followed them for 4 years. At the end of 4 years, angiographic evidence of disease, deaths, CHD events, and hospitalizations were all improved in the treatment group compared to control. In 2009, the COURAGE trial showed that intensive CHD risk factor reduction was equivalent to intensive risk factor reduction plus PCI in selected patients.[10] These important health outcomes have also been documented in numerous studies worldwide and in diverse populations.[11,12]

In a recent presidential advisory from the American Heart Association (AHA), Balady and coauthors[13] made a clear and compelling case for the importance of CR programs as secondary prevention centers. "Given the significant benefits that CR/SP programs bring CV disease prevention, every recent major evidence-based guideline from the AHA and the American College of Cardiology (ACC) Foundation about the management and prevention of CHD provides a Class I–level recommendation (i.e., procedure or treatment should be performed or administered) for referral to CR/SP for those patients with recent MI or ACS, chronic stable angina, heart failure, or after coronary artery bypass surgery or PCI. CR/SP is also indicated for those patients after valve surgery or cardiac transplantation."

The current system of medical practice is fast evolving to include accountable care organizations, shared decision making, and patient-centered medical homes.[14] Traditional CR/SP is well positioned to integrate into these new systems and greatly improve CHD-related outcomes.[13,15] In this expanded model of care, CR/SP has the potential to provide important medical services to other high-risk populations such as patients with type 2 diabetes and patients with multiple CHD risk factors who are at high lifetime risk of a CHD event. Cost-effective interventions that improve adherence to lifestyle and medical therapy—therapy that reduces hospitalizations and procedures and improves health care outcomes—will be vital to health care systems and patients.

Cardiac Rehabilitation: Finding Its Place in the Evolving Health Care Arena

CR programs must continue to evolve to provide evidence of value to patients and health systems. New scientific findings must be embraced and practice adapted accordingly to provide effective and efficient services. Medical interventions will be increasingly scrutinized and reimbursement tied to efficacy.

CR/SP providers have been mandated by private and public insurance payers, including the Centers for Medicare and Medicaid Services (CMS), to individualize the services that are delivered. Patient care should be individualized to provide the most effective and efficient care. No longer do all patients receive all components offered as part of a CR/SP. Each patient must be an active participant in the process of determining and focusing on what is most important and necessary to the individual. Such an approach has been shown to lead to improved patient outcomes, the ultimate goal of every CR program.[16]

How does our profession stay ahead of the curve in such a rapidly changing health care environment? Four critical components are (1) current and evidence-based science, (2) sound practice that incorporates the science, (3) advocacy that promotes both the science and practice, and (4) fiscal accountability. These key elements work synergistically and are equally important if the profession is to sustain long-term viability.

The science of CR has advanced over the past 50 years. The original question was whether exercise was safe for cardiac patients; now it is known that CR significantly reduces mortality and morbidity and improves a variety of health outcomes.[17-19] The foundation of CR/SP is dependent on scientific statements and practice guidelines. As such, it is the responsibility of every CR/SP program to remain current with these documents and update practices accordingly.

As challenging as it is for individual programs to continually change how CR/SP is delivered in order to improve effectiveness, it is even more difficult for private and public payers, such as Medicare, to integrate science into policy. The field of CR/SP will be unable to make positive changes based on emerging research if coverage policies arbitrarily limit program delivery paradigms. Therefore, it is imperative that the profession share clinical expertise with decision makers at the payer level. This becomes more critical as all partners (payers, providers, and patients) increasingly seek more efficacious treatments that are also less costly. Coverage policies and new delivery options are accepting evidence-based research to obtain improved outcomes. One example of this was the decision by CMS to extend the window of completion for a CR program from 12 to 18 weeks to 36 weeks for Medicare beneficiaries. This decision was based on evidence that clinical outcomes are improved with extended program duration.[20]

Advocacy for CR/SP extends beyond bureaucratic decision makers. The promotion of best practices to CR/SP is a primary role of our professional organizations such as the American Association of Cardiovascular and Pulmonary Rehabilitation, AHA, ACC, and the American College of Sports Medicine. As practitioners, we should expect assistance from professional organizations in keeping current with the scientific literature. In addition, it is our responsibility to volunteer and participate in the development of best practices and guidelines to improve our care and outcomes. This educational process is ongoing and requires commitment on the part of individual professionals in the field as well as the organizations representing those who provide CR/SP.

Fiscal sustainability is fundamental and should be a priority for every program. CR/SP cannot risk being operationally inefficient. Health care systems insist on evidence of the value each service provides. CR/SP has a huge opportunity to play a larger role with the focus of hospitals and payers shifting to quality patient care and meaningful patient outcomes. CR/SP would do well to ask three introspective yet critical questions:

1. With each component of service that is delivered, what is the scientific basis for efficacy and safety?
2. How can our practice change to better reflect current research?
3. Which patient populations will benefit most from active participation in CR/SP?

The benefit of collaboration between payers, scientists, and practitioners is evident in the progress that has been made in the field of CR/SP. Communication between researchers and practitioners, researchers and payers, and practitioners and payers will continue to be instrumental in continued growth of the service with the ultimate goal of enhanced patient outcomes.

Cardiac Rehabilitation Programs as Secondary Prevention Centers

The 2011 update to "Secondary Prevention and Risk Reduction Therapy for Patients with Coronary and Other Atherosclerotic Vascular Disease"[21] documented Class 1 and Class IIa recommendations stressing the role of intensive secondary prevention through intensive risk factor reduction and CR. The specific recommendations are outlined in guideline 1.1.

Guideline 1.1   Recommendations for Stressing the Role of Intensive Secondary Prevention Through Intensive Risk Factor Reduction and Cardiac Rehabilitation

Class I

• All eligible patients with acute coronary syndrome or whose status is immediately post-coronary artery bypass surgery or post-PCI *should be referred to a comprehensive outpatient cardiovascular rehabilitation program* either before hospital discharge or during the first follow-up office visit *(Level of Evidence: A).*

• All eligible outpatients with the diagnosis of ACS, coronary artery bypass surgery, or PCI *(Level of Evidence: A)*, chronic angina *(Level of Evidence: B)*, and/or peripheral artery disease *(Level of Evidence: A)* within the past year *should be referred to a comprehensive outpatient cardiovascular rehabilitation program.*

• A home-based cardiac rehabilitation program can be substituted for a supervised, center-based program for low-risk patients *(Level of Evidence: A).*

Class IIa

• A comprehensive exercise-based outpatient cardiac rehabilitation program can be safe and beneficial for clinically stable outpatients with a history of heart failure *(Level of Evidence: B).*

Adapted, by permission, from S.C. Smith et al., 2011, "AHA/ACCF secondary prevention and risk Reduction therapy for patients with coronary and other atherosclerotic vascular disease," *Circulation* 124: 2458-2473.

Summary

The science and the guidelines support CR/SP efforts. Systematic approaches to guideline-based care, such as Get With the Guidelines and multifactor case management, are examples of successful models.[22] These models rely on a team-based approach; information technology for tracking and information; regular assessment and titration of therapies to achieve risk reduction goals; use of behavioral therapies for lifestyle change; ongoing health education; use of telephone, e-mail, and written and online materials for regular assessment; and ongoing patient support. Outcome measures are critical to the evaluation of a programs' success and to implementation of quality improvement measures.[23-26]

It is time for CR programs to become secondary prevention centers and to expand the scope of patients cared for in CR/SP. A center for the provision of individualized lifestyle and medical therapies, for monitoring symptoms and managing risk factors, for measuring outcomes and adjusting therapies to achieve guideline-based care—and one that can provide ongoing health education, as well as social and psychological support, to reduce morbidity and mortality and improve quality of life to people across the life span—has real value in the future of health care.

The Continuum of Care

From Inpatient and Outpatient Cardiac Rehabilitation to Long-Term Secondary Prevention

A significant paradigm shift has occurred in health care over the past decade. In the past, health care focused largely on episodic care—the provision of health care during an episode of acute illness or injury. In recent years, health care has incorporated an additional focus on the continuum of care—the provision of care not only during an acute illness or injury, but afterward as well.[1-3] This increased emphasis on providing patient care along a continuum has occurred with particular vigor in the field of cardiovascular (CV) medicine.[4-7] Several factors help explain this growing focus, including the following:

- Survival of patients suffering an acute myocardial infarction has improved, resulting in more patients with chronic coronary artery disease.
- Effective medical and lifestyle therapies have been developed that improve long-term survival of patients with cardiovascular disease (CVD) who receive appropriate secondary prevention (SP) therapies and follow-up services.
- The clear realization is that the majority of patients with chronic CVD do not receive optimal care throughout the continuum of care. In fact, only a small minority of patients actually receive appropriate SP treatments and follow-up services.
- Private and governmental organizations have taken notice of the significant gaps in the continuum of care for patients with CVD, and have taken steps to reduce those gaps by establishing policies to bridge important gaps in the continuum of CV care.

OBJECTIVES

This chapter
- provides an overview of the operational structure and sequence of cardiac rehabilitation (CR) programming,
- describes practical tools that can be useful in the delivery of contemporary outpatient CR/SP programming, and
- identifies opportunities to redesign existing programs to optimize performance within an evolving continuum.

Cardiovascular Continuum of Care

While the continuum of care for CVD should begin early in life, before the clinical manifestation of CVD,[8,9] for the purposes of this discussion it is assumed that the continuum of care for the patient with CVD begins at the time of the clinical diagnosis or event. Steps in the CV continuum of care include (figure 2.1) the following:

1. Treatment of acute event: An initial step in the CV care continuum occurs when treatments are given to address the acute CVD event at hand. For an acute coronary syndrome, prompt provision of antiplatelet therapy, thrombolytic therapy, percutaneous coronary intervention, or some combination of these is critically important to help patients survive the acute event and to do so with minimal damage to the heart.[10]

2. Initiation of Secondary Prevention (SP) therapies: A second step in the care continuum occurs shortly after the acute event has resolved and a longer-term treatment plan is initiated. This long-term plan generally includes lifesaving lifestyle and medical therapies and is ideally started before discharge. In fact, evidence shows that when SP treatments are started in the hos-

pital, patients are more likely to adhere to those treatments in the long term, and are more likely to remain free from recurrent CV events than when those treatments were not started before discharge.[11]

3. Early outpatient CR: One to 36 sessions over a period of up to 36 weeks following a CVD event. An important "hand-off" occurs at the time of patient discharge from the hospital, when the patient leaves the acute care setting and begins taking steps toward CR and restorative health in the outpatient setting, under the supervision and guidance of health care professionals. Unfortunately, this important step is often a misstep, when prescribed therapies are not taken and follow-up visits are delayed or even missed.[12,13] These gaps in adherence to the secondary treatment plan can occur for a variety of reasons, including patient, provider, and health care system factors.[14-18]

From the patient perspective, the time following hospitalization for a CVD event is filled with concerns, questions, and confusion. Patients have been diagnosed with a serious heart condition and have been prescribed an array of new therapies. Concerns about costs and potential side effects, as well as uncertainty about treatment benefits, may lead patients to avoid prescribed treatments.[12,13] In addition, depression and anxiety, commonly

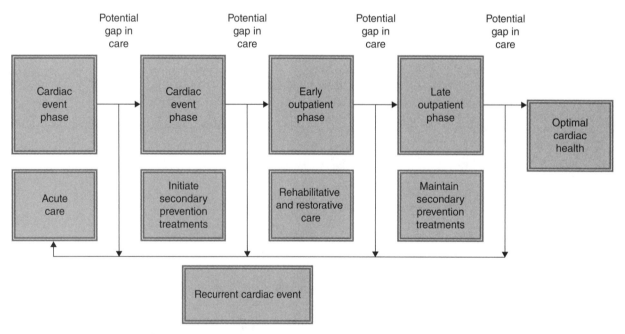

Figure 2.1 Continuum of cardiovascular care following a cardiac event, highlighting important potential gaps in the care continuum.

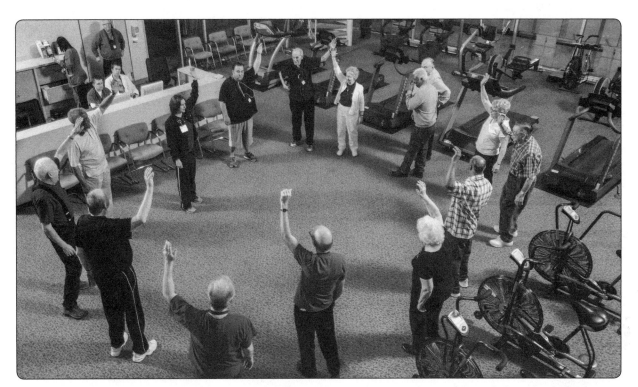

CR services help bridge the divide between the hospital and outpatient settings and are a key reason why CR helps improve patient care and outcomes.

experienced following a CVD event, make it even more challenging for patients to maneuver through this difficult time.[19] CR services can help bridge the divide between the hospital and outpatient settings. Patient education and counseling services are provided and give needed guidance and trouble-shooting resources to help initiate and maintain the secondary treatment plan. In addition, outpatient CR programs help promote coordination of care between health care providers, a key reason why CR helps to improve patient

care and outcomes throughout the continuum of care.[20,21]

4. Long-term CR/SP: The period following completion of early outpatient CR. Following the early rehabilitation phase after a CVD event, patients shift into long-term CR/SP, another step that is prone to missteps and subsequent gaps in the CV care continuum. Patients who have participated in an early outpatient CR program and continue with long-term maintenance CR/SP are likely to continue to receive effective therapies

Guideline 2.1

To demonstrate its place in the continuum of care, each program should have available

- an outline or illustration of the structure or sequence of cardiovascular care and CR/SP within its operation;
- a written description of the scope of services, based on the American Association of Cardiovas-

cular and Pulmonary Rehabilitation (AACVPR) Core Components of Cardiac Rehabilitation/Secondary Prevention Programs[31] (tables 2.1 and 2.2), that are provided to patients, including exercise, risk intervention, and education and counseling; and

- standards of care that outline how each service will be delivered and evaluated.

and the associated morbidity and mortality benefits.[22-29] However, many patients who complete an early outpatient CR program fail to continue with a long-term follow-up program and fail to continue with the recommended SP therapies.[13,30]

Even worse, patients who do not participate in an early outpatient CR program are less likely to receive effective SP therapies in the long term as well.[27]

Table 2.1 Core Components of Cardiac Rehabilitation/Secondary Prevention Programs: Patient Assessment, Nutritional Counseling, and Weight Management

PATIENT ASSESSMENT	
Evaluation	• Medical history: Review current and prior CV medical and surgical diagnoses and procedures (including assessment of left ventricular function); comorbidities (including peripheral arterial disease, cerebral vascular disease, pulmonary disease, kidney disease, diabetes mellitus, musculoskeletal and neuromuscular disorders, depression, and other pertinent diseases); symptoms of CV disease; medications (including dose, frequency, and compliance); date of most recent influenza vaccination; CV risk profile; and educational barriers and preferences. Refer to each core component of care for relevant assessment measures. • Physical examination: Assess cardiopulmonary systems (including pulse rate and regularity, blood pressure, auscultation of heart and lungs, palpation and inspection of lower extremities for edema and presence of arterial pulses); post-CV procedure wound sites; orthopedic and neuromuscular status; and cognitive function. Refer to each core component for respective additional physical measures. • Testing: Obtain resting 12-lead electrocardiogram (ECG); assess patient's perceived health-related quality of life or health status. Refer to each core component for additional specified tests.
Interventions	• Document the patient assessment information that reflects the patient's current status and guides the development and implementation of (1) a patient treatment plan that prioritizes goals and outlines intervention strategies for risk reduction, and (2) a discharge and follow-up plan that reflects progress toward goals and guides long-term SP plans. • Interactively, communicate the treatment and follow-up plans with the patient and appropriate family members or domestic partner in collaboration with the primary health care provider. • In concert with the primary care provider, cardiologist, or both, ensure that the patient is taking appropriate doses of aspirin, clopidogrel, beta-blockers, lipid-lowering agents, and angiotensin-converting enzyme (ACE) inhibitors or angiotensin receptor blockers as recommended by the American Heart Association/American College of Cardiology (AHA/ACC), and that the patient has had an annual influenza vaccination.
Expected outcomes	• Patient treatment plan: Documented evidence of patient assessment and priority short-term (i.e., weeks to months) goals within the core components of care that guide intervention strategies. Discussion and provision of the initial and follow-up plans to the patient in collaboration with the primary health care provider. • Outcome report: Documented evidence of patient outcomes within the core components of care that reflects progress toward goals, including whether the patient is taking appropriate doses of aspirin, clopidogrel, beta-blockers, and ACE inhibitors or angiotensin receptor blockers as recommended by AHA/ACC; reflects whether the patient has had an annual influenza vaccination (and if not, documented evidence for why not); and identifies specific areas that require further intervention and monitoring. • Discharge plan: Documented discharge plan summarizing long-term goals and strategies for success.
NUTRITIONAL COUNSELING	
Evaluation	• Obtain estimates of total daily caloric intake and dietary content of saturated fat, trans fat, cholesterol, sodium, and nutrients. • Assess eating habits, including fruit and vegetable, whole grain, and fish consumption; number of meals and snacks; frequency of dining out; and alcohol consumption. • Determine target areas for nutrition intervention as outlined in the core components of weight, hypertension, and diabetes, as well as heart failure, kidney disease, and other comorbidities.
Interventions	• Prescribe specific dietary modifications aiming to at least attain the saturated fat and cholesterol content limits of the Therapeutic Lifestyle Changes diet. Individualize diet plan according to specific target areas as outlined in the core components of weight, hypertension, and diabetes, as well as heart failure and other comorbidities. Recommendations should be sensitive and relevant to cultural preferences. • Educate and counsel patient (and appropriate family members or domestic partner) on dietary goals and how to attain them. • Incorporate behavior change models and compliance strategies into counseling sessions.
Expected outcomes	• Patient adheres to prescribed diet. • Patient understands basic principles of dietary content, such as calories, fat, cholesterol, and nutrients. • A plan has been provided to address eating behavior problems.

WEIGHT MANAGEMENT	
Evaluation	• Measure weight, height, and waist circumference. Calculate body mass index (BMI).

Interventions	• In patients with BMI >25 kg/m² and/or waist >40 inches in men (102 cm) and >35 inches (88 cm) in women:
	  • Establish reasonable short-term and long-term weight goals individualized to the patient and his associated risk factors (e.g., reduce body weight by at least 5% and preferably by >10% at a rate of 1 to 2 lb/week over a period of time up to 6 months).
	  • Develop a combined diet, physical activity or exercise, and behavioral program designed to reduce total caloric intake, maintain appropriate intake of nutrients and fiber, and increase energy expenditure. The exercise component should strive to include daily longer-distance or -duration walking (e.g., 60-90 min).
	  • Aim for an energy deficit tailored to achieve weight goals (e.g., 500-1000 kcal/day).

Expected outcomes	• Short-term: Continue to assess and modify interventions until progressive weight loss is achieved. Provide referral to specialized, validated nutrition weight loss programs if weight goals are not achieved. • Long-term: Patient adheres to diet and physical activity or exercise program aimed toward attainment of established weight goal.

BMI definitions for overweight and obesity may differ by race-ethnicity and region of the world. Relevant definitions, when available, should be respectively applied.

Reprinted with permission *Circulation*. 2007; 115:2675-2682 ©2007 American Heart Association, Inc.

Table 2.2 Core Components of Cardiac Rehabilitation/Secondary Prevention Programs: Blood Pressure Management, Lipid Management, Diabetes Management, Tobacco Cessation, Psychosocial Management, Physical Activity Counseling, and Exercise Training

BLOOD PRESSURE MANAGEMENT	
Evaluation	• Measure blood pressure in both arms at program entry. • Measure seated resting blood pressure on two or more visits. • To rule out orthostatic hypotension, measure lying, seated, and standing blood pressure at program entry and after adjustments in antihypertensive drug therapy. • Assess current treatment and compliance. • Assess use of nonprescription drugs that may adversely affect blood pressure.

Interventions	• Provide or monitor drug therapy (or do both) in concert with primary health care provider as follows:
	• If blood pressure is 120 to 139 mm Hg systolic or 80 to 89 mm Hg diastolic:
	  • Provide lifestyle modifications, including regular physical activity or exercise; weight management; moderate sodium restriction and increased consumption of fresh fruits, vegetables, and low-fat dairy products; alcohol moderation; and smoking cessation.
	  • Provide drug therapy for patients with chronic kidney disease, heart failure, or diabetes if blood pressure is ≥130/ ≥80 mm Hg after lifestyle modification.
	• If blood pressure is ≥40 mm Hg systolic or ≥90 mm Hg diastolic:
	  • Provide lifestyle modification and drug therapy.

Expected outcomes	• Short-term: Continue to assess and modify intervention until normalization of blood pressure in prehypertensive patients, that is, <140 mm Hg systolic and <90 mm Hg diastolic in hypertensive patients; <130 mm Hg systolic and <80 mm Hg diastolic in hypertensive patients with diabetes, heart failure, or chronic kidney disease. • Long-term: Maintain blood pressure at goal levels.
LIPID MANAGEMENT	
Evaluation	• Obtain fasting measures of total cholesterol, high-density lipoprotein, low-density lipoprotein, and triglycerides. In patients with abnormal levels, obtain a detailed history to determine whether diet, drug, or other conditions that may affect lipid levels can be altered. • Assess current treatment and compliance. • Repeat lipid profiles at 4 to 6 weeks after hospitalization and at 2 months after initiation of or change in lipid-lowering medications. • Assess creatine kinase levels and liver function in patients taking lipid-lowering medications as recommended by the National Cholesterol Education Program (NCEP).

(continued)

LIPID MANAGEMENT (CONTINUED)

Interventions	• Provide nutritional counseling consistent with the Therapeutic Lifestyle Changes diet, such as the recommendation to add plant stanols/sterols and viscous fiber and encouragement to consume more omega-3 fatty acids, as well as weight management counseling, as needed, in all patients. Add or intensify drug treatment in those with low-density lipoprotein >100 mg/dL; consider adding drug treatment in those with low-density lipoprotein >70 mg/dL. • Provide interventions directed toward management of triglycerides to attain non-high-density lipoprotein cholesterol of <130 mg/dL. These include nutritional counseling and weight management, exercise, smoking cessation, alcohol moderation, and drug therapy as recommended by NCEP and AHA/ACC. • Provide or monitor drug treatment (or do both) in concert with primary health care provider.
Expected outcomes	• Short-term: Continue to assess and modify intervention until low-density lipoprotein is <100 mg/dL (further reduction to a goal of <70 mg/dL is considered reasonable) and non-high-density lipoprotein cholesterol is <130 mg/dL (further reduction to a goal of <100 mg/dL is considered reasonable). • Long-term: Low-density lipoprotein cholesterol of <100 mg/dL (further reduction to a goal of <70 mg/dL is considered reasonable). Non-high-density lipoprotein cholesterol of <130 mg/dL (further reduction to a goal of <100 mg/dL is considered reasonable).

DIABETES MANAGEMENT

Evaluation	• From medical record review:
	  • Confirm presence or absence of diabetes in all patients.
	  • If a patient is known to be diabetic, identify history of complications such as findings related to heart disease; vascular disease; problems with eyes, kidneys, or feet; or autonomic or peripheral neuropathy.
	• From initial patient interview:
	  • Obtain history of signs and symptoms related to these complications and any reports of episodes of hypoglycemia or hyperglycemia.
	  • Identify physician managing diabetic condition and prescribed treatment regimen, including:
	    • Medications and extent of compliance.
	    • Diet and extent of compliance.
	    • Blood sugar monitoring method and extent of compliance.
	• Before starting exercise:
	  • Obtain latest fasting plasma glucose (FPG) and glycosylated hemoglobin (HbA1c).
	  • Consider stratifying patient to high-risk category because of the greater likelihood of exercise-induced complications.

Interventions	• Educate patient and staff to be alert to signs or symptoms of hypoglycemia or hyperglycemia and provide appropriate assessment and interventions as recommended by the American Diabetes Association.
	• In those taking insulin or insulin secretagogues:
	  • Avoid exercise at peak insulin times.
	  • Advise that insulin be injected in abdomen, not muscle to be exercised.
	  • Test blood sugar levels pre- and postexercise at each session. If blood sugar value is <100 mg/dL, delay exercise and provide patient 15 g carbohydrate; retest in 15 min; proceed if blood sugar value is >100 mg/dL. In patients with Type 2 diabetes, if blood sugar value is >300 mg/dL, patient may exercise with caution if she feels well, is adequately hydrated, and blood or urine ketones (or both) are negative; otherwise, contact patient's physician for further treatment.
	  • Encourage adequate hydration to avoid effects of fluid shifts on blood sugar levels.
	  • Caution patient that blood sugar may continue to drop for 24 to 48 h after exercise.
	• In those treated with diet, metformin, alpha glucosidase inhibitors, or thiozolidinediones, without insulin or insulin secretagogues, test blood sugar levels before exercise for first 6 to 10 sessions to assess glycemic control; exercise is generally unlikely to cause hypoglycemia.
	• Education
	  • Teach and practice self-monitoring skills for use during unsupervised exercise.
	  • Refer to registered dietitian for medical nutrition therapy.
	  • Consider referral to certified diabetic educator for skill training, medication instruction, and support groups.

Expected outcomes	• Short-term:
	  • Communicate with primary physician or endocrinologist about signs and symptoms and medication adjustments.
	  • Confirm patient's ability to recognize signs and symptoms, self-monitor blood sugar status, and self-manage activities.
	• Long-term:
	  • Attain FPG levels of 90 to 130 mg/dL and HbA1c <7%.
	  • Minimize complications and reduce episodes of hypoglycemia or hyperglycemia at rest, with exercise, or both.
	  • Maintain blood pressure at <130/<80 mm Hg.

	TOBACCO CESSATION

Evaluation	• Initial encounter:
	  • Ask the patient about his smoking status and use of other tobacco products. Document status as never smoked, former smoker, current smoker (includes those who have quit in the last 12 months because of the high probability of relapse). Specify both amount of smoking (cigarettes per day) and duration of smoking (number of years). Quantify use and type of other tobacco products. Ask about exposure to secondhand smoke at home and at work.
	  • Determine readiness to change by asking every smoker or tobacco user if she is now ready to quit.
	  • Assess for psychosocial factors that may impede success.
	  • Ongoing contact: Update status at each visit during first 2 weeks of cessation, periodically thereafter.

Interventions	• When readiness to change is not expressed, provide a brief motivational message containing the "5 Rs": Relevance, Risks, Rewards, Roadblocks, and Repetition.
	• When readiness to change is confirmed, continue with the "5 As": Ask, Advise, Assess, Assist, and Arrange. Assist the smoker or tobacco user to set a quit date, and select appropriate treatment strategies (preparation):
	Minimal (brief):
	  • Individual education and counseling by program staff supplemented with self-teaching materials.
	  • Social support provided by physician, program staff, and family or domestic partner; identify other smokers in the house; discuss how to engage them in the patient's cessation efforts.
	  • Relapse prevention: problem solving, anticipated threats, practice scenarios.
	Optimal (intense):
	  • Longer individual counseling or group involvement.
	  • Pharmacological support (in concert with primary physician): nicotine replacement therapy, bupropion hydrochloride.
	  • Supplemental strategies if desired (e.g., acupuncture, hypnosis).
	• If patient has recently quit, emphasize relapse prevention skills.
	• Urge avoidance of exposure to secondhand smoke at work and home.

Expected outcomes	Note: Patients who continue to smoke upon enrollment are subsequently more likely to drop out of CR/SP programs. • Short-term: Patient will demonstrate readiness to change by initially expressing decision to quit and selecting a quit date. Subsequently, patient will quit smoking and all tobacco use and adhere to pharmacological therapy (if prescribed) while practicing relapse prevention strategies; patient will resume cessation plan as quickly as possible when temporary relapse occurs. • Long-term: Complete abstinence from smoking and use of all tobacco products for at least 12 months (maintenance) from quit date. No exposure to environmental tobacco smoke at work and home.
	PSYCHOSOCIAL MANAGEMENT
Evaluation	• Identify psychological distress as indicated by clinically significant levels of depression, anxiety, anger or hostility, social isolation, marital or family distress, sexual dysfunction or adjustment, and substance abuse (alcohol or other psychotropic agents), using interview, standardized measurement tools, or both. • Identify use of psychotropic medications.
Interventions	• Offer individual or small-group education and counseling (or both) on adjustment to heart disease, stress management, and health-related lifestyle change. When possible, include family members, domestic partners, or significant others in such sessions. • Develop supportive rehabilitation environment and community resources to enhance the patient's and the family's level of social support. • Teach and support self-help strategies. • In concert with primary health care provider, refer patients experiencing clinically significant psychosocial distress to appropriate mental health specialists for further evaluation and treatment.
Expected outcomes	• Emotional well-being is indicated by the absence of clinically significant psychological distress, social isolation, or drug dependency. • Patient demonstrates responsibility for health-related behavior change, relaxation, and other stress management skills; ability to obtain effective social support; compliance with psychotropic medications if prescribed; and reduction or elimination of alcohol, tobacco, caffeine, or other nonprescription psychoactive drugs. • Arrange for ongoing management if important psychosocial issues are present.
	PHYSICAL ACTIVITY COUNSELING
Evaluation	• Assess current physical activity level (e.g., questionnaire, pedometer) and determine domestic, occupational, and recreational needs. • Evaluate activities relevant to age, gender, and daily life, such as driving, sexual activity, sports, gardening, and household tasks. • Assess readiness to change behavior, self-confidence, barriers to increased physical activity, and social support in making positive changes.

(continued)

PHYSICAL ACTIVITY COUNSELING *(CONTINUED)*	
Interventions	• Provide advice, support, and counseling about physical activity needs on initial evaluation and in follow-up. Target exercise program to meet individual needs (see exercise training section of table). Provide educational materials as part of counseling efforts. Consider exercise tolerance or simulated work testing for patients with heavy-labor jobs. • Consistently encourage patients to accumulate 30 to 60 min per day of moderate-intensity physical activity on ≥5 (preferably most) days of the week. Explore daily schedules to suggest how to incorporate increased activity into usual routine (e.g., parking farther away from entrances, walking two or more flights of stairs, walking during lunch break). • Advise low-impact aerobic activity to minimize risk of musculoskeletal injury. • Recommend gradual increases in the volume of physical activity over time. • Caution patients to avoid performing unaccustomed vigorous physical activity (e.g., racket sports and manual snow removal). • Reassess the patient's ability to perform such activities as exercise training program progresses.
Expected outcomes	• Patient shows increased participation in domestic, occupational, and recreational activities. • Patient shows improved psychosocial well-being, reduction in stress, facilitation of functional independence, prevention of disability, and enhancement of opportunities for independent self-care to achieve recommended goals. • Patient shows improved aerobic fitness and body composition and lessens coronary risk factors (particularly for the sedentary patient who has adopted a lifestyle approach to regular physical activity).
EXERCISE TRAINING	
Evaluation	• Symptom-limited exercise testing before participation in an exercise-based CR program is strongly recommended. The evaluation may be repeated as changes in clinical condition warrant. Test parameters should include assessment of heart rate and rhythm, signs, symptoms, ST-segment changes, hemodynamics, perceived exertion, and exercise capacity. • On the basis of patient assessment and the exercise test if performed, risk stratify the patient to determine the level of supervision and monitoring required during exercise training. Use risk stratification schema as recommended by AHA and AACVPR.

Interventions	• Develop an individualized exercise prescription for aerobic and resistance training that is based on evaluation findings, risk stratification, comorbidities (e.g., peripheral arterial disease and musculoskeletal conditions), and patient and program goals. The exercise regimen should be reviewed by the program medical director or referring physician, modified if necessary, and approved. Exercise prescription should specify frequency (F), intensity (I), duration (D), modalities (M), and progression (P).
	  • For aerobic exercise: F = 3 to 5 days/week; I = 50% to 80% of exercise capacity; D = 20 to 60 min; and M = walking, treadmill, cycling, rowing, stair climbing, arm and leg ergometry, and others using continuous or interval training as appropriate.
	  • For resistance exercise: F = 2 or 3 days/week; I = 10 to 15 repetitions per set to moderate fatigue; D = one to three sets of 8 to 10 different upper and lower body exercises; and M = calisthenics, elastic bands, cuff or hand weights, dumbbells, free weights, wall pulleys, or weight machines.
	• Include warm-up, cool-down, and flexibility exercises in each exercise session.
	• Provide progressive updates to the exercise prescription and modify further if clinical status changes.
	• Supplement the formal exercise regimen with activity guidelines as outlined in the physical activity counseling section of this table.

Expected outcomes	• Patient understands safety issues during exercise, including warning signs and symptoms. • Patient achieves increased cardiorespiratory fitness and enhanced flexibility, muscular endurance, and strength. • Patient achieves reduced symptoms, attenuated physiological responses to physical challenges, and improved psychosocial well-being. • Patient achieves reduced global CV risk and mortality resulting from an overall program of CR/SP that includes exercise training.

Reprinted with permission *Circulation*. 2007; 115:2675-2682. ©2007 American Heart Association, Inc.

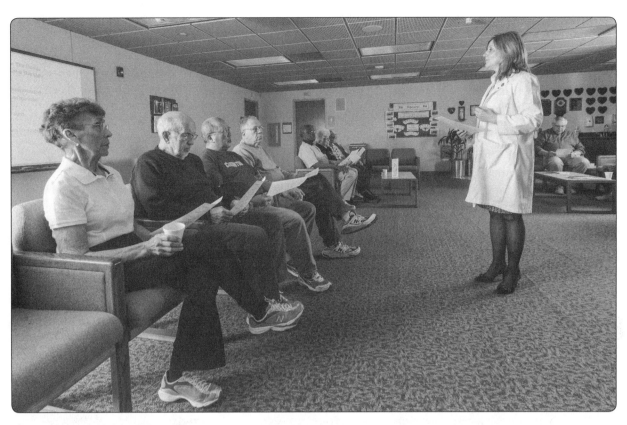

Offering small-group education and counseling on adjustment to heart disease, stress management, and health-related lifestyle change is one facet of effective psychosocial management.

Efforts to Reduce Gaps in the Continuum of Care

Considerable effort has been made over the past two decades to identify, understand, and reduce the gaps in SP of CVD. Gaps in inpatient care, commonly due to systematic barriers and inefficiencies, have been reduced with organized approaches to quality improvement. For instance, critical pathways of care and standing orders have been found to improve the inpatient provision of SP therapies.[11,32] Furthermore, the use of automatic referral systems has been found to improve referral to outpatient CR.[17,33,34] Likewise, systematic approaches to enrollment of patients in outpatient CR have been fruitful.[33] However, despite these advances, only a minority of patients receive appropriate CR and SP services. Women, the elderly, underserved minorities, and uninsured patients are particularly at risk for falling into the SP gaps that occur in the continuum of care.[35,36]

Clinical practice guidelines have been developed and disseminated by experts from various national health care organizations with the intent to improve the delivery of care. Unfortunately, clinical practice guidelines alone have not been sufficient to reduce the gaps in CVD secondary preventive care, due at least in part to the variable rates at which guidelines are adopted and maintained by clinicians.[37] However, such guidelines have been important in their influence on establishing standards of care and decisions in health care policy.[38]

In recent years, various organizations have made new efforts to improve the quality of health care services, including the Institute of Medicine, the Joint Commission, the Institute for Healthcare Improvement, the Physician Consortium for Practice Improvement, and the National Quality Forum (NQF). These organizations have promoted improvements in health care quality by increasing the national focus on transparency and accountability in health care delivery. One quality improvement method that has been promoted by these and other organizations is the use of quality indicators or performance measures. Performance measures are designed to promote high-quality care through three steps: (1) measurement of important processes and outcomes of care that are provided by a health care provider or organization, (2) identification of performance gaps in the processes and outcomes measured, and (3) use of quality improvement methods to revise and improve the processes of care and thereby reduce gaps in care. A standard approach to developing performance measures has been published by the ACC and the AHA.[39]

Early enthusiasm for the use of performance measures was tempered somewhat by evidence suggesting minimal effects of some performance measures on patient outcomes.[40] However, the use of performance measures that have been highly correlated with desired outcomes appears to improve the likelihood of success.[41] Refined methods for development of performance measures have recently been published and are likely to help improve the impact of performance measures on reducing treatment gaps in the CV continuum of care.[42]

Performance measures for the referral to and delivery of CR/SP have been developed and published by AACVPR, ACC, and AHA.[43,44] These measures are grouped into two sets: one set (Set A) that covers the referral of eligible patients to outpatient CR programs and a second set (Set B) that covers the delivery of CR services by CR programs. The referral measures (Set A) are designed to help improve the referral of eligible patients to early outpatient CR programs, holding health care providers accountable in both the inpatient and outpatient settings (table 2.3). The

Table 2.3 Performance Measures for Referral to Cardiac Rehabilitation/Secondary Prevention Programs From an Inpatient Setting (A-1) and an Outpatient Setting (A-2)[44]

PERFORMANCE MEASURE A-1: CARDIAC REHABILITATION PATIENT REFERRAL FROM AN INPATIENT SETTING	
All patients hospitalized with a primary diagnosis of an acute myocardial infarction (MI) or chronic stable angina (CSA), or who during hospitalization have undergone coronary artery bypass graft (CABG) surgery, a percutaneous coronary intervention (PCI), cardiac valve surgery, or cardiac transplantation, are to be referred to an early outpatient cardiac rehabilitation/secondary prevention (CR) program.	
Numerator	Number of eligible patients with a qualifying event or diagnosis who have been referred to an outpatient CR program before hospital discharge or have a documented medical or patient-centered reason why such a referral was not made.
	(Note: The program may include a traditional CR program based on face-to-face interactions and training sessions or may include other options such as home-based approaches. If alternative CR approaches are used, they should be designed to meet appropriate safety standards.)
	A referral is defined as an official communication between the health care provider and the patient to recommend and carry out a referral order to an early outpatient CR program. This includes the provision of all necessary information to the patient that will allow the patient to enroll in an early outpatient CR program. This also includes a written or electronic communication between the health care provider or health care system and the cardiac rehabilitation program that includes the patient's enrollment information for the program. A hospital discharge summary or office note may potentially be formatted to include the necessary patient information to communicate to the CR program (e.g., the patient's cardiovascular history, testing, and treatments). All communications must maintain appropriate confidentiality as outlined by the 1996 Health Insurance Portability and Accountability Act (HIPAA).
	Exclusion criteria:
	• Patient factors (e.g., patient to be discharged to a nursing care facility for long-term care).
	• Medical factors (e.g., patient deemed by provider to have a medically unstable, life-threatening condition).
	• Health care system factors (e.g., no cardiac rehabilitation program available within 60 min of travel time from the patient's home).
Denominator	Number of hospitalized patients in the reporting period hospitalized with a qualifying event or diagnosis who do not meet any of the exclusion criteria listed in the numerator section.
	(Note: Patients with a qualifying event who are to be discharged for a short-term stay in an inpatient medical rehabilitation facility are still expected to be referred to an outpatient cardiac rehabilitation program by the inpatient team during the index hospitalization. This referral should be reinforced by the care team at the medical rehabilitation facility.)
Period of assessment	Inpatient hospitalization

PERFORMANCE MEASURE A-1: CARDIAC REHABILITATION PATIENT REFERRAL FROM AN INPATIENT SETTING *(CONTINUED)*	
Method of reporting	Proportion of health care system's patients with a qualifying event or diagnosis who had documentation of their referral to an outpatient CR program.
Sources of data	Administrative data, medical records, or data.
Rationale	A key component to outpatient CR program utilization is the appropriate and timely referral of patients. Generally, the most important time for this referral to take place is while the patient is hospitalized for a qualifying event or diagnosis (MI, CSA, CABG, PCI, cardiac valve surgery, or cardiac transplantation).
	This performance measure has been developed to help health care systems implement effective steps in their systems of care that will optimize the appropriate referral of a patient to an outpatient CR program.
	This measure is designed to serve as a stand-alone measure or, preferably, to be included within other performance measurement sets that involve disease states or other conditions for which CR services have been found to be appropriate and beneficial (e.g., following MI, CABG surgery). This performance measure is provided in a format that is meant to allow easy and flexible inclusion into such performance measurement sets.
	Effective referral of appropriate inpatients to an outpatient CR program is the responsibility of the health care team within a health care system that is primarily responsible for providing cardiovascular care to the patient during the hospitalization.
Corresponding guidelines and clinical recommendations	ACC/AHA 2004 Guideline Update for Coronary Artery Bypass Graft Surgery.
	Class I: Cardiac rehabilitation should be offered to all eligible patients after CABG *(Level of Evidence: B)*.
	ACC/AHA 2007 Update of the Guidelines for the Management of Patients With ST-Elevation Myocardial Infarction.
	Class I: Advising medically supervised programs (cardiac rehabilitation) for high-risk patients (e.g., recent acute coronary syndrome or revascularization, heart failure) is recommended *(Level of Evidence: B)*.
	ACC/AHA 2007 Guidelines for the Management of Patients With Unstable Angina and Non–ST-Segment Elevation Myocardial Infarction.
	Class I: Cardiac rehabilitation/secondary prevention programs, when available, are recommended for patients with unstable angina/non–ST-segment elevation MI, particularly those with multiple modifiable risk factors and those moderate- to high-risk patients in whom supervised or monitored exercise training is warranted *(Level of Evidence: B)*.
	ACC/AHA 2007 Chronic Angina Focused Update of the Guidelines for the Management of Patients With Chronic Stable Angina.
	Class I: Medically supervised programs (cardiac rehabilitation) are recommended for at-risk patients (e.g., recent acute coronary syndrome or revascularization, heart failure) *(Level of Evidence: B)*.
	ACC/AHA Guidelines for the Evaluation and Management of Chronic Heart Failure in the Adult.
	Class I: Exercise training is beneficial as an adjunctive approach to improve clinical status in ambulatory patients with current or prior symptoms of heart failure and reduced left ventricular ejection fraction (LVEF) *(Level of Evidence: B)*.
	AHA Evidence-Based Guidelines for Cardiovascular Disease Prevention in Women: 2007 Update.
	Class I: A comprehensive risk reduction regimen, such as cardiovascular or stroke rehabilitation or a physician-guided home- or community-based exercise training program, should be recommended to women with a recent acute coronary syndrome or coronary intervention, new-onset or chronic angina, recent cerebrovascular event, peripheral arterial disease *(Level of Evidence: A)*, or current or prior symptoms of heart failure and an LVEF <40% *(Level of Evidence: B)*.
	ACC/AHA/SCAI 2007 Focused Update of the Guidelines for Percutaneous Coronary Intervention.
	Class I: Advising medically supervised programs (cardiac rehabilitation) for high-risk patients (e.g., recent acute coronary syndrome or revascularization, heart failure) is recommended *(Level of Evidence: B)*.
Challenges to implementation	Identification of all eligible patients in an inpatient setting will require that a timely, accurate, and effective system be in place. Communication of referral information by the inpatient hospital service team to the outpatient CR program represents a potential challenge to the implementation of this performance measure. However, this task is generally performed by an inpatient cardiovascular care team member, such as an inpatient CR team member or a hospital discharge planning team member.

(continued)

PERFORMANCE MEASURE A-2: CARDIAC REHABILITATION PATIENT REFERRAL FROM AN OUTPATIENT SETTING *(CONTINUED)*	
All patients evaluated in an outpatient setting who within the past 12 months have experienced an acute myocardial infarction (MI), coronary artery bypass graft (CABG) surgery, a percutaneous coronary intervention (PCI), cardiac valve surgery, or cardiac transplantation, or who have chronic stable angina (CSA) and have not already participated in an early outpatient cardiac rehabilitation/secondary prevention (CR) program for the qualifying event or diagnosis, are to be referred to such a program.	
Numerator	Number of patients in an outpatient clinical practice who have had a qualifying event or diagnosis during the previous 12 months and who have been referred to an outpatient CR program.
	(Note: The program may include a traditional CR program based on face-to-face interactions and training sessions or other options that include home-based approaches. If alternative CR approaches are used, they should be designed to meet appropriate safety standards.)
	A referral is defined as an official communication between the health care provider and the patient to recommend and carry out a referral order to an outpatient CR program. This includes the provision of all necessary information to the patient that will allow the patient to enroll in an outpatient CR program. This also includes a written or electronic communication between the health care provider or health care system and the cardiac rehabilitation program that includes the patient's enrollment information for the program. A hospital discharge summary or office note may potentially be formatted to include the necessary patient information to communicate to the CR program (e.g., the patient's cardiovascular history, testing, and treatments). According to standards of practice for cardiac rehabilitation programs, care coordination communications are sent to the referring provider, including any issues regarding treatment changes, adverse treatment responses, or new nonemergency conditions (e.g., new symptoms, patient care questions) that need attention by the referring provider. These communications also include a progress report once the patient has completed the program. All communications must maintain an appropriate level of confidentiality as outlined by the 1996 Health Insurance Portability and Accountability Act (HIPAA).
	Exclusion criteria:
	• Patient factors (e.g., patient resides in a long-term nursing care facility).
	• Medical factors (e.g., patient deemed by provider to have a medically unstable, life-threatening condition).
	• Health care system factors (e.g., no cardiac rehabilitation program available within 60 min of travel time from the patient's home).
Denominator	Number of patients in an outpatient clinical practice who have had a qualifying event or diagnosis during the previous 12 months and who do not meet any of the exclusion criteria mentioned in the numerator section, and who have not participated in an outpatient cardiac rehabilitation program since the qualifying event or diagnosis.
Period of assessment	Twelve months following a qualifying event or diagnosis.
Method of reporting	Proportion of patients in an outpatient practice who have had a qualifying event or diagnosis during the past 12 months and have been referred to a CR program.
Sources of data	Administrative data, medical records, or both.
Attribution/ aggregation	This measure should be reported by the clinician who provides the primary cardiovascular-related care for the patient. In general, this would be the patient's cardiologist, but in some cases it might be a family physician, internist, nurse practitioner, or other health care provider. The level of "aggregation" (clinician vs. practice) will depend on the availability of adequate sample sizes to provide stable estimates of performance.
Rationale	Cardiac rehabilitation services have been shown to help reduce morbidity and mortality in persons who have experienced a recent coronary artery disease event, but these services are used in less than 30% of eligible patients. A key component to cardiac rehabilitation utilization is the appropriate and timely referral of patients to an outpatient CR program. While referral takes place generally while the patient is hospitalized for a qualifying event (MI, CSA, CABG, PCI, cardiac valve surgery, or heart transplantation), there are many instances in which a patient can and should be referred from an outpatient clinical practice setting (e.g., when a patient does not receive such a referral while in the hospital, or when the patient fails to follow through with the referral for whatever reason).
	This performance measure has been developed to help health care systems implement effective steps in their systems of care that will optimize the appropriate referral of a patient to an outpatient CR program.
	This measure is designed to serve as a stand-alone measure or, preferably, to be included within other performance measurement sets that involve disease states or other conditions for which CR services have been found to be appropriate and beneficial (e.g., following MI, CABG surgery). This performance measure is provided in a format that is meant to allow easy and flexible inclusion into such performance measurement sets.
	Referral of appropriate outpatients to a CR program is the responsibility of the health care provider within a health care system that is providing the primary cardiovascular care to the patient in the outpatient setting.

PERFORMANCE MEASURE A-2: CARDIAC REHABILITATION PATIENT REFERRAL FROM AN OUTPATIENT SETTING *(CONTINUED)*	
Corresponding guidelines and clinical recommendations	See clinical recommendations section from Performance Measure A-1.
Challenges to implementation	Identification of all eligible patients in an outpatient clinical practice will require that a timely, accurate, and effective system be in place. Communication of referral information by the outpatient clinical practice team to the outpatient CR program represents a potential challenge to the implementation of this performance measure.

Reprinted, by permission, from R.J. Thomas et al., 2010, "AACVPR/ACCF/AHA 2010 Update: Performance measures on cardiac rehabilitation for referral to cardiac rehabilitation/secondary prevention services," *Journal of Cardiopulmonary Rehabilitation Prevention* 30: 279-388.

NQF has endorsed these measures (Set A), an important step toward their widespread acceptance and implementation. Subsequent to the endorsement by NQF, other organizations have included the CR referral performance measures in their performance measure sets for the care of patients with CVD, including performance measure sets developed by the Physician Consortium for Practice Improvement and ACC/AHA.[45]

The CR delivery performance measures (Set B) are incorporated into standards for CR programs as specified by AACVPR publications and its program certification process. These CR program delivery performance measures are currently being revised and retested in order to identify those measures that meet NQF standards for validation and correlation with desired patient outcomes. AACVPR has developed resources to assist CR programs and other groups to help guide clinicians in the implementation of the CR performance measures into their local practices.

The Role of CR/SP in the Continuum of Care

In endorsing the CR referral performance measures in May 2010, the National Quality Forum has identified CR/SP as critically important steps in the continuum of care for patients with CVD. The decision by NQF to endorse the CR referral performance measures was based on several factors, including a growing body of published evidence showing that CR services reduce gaps in the delivery of CR/SP therapies and thereby improve the care and outcomes of patients who have had a CVD event.[22-29]

A number of reasons have been suggested to explain the beneficial effects of CR/SP, including the following:

- Positive vascular, metabolic, and rheologic changes related to exercise training[28]
- Improvement in patient adherence to medical and lifestyle therapies for SP[13]
- Improvement in the control of CVD risk factors[27]
- Identification and management of comorbid conditions, including depression and other psychological disorders, resulting in improved quality of life[46-48]
- Coordination of care between a patient's health care providers, helping patients understand, receive, and continue with appropriate SP treaments[20]

Although CR/SP fills an important role in the continuum of CV care, there continues to be a gap in the utilization of CR/SP due to relatively low referral and enrollment rates.[35,36] The future success of efforts to improve the delivery and impact of CR/SP throughout the continuum of CV care will depend directly on how well those efforts can extend CR/SP to all eligible patients. This is most likely to occur as new, effective models are added to current delivery models for CR/SP, and as federal and private health insurance plans provide coverage for those expanded services.[49-53]

Putting It All Together

Several important factors are essential as health care organizations seek to bridge gaps in the continuum of CV care and provide high-quality SP care to patients. These factors reflect an organizational culture that supports quality improvement efforts through the following common threads[54,55]:

- Organizational values and goals
- Involvement of key leaders

- Staff expertise and participation
- Systems and tools that support collaboration, problem solving, and learning

Professionals in the field of CR/SP can play a valuable role in improving the continuum of SP care that is provided to patients with CVD. Specific steps that can be taken to promote a culture of quality improvement in their practice area include the following:

1. Gain an understanding about and experience with important quality improvement issues and strategies that involve CR/SP.

2. Establish a culture of quality improvement in your CR/SP program and develop effective delivery models that address the needs of all patients who are eligible for CR/SP, both in the early outpatient phase and over the longer term of CR/SP.

3. Develop collaborative relationships with leaders in the hospitals and practices who care for patients with CVD in the local area.

4. Communicate with local health care leaders and other key partners about the important gaps in CR/SP that exist, using local data if available.

5. Work with local leaders to establish common goals for quality improvement efforts in CR/SP.

6. Work together with leaders and key staff members to develop and carry out quality improvement projects that are in alignment with the quality improvement goals of the organization(s).

7. Communicate results of quality improvement efforts and continually work to improve upon those efforts to attain quality improvement goals.

Summary

In health care today, there is an increasing focus on meeting patient needs along the entire continuum of CV care, from inpatient to outpatient settings. Gaps exist along that continuum, especially in the provision of CR/SP. These gaps in care ultimately result in suboptimal patient outcomes. Various efforts are under way to reduce the gaps that exist along the care continuum, including the gaps in the use of CR/SP performance measures. Quality improvement strategies, including the use of performance measures for the referral of eligible patients to CR/SP programs, increase the accountability of health care organizations and providers for the referral of patients to CR/SP.

CR programs are ideally positioned to deliver all phases of CR and SP services to eligible patients. To do so, CR programs must be actively involved in local and national efforts to implement new strategies that improve the reach and impact of SP services. CR programs will be successful in bridging gaps in the continuum of SP as they develop and implement a variety of delivery models and options to meet individual patient circumstances and needs. Changes must also continue to occur in the arena of health care policy and reimbursement to promote and cover effective models of care that can bridge the current gaps in CR/SP.

Behavior Modification and Risk Factor Reduction

Guiding Principles and Practices

The aim of this chapter is to provide the cardiac rehabilitation/secondary prevention (CR/SP) health professional with guiding principles and related practices to deliver effective patient education and behavior change programs within the context of secondary prevention of heart disease.

OBJECTIVES

This chapter provides an overview of

- patient education and health behavior change,
- basic counseling skills, and
- theoretical models of social learning and readiness for change.

Overview of Patient Education and Health Behavior Change

A primary goal of patient education is to facilitate behavior change known to improve health outcomes.[1] Changing health behaviors involves a process that may alter how people think (cognitive factors such as knowledge, attitudes, and beliefs related to the behavior) and feel (such as emotions, anxiety, or depression). In order to promote long-term and sustainable behavior change, health professionals must be aware of the meaning a target behavior has to a patient, the patient's understanding of the benefits and consequences of specific health-related activities, and how the patient evaluates the outcomes in association with a change (socially, emotionally, physically, financially). The health behavior literature[1,2] predominantly describes the factors that influence behavior change as a series of steps, stages, or concepts that are largely based on how a person thinks (cognitions) about the outcomes associated with a behavior. Specifically, a primary part of the change process is for the individual to evaluate the expected outcomes from doing (or not doing) a behavior, weigh the expected benefits and consequences, estimate the probability that an expected outcome will occur, and appraise his ability to perform a specific activity to achieve the desired outcome.[3,4]

Some health behavior change theories[3,4] include factors external to the individual and address the interplay between individual and environmental characteristics (e.g., availability, accessibility, and acceptability of cardiac rehabilitation/secondary prevention [CR/SP] program services). In most health behavior theories and models,[5-10] how a person thinks about the behavior (cognitions) is the primary determinant to explain or predict adoption of a behavior. This cognitive approach to health behavior change is a weakness to the extent that patients often engage in behaviors for nonrational (as well as nonhealth motivated) reasons. It is not sufficient to merely target a change in what people know in order to bring about a sustained change in behavior. In reality, patients may be influenced by emotions that are often associated with surviving a cardiac event (depressive mood,[11] anxiety, anger, fear), which may bias their ability to systematically process information[12,13] and to successfully implement a behavior change program. It is critical that health professionals design risk factor modification programs to meet the specific cognitive abilities and well-being of the patient, including an understanding of how patients view their behavior as a part of their overall recovery and their role as an active participant in a CR/SP program and the behavior change process.

The following summary of principles and related practices integrate cross-cutting themes and concepts that have been developed and tested extensively by health behavior scholars. Sources are largely derived from social cognitive theory[3,4]; the Transtheoretical Model (TTM), also known as Stages of Change[5,6]; Protection Motivation Theory[7]; the Health Belief Model[8]; and the Theory of Reasoned Action/Planned Behavior.[9,10] Health professionals who seek more information than can be provided here are encouraged to review the references for further reading on the theories and models included in this summary. To achieve an optimal program of education and behavior modification, CR/SP professionals should address the following points (guideline 3.1):

Principle 1: Provide a Tailored and Individualized Approach

One size does not fit all. Human behavior is complex, and so is behavior change as an element of promoting cardiovascular disease risk factor reduction. People differ in their ability to process information, their existing knowledge and ability to learn, and the skills required to be successful with a change in health behavior. One size does not fit all when it comes to designing new educational or behavioral change programs or selecting prepackaged materials that are well suited to individuals or groups. Risk reduction strategies work best when individually targeting key characteristics that are relevant to readiness and ability to change. These characteristics include the following:

• Cognitive characteristics—consider existing knowledge of the disease process, ability to learn (attend to, process, retain, and apply new knowledge), and the presence of distractions to cognitive processing (such as fear, anxiety, hostility, and depressive symptoms).

Guideline 3.1   Delivery of Education and Behavioral Modification Programming

An optimal program of education and behavior modification is based on the following:

- Allocate resources for *all* modifiable risk factors.
- Develop plans for risk factor modification using current clinical practice methodologies.
- Train staff in health counseling skills.
- Employ a variety of strategies and materials that take into account the individual patient and family needs and preferences, culture, and spiritual beliefs.
- Foster patient independence.
- Allocate resources to facilitate transition to full independence postdischarge.

- Evaluate the potential for social isolation prior to discharge from the hospital.
- Include written teaching plans and documentation of progress toward goals.
- Address smoking cessation immediately on an inpatient basis.
- Address all risk factors, disease processes, management of cardiac emergencies, maintenance of psychosocial health, and adaptation to limitations on an outpatient basis.
- Address and formulate a plan for returning to work and the need for job retraining, where appropriate, on an outpatient basis.

- Behavioral characteristics—identify which risk behavior(s) to target, with consideration of the complexity of enacting a sustained change in the target behavior and an understanding of the consequences and outcomes associated with success and failure.

- Psychosocial or motivational characteristics—consider the sense of self-confidence in the ability to perform the behavior,[3,4,14] including prior experiences with the behavior and related successes or failures; readiness to change; limitations imposed by illness such as functioning at work, at home, and in recreational activities; priorities; and values.

- Demographic characteristics—be aware of the influence of age, gender, education and literacy level, race-ethnicity, culture, and linguistic differences.

- Environmental characteristics—these include the support of family, friends, social networks, and powerful others; the involvement of health professionals and CR/SP professional staff; and access to a quality risk factor management program.

At the time of the initial assessment in CR/SP, health professionals are encouraged to assess patients across these dimensions and to match programmatic components to identified needs (see "Sample Behavioral Diagnosis and Steps in Developing a Plan" for a sample behavioral diagnosis[15]). During the change process, health professionals must also be able to adjust over time since the balance of these factors may change during the course of treatment.

Principle 2: Recognize That Knowledge Is Necessary but Not Sufficient for Behavior Change

It is critical for CR/SP professionals to ensure that patients have the requisite knowledge of behavioral factors that increase their risk of a secondary event or procedure and ways to effectively prevent or reduce that risk. Knowledge gain (learning what to do and how to do it) is a component of many health behavior change models. Patients must have sufficient knowledge of health risks and benefits of different health practices. They must understand what positive and adverse consequences can be expected from success as well as failure (and understand how to reframe a failure into an opportunity to reappraise goals and problem-solve strategies to overcome obstacles to success). Health professionals should prepare patients for outcomes associated with behavior change, including[14]:

- The physical effects a behavior is likely to produce (e.g., weight loss, functional improvements, muscle soreness due to exertion)

Sample Behavioral Diagnosis and Steps in Developing a Plan[15]

1. What is the problem, and what are the modifiable (behavior related) causes of the problem?
   - List behavior(s) that must be modified for risk reduction and management.
2. Discuss the list of behaviors with the patient.
   - Rank in order of importance for health improvements.
   - Discuss list with patient. What does the patient believe she can change? What is the patient ready to change?
   - Prioritize behaviors in order of importance and changeability. Select behavior(s) that will be the target for short-term goals.
   - Discuss past experiences with the selected behavior(s), expected outcomes, barriers that must be overcome (transportation, triggers for relapse), and required support.
3. Develop specific goals (short-term and long-term) and the strategies to achieve them.
4. Discuss what is necessary to learn (knowledge, skills) and do for success.
   - Consider learning needs and potential and adjust materials appropriately.
   - Discuss program components; break down timeline and actions into manageable steps.
   - Discuss patient and professional staff responsibility.
   - Engage support from positive influences (family, friends, peer role models).
5. Define how success will be measured.
   - Discuss self-monitoring and feedback plan.
   - Discuss time frame and plan for review of behavioral goals and clinical outcomes.

- Social effects (approval or disapproval of significant or powerful others)
- Self-evaluative effects (self-satisfaction, self-esteem)

However, though knowledge gain is necessary, it is not sufficient by itself to ensure such change.[1] Well-informed people may have low motivation or poor self-concept or may lack the skills and personal resources necessary to bring about a positive behavior change. As pointed out previously, it is important for CR/SP professionals to perform baseline assessments (see sidebar "Sample Behavioral Diagnosis and Steps in Developing a Plan") and provide tailored interventions to appropriately address the cognitive, emotional, and behavioral needs, values, and priorities of each patient.

Selecting and developing materials to promote knowledge among patients requires careful consideration. The average reading level in the United States is between the 8th and 9th grade level, and one in five adults reads at the 5th grade level and below.[16,17] Almost two of five older Americans (65 and over) read below the 5th grade level. Most people with a reading problem do not tell a health professional that they cannot read due to the strong social stigma attached to illiteracy. It is important to note that years of education is not a good indicator of literacy level because adults tend to read three to five grade levels lower than the years of education completed. Research has demonstrated that many patient education materials are written at or above the college reading level.[18] If print materials are used, technical words should be reviewed separately with patients to reduce their anxiety and improve comprehension. Elderly patients generally find materials with large print on nonglossy paper more readable. Another issue is that many patients do not speak or read English or that English is a second language for them. For this reason, it is helpful to have some materials in other languages, appropriate to the community served. Many publishers and pharmaceutical companies can readily supply these types of materials. The American Heart Association and other producers of educational materials have translated their products into Spanish and

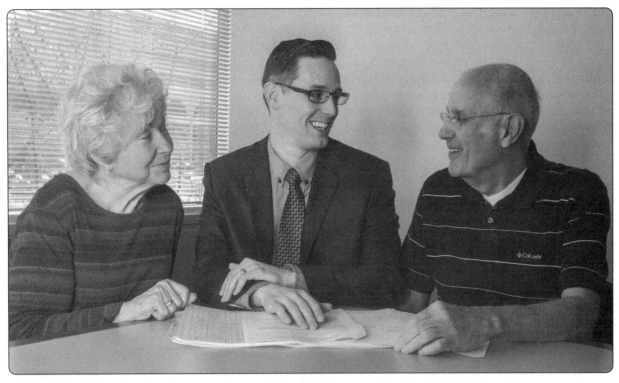

During the initial assessment, remember that one size does not fit all and match programmatic components to individual needs.

Chinese and have produced materials tailored to women and African American patients. For CR/SP professionals interested in developing new health education materials rather than using existing products, an exceptionally well-produced step-by-step tool is available to guide the development of effective communication products. *Making Health Communication Programs Work* can be obtained at no cost from the National Cancer Institute.[19]

Principle 3: Promote a Positive Sense of Self and the Personal Relevance of Risk Reduction

The self-esteem and risk perception literature suggests that people tend to protect self-esteem under conditions in which a negative outcome is regarded as controllable.[20-23] Acknowledgment of the role of high-risk behavior (e.g., smoking) in an adverse occurrence (e.g., a heart attack) may threaten self-esteem. Attributing a negative outcome to a factor beyond personal control (e.g., heredity, age) poses no threat to sense of self. Similarly, patients who undergo a surgical

intervention, such as cardiovascular bypass graft surgery, may believe that risk factor modification is not relevant to them because "the surgeon fixed me." The implications of such a belief are that risk factor modification is not worth the effort, is not personally relevant, or will not be necessary to achieve the desired outcome of health improvement.

When counseling patients about behavioral risk factors, it is advisable to avoid strategies that threaten self-esteem; instead, emphasize the link between behavior and the personal relevance[24] of risk factor reduction. In addition, it is important that all members of the team (primary care physician, cardiologist, and CR/SP professional staff) provide consistent and repeated verbal instructions and reinforcements of the need for specific behavior changes.

Principle 4: Promote Self-Efficacy and the Power of Control

It is critical to assess and to promote self-efficacy for successful behavior change.[3,4] Self-efficacy is the belief in one's ability to exercise control of health and to successfully perform the behaviors required to achieve the desired outcomes. "Efficacy belief is the foundation of human motivation and action. Unless people believe they can produce desired effects by their actions they have little incentive to act or to persevere in the face of difficulties."[14] Patients must be encouraged to believe that changes in one or more behaviors will achieve the desired outcomes and that they are able to implement the changes successfully.

Experiencing success in performing a particular behavior makes that behavior much easier to perform at a future time. Conversely, failures, including those in the near or distant past, can be barriers to beginning a behavior change program. For this reason, it is crucial that CR/SP professionals inquire about previous experiences with specific behavior changes and address the issues that led to past failures so that patients are guided through a problem-solving process. Additionally, to ensure successful performance, health professionals should encourage realistic goals and make changes in small, achievable steps (see principle 6 for more information about setting goals).

Principle 5: Promote Readiness to Change

Five ordered categories of readiness to change behavior have been identified to describe the process of modifying health behaviors. These categories are referred to as the stages of change[5,6,25] and should be considered and assessed in order to match a patient to stage-appropriate behavior modification strategies:

• Precontemplation stage: There is no intention to change the behavior in the near future (usually defined as within the next 6 months). Patients in this stage may believe that they do not have a problem or that the behavior is not serious enough to warrant attention. They may lack understanding of the potential consequences of not changing. It also is possible that patients in this stage recognize the need to change their behavior but have no serious intention of trying to do so. They may lack self-efficacy about their ability to be successful due to past unsuccessful attempts to change. People in this stage believe that the costs of change significantly outweigh the benefits. At the precontemplation stage, when

patients may have little or no interest in changing, repeated, gentle confrontation may be helpful.

Gentle confrontation helps patients see discrepancies in their beliefs and actions. Confronting patients does not imply that health professionals take an adversary role. Rather, it means that a statement such as "I see you've missed several sessions" allows for honest feedback, giving the patient an opportunity to respond. Confrontation should not take the form of a question like "Why are you missing appointments?" Such a question could put the patient on the defensive.[15] Strategies that might help patients progress to the next stage include the use of brochures, books, newsletters, videos, newspaper articles, and guest speakers who are positive role models of success.

• Contemplation stage: Patients are giving serious consideration to changing the health behavior within the next 6 months. They are thinking but are indecisive and lack commitment to make a plan of action. In the contemplation stage, interventions should be aimed at providing information in the form of written materials, videotapes, and persuasive role models (such as graduates of the program, ideally of similar gender and age) that can demonstrate the benefits of change (outweighing the costs).

Discussions with the patient regarding the particular behavior should include an appeal to what seems to be a motivating force for that person. Common examples include a desire to engage in a favorite recreational activity or to return to work, family, or social activities. In addition, at this stage a cost–benefit analysis is often quite useful. Accomplish this by helping the patient write down all the costs (negative consequences, such as fear of failure, giving up favorite foods, or time required to attend the program) and benefits (positive consequences, such as improved fitness and functioning) of making a particular change. Professional staff should be aware that most patients need help listing immediate benefits and may need counseling to minimize the influence of costs. However, this is probably time well spent. A patient may conclude that the behavior is not worth changing unless it is apparent that the short- and long-term benefits truly outweigh the costs. Once this cost–benefit list is developed, it is useful to have the patient keep the list for reference during difficult times.

• Preparation stage: The person intends to act on the health behavior change in the immediate future, usually within the next 30 days. Patients in this stage may make a plan of action and take small steps toward action, such as talking to health professionals and seeking advice and trying out the new behavior (e.g., such as acquiring low-fat diet recipes, joining a health club, quitting smoking for a day). The combination of intending to change and having enacted recent attempts to change is the hallmark characteristic of the preparation stage. Details on strategies to help a patient make a plan are provided as a part of principle 6.

• Action stage: The patient has a plan and is in the act of changing the health behavior or has made specific changes within the last 6 months or less. In order to qualify as action, the behavior must occur at a level that is acceptable for optimal health benefits according to current knowledge and standards. For example, only the time period in which total abstinence from smoking was achieved is counted within the action stage. The period of time in which the number of cigarettes was reduced, but abstinence was not total, falls within the preparation phase.

Most interventions are designed for the preparation and action stages. These stages are the skills-building stages, when staff and patients begin to set goals and to problem solve barriers and obstacles to continuous success (preparation), and then implement plans (action) and make adjustments as required. The action stage includes implementation of the new behavior and requires strategies to promote independence, feedback and reinforcement, and environmental supports (described in greater detail as part of the following maintenance stage).

• Maintenance stage: The health behavior has been successfully maintained continuously for more than 6 months. For some behaviors, the maintenance stage is a lifelong struggle and not a discrete period of time. The focus for health professionals who support patients at this stage of change is to assist with relapse prevention by promoting self-efficacy beliefs and problem-solving and coping skills to overcome challenging situations that may trigger relapse. Most people who relapse at a later stage do not return to precontemplation.

• Lapse and relapse: It is important for health professionals to counsel their patients that experiencing a lapse (a temporary slip, such as a discontinuation of a behavior) is a common and normal part of behavior change. Lapsed behavior does not necessarily lead to relapse (a long-term discontinuation of the behavior). Patients who lapse or relapse should be encouraged not to view this as a failure but rather as an opportunity to learn and try new strategies. Focusing on positive aspects of the behavior change process such as the physical, social, and emotional benefits is a more positive approach.

Program staff and patients should discuss situations in which the patient is most at risk for lapse or relapse and develop a coping strategy or plan of action for those particular high-risk situations to prevent or minimize the impact. One example is providing a telephone number to call, or a card with positive affirmation statements to read, that prompts the patient not to let the lapse become a relapse. Stress is a common reason for lapse and relapse, so it is important to include relaxation training and stress management at this stage. Finally, the patient should be encouraged to take ownership of and responsibility for his actions to promote the maintenance of behavior change after program discharge and the ability to sustain it indefinitely. Family and friends should be enlisted to provide social support outside the program to facilitate long-term adherence to desired behavior changes (see principle 10 for strategies related to environmental supports).

Program staff should assess readiness to change, because educational and behavioral strategies vary accordingly. An answer to a single question[26,27] that focuses on readiness to change exercise behavior usually provides a reasonable estimate. The example in the sidebar "Using Readiness to Change Directed at Exercise Behavior" uses readiness to change directed at exercise behavior.

Once determined, the stage can guide the professional in choosing appropriate strategies. Program staff should be aware that patients can move quickly and unexpectedly forward or backward in the change process due to influences within and outside the rehabilitation program; therefore ongoing monitoring of progress and adjustments are required to optimize effectiveness.

Using Readiness to Change Directed at Exercise Behavior

Question to a Patient From a Health Professional[26,27]:

"Do you exercise regularly? By regular exercise, I mean any planned physical activity (e.g., brisk walking, aerobics, jogging, bicycling, swimming, rowing) performed at a level that increases your breathing rate and causes you to break a sweat. Such activity, if performed regularly, is done three to five times per week for 20 to 60 minutes per session. According to this definition, do you exercise regularly?"

Response Options:

1. Yes, I have been for more than 6 months. (Patient is in maintenance.)
2. Yes, I have been for less than 6 months. (Patient is in action.)
3. No, but I intend to in the next 30 days. (Patient is in preparation.)
4. No, but I intend to in the next 6 months. (Patient is in contemplation.)
5. No, and I do not intend to in the next 6 months. (Patient is in precontemplation.)[26,27]

Principle 6: Set Goals to Promote a S.M.A.R.T. Plan of Action

Staff should encourage patients to set Specific, Measurable, Achievable, Realistic/Relevant, and Time-framed (S.M.A.R.T.) goals for both the short-term and the long term.[28] Risk reduction programs should begin with goals that a patient strongly believes *can* (self-efficacy[3,4]) and *will* (behavioral intent[9]) be put into motion. Behavior change targets should reflect the most current clinical practice recommendations based on local, regional, and national consensus. As a part of this principle, it is important to assist patients to prioritize which behaviors they are willing to change. As a part of developing a plan, patients require counseling to identify and problem-solve potential obstacles and how they will cope with temptations or make adjustments to promote the likelihood of success. Patients should be encouraged to develop both short-term and long-term goals. Short-term goals focus on small incremental changes in behaviors that will break down larger skills and build mastery for actions required to achieve the overall long-term goal. Long-term goals are those that the immediate short-term goals are directed toward; the ultimate goal is improvement in personal health through sustained risk factor modification and management. An example of a long-term goal is "I will walk 5 days a week for 30 minutes each day, within 6 months"; an example of a short-term goal is "This week I will walk 3 days a week for 10 minutes a day." It is important that the short-term goals be achievable so that the patient can experience success. By setting achievable short-term goals in small, gradually increasing steps, the patient can eventually attain his long-term goal. If the short-term goals are not achieved, the patient and professional staff should reappraise and adapt as needed.

One way to counsel a patient to set realistic goals and create an action plan to achieve those goals is to ask the patient, "How do you rate, on a scale of 0% (not at all confident) to 100% (completely confident), how confident you are of achieving the goal?"[3,4] If the patient is less than completely confident, discuss with the patient what she needs to be more confident (such as problem solving to reduce barriers that must be overcome as a part of the program plan). Similar scales can be used to rate the strength of a patient's belief in the likelihood of implementing specific aspects of the plan, from 0% (not at all likely) to 100% (completely likely), within the next week or the next 30 days. If despite achieving behavioral goals (e.g., improvement in intensity or duration of regular physical activity) a patient continues to be unable to reach health outcomes (e.g., control of hypertension, achievement of weight loss goal), the clinical team should work collaboratively to discuss a potential change in approach such as adjustments in exercise prescription, pharmacotherapy, or both.

Principle 7: Promote Independence Through Consciousness Raising and Self-Monitoring Skills

Skills and resources that help facilitate independence are critical to successful behavior change. Promoting heightened self-awareness and self-monitoring behaviors that track (and reflect on) the health behavior change process is one important strategy that is consistent with the principle of promoting independence. Self-monitoring involves recording intrinsic feedback (feedback encountered as a natural consequence of behavior) and extrinsic feedback (external feedback from health professionals and significant others) about progress throughout the behavior change program. Feedback can be psychological, social, physiological, and clinical and requires health counseling from professional staff about how to recognize and positively frame behavioral outcomes to improve chances of success.

Patients should be encouraged to self-monitor health behaviors with written records, logs, or diaries that record health behaviors and feedback. People can self-monitor using a wide range of tracking mechanisms, from low-tech (paper and pen) to high-tech (mobile devices, computer-assisted self-management systems).[3,14,29] Self-monitoring can track compliance and provide feedback. Records to monitor progress should be simple to use and readily accessible.

As an example of monitoring feedback, consider a patient who experiences muscle soreness after an exercise session. Assuming that muscle soreness may be an expected result of starting an exercise program, one may use this specific symptom in counseling the patient that it is not unusual, is temporary, and is a positive consequence of exercise. Staff can reinforce the training effort and advise that the discomfort is likely to decrease over time. Similarly, a patient who is reducing dietary fat intake could be counseled to frame gastrointestinal distress after eating a high-fat meal as an unpleasant consequence of the fat content. Contrasting this to the feelings after a different, more healthful meal may reinforce the healthier choice. Staff members who serve as behavior change specialists must suggest methods to aid patients in their ability to understand the immediate and long-term physical or psychological effects of changes in health behavior. Informing patients about the potential effects will bolster success.

Encouraging patient independence during active participation in the program helps facilitate full independence from the program after discharge. One way to accomplish this transition is for staff to e-mail or make telephone calls to discharged patients at regular intervals (for example, every week for 1 month, every month for 3 months, and once at 12 months postdischarge) to offer additional support and encouragement. Telephone calls or e-mails may also facilitate collection of follow-up outcome data. It is important that cardiac rehabilitation/secondary prevention (CR/SP) staff follow institution policy on using e-mail for patient contact. Typically, e-mail is not the most secure mode of communication and therefore may not be appropriate for relaying confidential information without obtaining patient authorization.

Principle 8: Provide Routine Feedback and Rewards to Celebrate Success

Provide patients with regular feedback that details progress toward goals. These progress reports may include information related to their risk reduction goals, such as lipids, blood pressure, weight and body composition measures, functional capacity, and other measures of cardiopulmonary function. Progress reports must be presented in a format that is clear and understandable, and the meaning of values must be explained (ranges in categories such as "normal" and "high" are helpful for interpretation). Trend graphs can be used to illustrate changes in performance over time (decrease, increase, unchanged). Regular feedback is especially important to reinforce patients who have doubts about self-efficacy and control over the change process, who may be at risk of lapse or relapse.

Rewards (self-rewards as well as rewards by program staff) for achieving short- or long-term goals are very important for reinforcing adherence to health behavior change. Rewards such as a certificate of excellence or a T-shirt need not be expensive; what is important is that they be connected with specific milestone achievements. Patients should be encouraged to be aware of the personal rewards inherent in improved health and quality of life, regardless of whether improvements are noticeable by others or are intrinsic (e.g., ability to play with a grandchild or perform a desired recreational physical activity).

Principle 9: Help Patients Create Positive Environmental Cues to Action

Cues that promote or remind patients of healthy behaviors and that reinforce healthful choices are particularly helpful.[8] Examples of reminders to comply with a scheduled appointment at a rehabilitation program are a phone call or an automated e-mail the day before a session and programmed reminders on personal handheld devices. Prompts can be as simple as a daily log on the refrigerator to track dietary intake, an inspirational photograph (of a loved one such as a special family member or of the self at a desired weight), or a motivating written expression in a place of prominence in the kitchen. In addition to helpful cues to prompt desired behaviors, patients may need support to (1) remove cues for unhealthy behaviors from the environment (e.g., remove unhealthy foods from the kitchen, throw out all tobacco products), (2) avoid challenging social situations (such as areas at work or other gathering places where smoking is permitted), and (3) seek alternative environments that provide support for healthy behaviors.

Principle 10: Promote Helping Relationships and Engage Role Models

Support from the referring physician as well as program staff, family, friends, and successful graduates of the program is a critical component in any behavior change process. Staff can encourage social support by allowing spouses, other family members, or friends who are a positive influence to participate in the program (for example, by coattending educational sessions). Before enlisting the help of family or friends, health professionals are cautioned to take note of the relationship between the significant others and the patient. Avoid placing patients in a situation in which reminders become unpleasant "nagging" rather than positive reinforcement.[15]

Program staff can also create opportunities for peer-to-peer helping, for example by instituting a buddy system (e.g., car pool to program sessions) or behavioral contracts, or by providing patients with contact information for informal interactions (with their permission). Developing a contract between a patient and another support person can help identify potential barriers the patient may encounter. Contracts should specify the behavior to be performed (the goal) and the responsibilities between the parties involved, outlining what each will contribute.

Patients learn about outcome expectations not only from personal experience but also from observation of others,[4] particularly those who are in a similar situation and to whom they relate. Peer role models such as guest speakers or audiovisual recordings of patients who have been successful can be integrated into sessions. In addition, persons in positions of authority (such as physicians and program staff) can function as powerful change agents. It is extremely important for program staff to model heart-healthy behavior and to positively reinforce those behaviors in patients. Finally, social networks (e.g., Facebook, Twitter) are major sources of information and social support for people of all ages and life experiences to connect on shared experiences. Since many social networking and other health education websites are unregulated for accuracy of information, health professionals should be available to answer questions about material that patients encounter. Staff should advise caution and should inform patients regarding websites that provide accurate patient education information such as the American Heart Association (www.americanheart.org) and the Centers for Disease Control and Prevention (www.cdc.gov).

Summary

This chapter summarizes several evidence-based principles and related strategies for health behavior change targeting risk factor reduction for secondary prevention of heart disease. These principles can be used to assess the needs of patients who are beginning a risk factor modification program and to guide the design, implementation, and evaluation of progress to achieve stated behavior change goals for personal health improvements. Program components can be delivered individually to patients for whom more intensive intervention is appropriate (such as one-on-one group counseling to assist with problem solving and goal setting), in group settings, or in combination (individual and group sessions). Home-based telemonitoring programs as well as Internet-based self-management programs may also be used to assist highly motivated patients. The mode of program delivery largely depends on the available resources (program, patient, family), particularly if a structured comprehensive outpatient CR/SP program is not accessible (e.g., in remote rural areas[30]).

Many of the principles outlined in this chapter include behavior change support, which requires health professionals to have effective counseling skills to assist patients with lifestyle modification.

Professionals who need further training in counseling skills are encouraged to pursue techniques that have demonstrated effectiveness, such as motivational interviewing.[31-33]

CR/SP directors and staff are encouraged to devote intentional efforts to actively recruit and retain patient populations, particularly women and racial–ethnic minorities, who tend to be underrepresented in CR/SP due to low referral, enrollment, and completion rates.[34-42] Ultimately, all eligible patients should be given the opportunity to be informed and motivated and to participate in an evidence-based, comprehensive lifestyle modification program for secondary prevention of heart disease.

Nutrition Guidelines

The objective of this chapter is to provide nutrition recommendations for the prevention and treatment of cardiovascular disease (CVD). The most prominent recommendation is to adhere to a primarily plant-based diet, similar to what has been described as a prudent Mediterranean diet or the DASH (Dietary Approaches to Stop Hypertension) diet. Since 2004, many important studies reinforce the knowledge base for nutrition in the prevention of CVD, including such topics as low-carbohydrate ("low-carb") versus low-fat diets for weight loss, folic acid, dietary antioxidants as anti-inflammatory agents, and marine-based omega-3 supplements. The topic of obesity has been of great interest and importance over the last 7 years. The pathophysiology that accompanies excess adiposity (particularly insulin resistance), as well as the clinical and metabolic complications and adverse events associated with being obese or overweight, is central to the nutritional principles involved in prevention of CVD. The growing realization that sugar is directly related to the obesity epidemic and to insulin resistance is embedded in this research.[1-4] In addition to briefly reviewing the current knowledge base for these topics, this chapter summarizes some of the most important new research relevant to new national dietary recommendations, including the 2010 USDA Dietary Guidelines for Americans and the 2006 American Heart Association (AHA) diet and lifestyle recommendations.[5,6]

OBJECTIVES

This chapter includes discussion of

- dietary patterns,
- obesity and weight control,
- fat versus sugar intake,
- anti-inflammatory diet,
- dietary supplements, and
- relevant guideline updates.

Dietary Patterns

Although there have been substantial developments in the scientific evidence base for connections between nutrition and cardiovascular health over the last decade, the general approach to a healthy diet remains unchanged. Hu and colleagues[7] characterized a *prudent* diet pattern as having a higher intake of vegetables, fruit, legumes, whole grains, fish, and poultry; this is in contrast to a Western pattern characterized by higher intake of red and processed meat, refined grains, sweets, and desserts. While there are many variations in the specifics of a Mediterranean diet,[8,9] Willet and coauthors[9] used a Mediterranean diet score to characterize this dietary pattern. Higher scores reflect greater consumption (more than the median) of vegetables, legumes, fruits and nuts, cereal, and fish and less (lower than the median) meat, poultry, and dairy. The DASH diet, originally demonstrated to effectively modify hypertension, has subsequently been shown to have beneficial effects on other CVD risk factors.[10-13] DASH is characterized by a food pattern rich in vegetables, fruits, and low-fat dairy products, with reduced saturated and total fat and sodium.

Plant-based is another term used to describe a similar nutritional pattern.[14-16] The three diets just discussed are plant-based. A plant-based diet is not the same as a vegetarian diet; while all vegetarian diets are plant-based, not all plant-based diets are vegetarian. In general, the term plant-based is intended to imply that the major portion of the diet comes from vegetables, legumes and beans, whole grains, and fruits and that only a minor portion is derived from animal-based foods.

Obesity and Weight Control

Excess adiposity has been linked to diabetes mellitus, cardiometabolic syndrome, CVD, and other chronic diseases and has been targeted as a

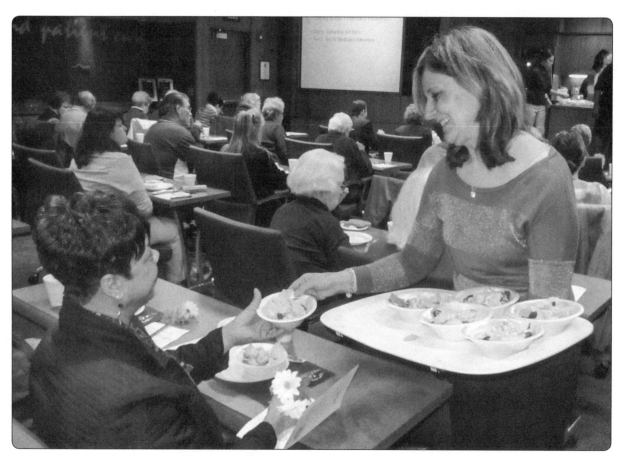

A prudent diet consists of vegetables, fruit, legumes, whole grains, fish, and poultry.

top public health priority.[17,18] The trend of rising obesity rates parallels the trend toward increased energy intake among Americans over the last 30 years.[19] National efforts to promote weight loss have been only nominally successful, and efforts to maintain weight loss have been an even bigger challenge.

Low Carbohydrate Versus Low Fat in the General Overweight or Obese Population

In 1998, a National Institutes of Health evidenced-based report on obesity evaluation and treatment recommended an energy-restricted diet that focused on a "low-fat" macronutrient approach for weight loss.[20] A low-fat dietary approach was used successfully in the landmark Diabetes Prevention Program (DPP) trial to achieve weight loss, and nearly 60 studies on diabetes prevention[21] as well as other evidence supported this approach.[22] However, data to support claims that a low-fat diet was superior to other approaches were limited.[23] An alternate hypothesis, that a low-carbohydrate diet might be an effective weight loss strategy, has emerged; but until 2003, the data to support this approach were limited. The primary overall conclusion of more than a dozen federally funded weight loss trials pitting low fat head-to-head against low carbohydrate was that low-carbohydrate diets were at least as effective for weight loss as low-fat diets. Some differences favor one or the other diet because of metabolic variables.[24-27] Another conclusion from these studies was that weight loss peaked at 6 months, followed by variable amounts of recidivism. Average weight loss among study participants who were initially 15 to 100 lb overweight was 5 to 10 lb at 12 to 24 months. Despite modest to nominal weight loss in these randomly assigned groups, there was substantial individual variability in weight change among study participants within all diet groups.[28-30]

Factors Affecting Variable Individual Weight Loss Results

Recently, at least two explanations have been hypothesized for variable weight loss among individuals assigned to the same weight loss diet. One involves the observation that adults shown to be relatively insulin resistant have been particularly unsuccessful with weight loss when assigned to a low-fat diet (which is, by definition, also high carbohydrate) and more successful when assigned to a low-carbohydrate diet (which is, by definition, also high fat).[31-34] Another, more tenuous explanation is the possibility of some level of genetic predisposition to differential success on various diets.[35] Before such findings of genetic predisposition can be considered of practical clinical relevance, they need to be further developed and replicated.

Low Carbohydrate for Weight Loss Among Those Who Are More Insulin Resistant

For the insulin resistance theory to be of practical use to health professionals, two important questions should be addressed:

1. What practical clinical assessments are available for diagnosing insulin resistance?

2. How low is low carbohydrate?

Insulin resistance is a relative term. There are no clinically validated cut points that distinguish people who are insulin resistant from those who are insulin sensitive. The simplest methods of assessing relative insulin resistance make use of fasting insulin level or a fasting triglyceride/high-density lipoprotein cholesterol (HDL-C) ratio; these correlate fairly well with the gold standard methods.[36] While there is no specific cut-point for fasting insulin levels to suggest higher risk, McLaughlin and colleagues[36] have proposed a cutoff of 3.5 for the triglyceride/HDL-C ratio; above 3.5 is strongly suggestive of relative insulin resistance. Finally, given the likelihood that insulin resistance is an important (or the most important) underlying factor in metabolic syndrome,[37,38] the established criteria for metabolic syndrome could be used.[39]

The second and related question that remains unresolved is how to best define and encourage patients to adhere to a low-carbohydrate diet. How "low" is "low carbohydrate"? Is it 40% or 30% or 20% of energy from carbohydrates? Although there is no formal consensus, an informal poll of experts in this field suggests that it is lower than 40% and higher than 20% (simply because less than that is difficult to maintain long-term). For most individuals, this boils down to a *lower*-carbohydrate diet, without imposing a specific percentage of energy value.

Conclusions for Obesity and Weight Control

The most important conclusion in the past decade in this area has been that a low-fat approach to weight control can no longer claim to be the single best choice. There is no single diet that is most successful for everyone, or even most people. If anything, the low-fat public health mantra that has dominated nutrition recommendations for the past few decades has likely been a less effective approach to weight loss than a *lower*-carbohydrate approach for the growing proportion of the population that is insulin resistant. It is more realistic to acknowledge that there will be a wide range of success among individuals with either low-carbohydrate or low-fat diets for weight loss. With either approach, it is not enough to simply recommend "low carbohydrate" or "low fat"; this advice needs to be accompanied by emphasis on high nutrient density and low energy density even when limiting carbohydrate-rich and fat-rich foods. Clearly, this will be difficult for patients, the general public, and health professionals to put into practice if the food environment offers primarily low nutrient density and high energy density foods. Because dietary adherence to these restrictive meal plans may be difficult, it is essential to refer patients to a registered dietitian to help individualize the plan whenever possible.

Fat Versus Sugar Intake

In the last 5 to 10 years, there has been increasing emphasis among many health professionals on simple sugar intake as a dietary target. This emphasis has gathered proponents from health professionals to national organizations.

Low Fat . . . Lower All Fat?

The low-fat mantra that dates back 50-plus years began to erode when the metabolic effects of different types of fats became evident. For example, it has been shown that for every 1% decrease in energy consumed as saturated fats, low-density lipoprotein cholesterol (LDL-C) is decreased by 1.83 mg/dL. Conversely, unsaturated fats (mono- and poly-) were shown to have beneficial effects on blood lipids[40] and were associated with lower rates of CVD relative to saturated and trans fats.[41] Marine omega-3 fats have been documented to be powerful agents for decreasing triglycerides and effective in at least one randomized controlled trial for the reduction of mortality and CVD events.[42,43] At this time, it is clear that all types of dietary fats should not be lowered. However, it can be difficult to succinctly and effectively communicate to patients what all the different kinds of fats are and what their different effects are, let alone what foods to choose or avoid in order to achieve an optimal fat intake balance. The evidence shows that it is prudent to limit intake of saturated and trans fats and to increase intake of poly- and mono-unsaturated fats. Whenever possible, referral to a registered dietitian who specializes in CVD prevention will greatly assist patients in recognizing and understanding the role of dietary fats.

More Calories, More Carbohydrates, More Added Sugars, More Fructose: A National Trend

During the last few decades, while attempts were ongoing to unravel the complexities of the science of "good fats versus bad fats," a striking shift was taking place in the eating patterns of Americans in a different section of the energy intake pie chart. This shift, as captured by national dietary surveillance data, has been characterized by a rise in total energy intake, which is explained primarily by increased intake of carbohydrate; in contrast, total fat intake (grams) and calories per day have remained relatively constant.[19] Data from the National Health and Nutrition Examination Survey indicate that from the 1970s to about 2000, self-reported daily carbohydrate intake increased by approximately 200 to 300 kcal/day. Most of the increase in carbohydrate intake was attributable to refined carbohydrate products and within this category, added sugars, especially beverages such as sodas.[44-47] A related change in consumption patterns has been the dramatic rise in fructose intake propelled by the addition of inexpensive high-fructose corn syrup (HFCS) to a staggeringly long list of processed foods.[48] A strong case can be made that the added sugars, and perhaps the high fructose intake in particular, contribute importantly to the obesity epidemic.

Resulting Shift in National Guidelines

The public health importance of all this has not escaped notice among those responsible for formulating national dietary guidelines. When the AHA diet and lifestyle recommendations were updated in 2006, one of the important additions or revisions made to the 2000 guidelines was a general recommendation to consume fewer sweetened beverages.[49] In 2009, an AHA position statement on dietary sugar intake and cardiovascular health recommended reductions in the intake of added sugars.[50] These recommendations are consistent with the 2010 USDA Dietary Guidelines for Americans, which highlighted significantly reducing the intake of foods containing added sugars (see guideline 4.1).[5]

Anti-Inflammatory Diet

The role of inflammation in chronic disease and the potential anti-inflammatory role(s) of various dietary components have generated great interest in the scientific community. The two categories of dietary components that have received the greatest attention are antioxidants and the marine-derived omega-3 fats.[51,52] Dietary antioxidants fall into broad classes, such as polyphenols or carotenoids (these broad classes include hundreds of individual types), or more specific molecules such as tocopherols and ascorbic acid. The most common food sources include vegetables and fruits, berries, nuts and seeds, and spices.[53] The two primary marine-derived omega-3 fats purported to have anti-inflammatory effects are eicosapentaenoic acid (EPA) and docosahexaenoic acid (DHA).[51] The increased availability of biomarkers to detect inflammation has led to a surge of both observational and intervention studies of dietary pattern or individual nutrients and inflammation.

Evidence From Observational Versus Intervention Studies

Findings from several observational studies support the hypothesis that dietary intakes or plasma levels of antioxidants (or both) and plasma levels of marine-derived omega-3 are inversely correlated with biomarkers of inflammation.[54-59] Similar beneficial associations have been reported for dietary patterns, such as a prudent versus a Western diet and for a more versus less Mediterranean diet.[60,61] Causal relationships can be determined only from randomized intervention trials.

Controlled intervention trials have been less consistent in their results. Trials using dietary supplements—vitamin C, tocopherols, folate, quercetin, resveratrol, green tea extract—have largely failed to observe a beneficial effect.[62-66] Most, but not all, of the trials examining foods high in antioxidants—soy products, tomatoes, almonds, cherries, raisins, and wine—have demonstrated a decrease in some but not all of the selected inflammatory markers assessed.[67-74] The few intervention studies of dietary patterns in this area have concluded that diets high in vegetables, fruits, almonds, soy, and other antioxidant-rich foods may lower biomarkers of inflammation.[76-81] But in these types of trials where the intervention involves combinations of different food types, it is not possible to attribute effects to any particular dietary component such as an antioxidant or a specific fatty acid.

Guideline 4.1   Dietary Recommendations for All Americans

- Consume less than 10% of calories from saturated fatty acids by replacing them with monounsaturated and polyunsaturated fatty acids.

- Consume less than 300 mg per day of dietary cholesterol.

- Keep trans fatty acid consumption as low as possible, especially by limiting foods that contain synthetic sources of trans fats, such as partially hydrogenated oils, and by limiting other solid fats.

- Reduce the intake of calories from solid fats and added sugars.

Data from Dietary Guidelines for Americans, 2010. www.cnpp.usda.gov/dietaryguidelines.htm.

Conclusions Regarding an Anti-Inflammatory Diet

While the importance of inflammation as an underlying causal factor in cardiovascular and other chronic diseases is well established,[82-84] it has been challenging to demonstrate that diet has a causal and beneficial impact on the prevention or treatment of inflammation. Further studies are needed to establish these effects and their magnitude. Given the large number of dietary components that may have anti-inflammatory effects, the range of doses that need to be tested for effects, and the large number of inflammatory markers that can be selected as study end points, this area of investigation will be complex and controversial for many years to come. There is evidence that a healthy dietary pattern has a positive influence on inflammation.[85,86] Should it turn out in the end that dietary components do not have a significant and beneficial effect on inflammation, it will still be important to promote vegetables, fruits, and other plant-based foods as excellent sources of dietary antioxidants and marine-based omega-3 fats.

Dietary Supplements

Dietary supplements have not been demonstrated to be effective for CVD prevention. Beneficial effects of beta-carotene, vitamin E, and B-vitamin supplements have all been disproven.[42,87-93] One of the last holdouts for promise remains marine-based omega-3 fats. The most widely cited study in this area has been the Italian GISSI study, which involved randomizing more than 11,000 survivors of myocardial infarction (MI) to 1 g/day of omega-3, or 300 mg vitamin E, or both, or neither for 3.5 years.[42] There was no significant benefit attributed to vitamin E, but for the fish oil a 20% to 30% decrease in morbidity and mortality was reported, including close to a 50% reduction in the risk of sudden cardiac death. However, several recent omega-3 trials have not replicated the beneficial effects of fish oil supplementation.[94,96]

Inherent Challenges in Dietary Supplement Trials With CVD Morbidity and Mortality Outcomes

It is important to acknowledge that there are several inherent and important challenges and limitations of dietary supplement intervention trials for CVD morbidity and mortality. Dose selection (typically, only a single dose is used in a large-scale trial) and appropriate chemical form of a dietary supplement (there may be multiple forms) are both difficult issues. Many of these trials are conducted as secondary prevention studies (i.e., among patients with existing disease) in patients in whom the disease process may be too advanced for a dietary supplement to have a clinically significant impact. Additionally these secondary prevention studies do not address the potential primary prevention effects of supplements. Finally, it is possible that some of these dietary supplements are effective in specific population subsets that are deficient in the particular nutrient but ineffective among those whose dietary status is adequate.

Given these inherent challenges in conducting dietary supplement studies for the prevention or treatment of CVD, it is not surprising that so many of these trials have failed to demonstrate a benefit. Nonetheless, that does not change the general conclusion that there currently are no dietary supplements with consistently proven beneficial effects for disease prevention (either primary or secondary).

Supplement Trials With CVD Risk Factors as Study End Points and Their Inherent Challenges

Lastly, it is appropriate to note that with CVD risk factors as outcomes, the evidence base for the beneficial effects of some dietary supplements is extensive and well documented. Stanol esters can be used effectively to lower elevated levels of LDL-C,[97] and marine-based omega-3 fats are effective in lowering elevated blood triglycerides.[98] Studying CVD risk factors that can potentially respond to a dietary supplement intervention in weeks or months (as opposed to many years) provides greater opportunity to conduct trials with different doses, different chemical forms, and a variety of population subsets. That is an important advantage in studying CVD risk factors versus hard outcomes such as CVD morbidity or mortality. The major limitation is that improving CVD risk factors does not always translate into reducing morbidity or mortality. Therefore, the potential beneficial role of dietary supplements in CVD risk factor management should be acknowledged, but the longer-term effects on morbidity and mortality should not be assumed simply on the basis of the risk factor effects until proven.

Relevant Guideline Updates

There have been several updates to nutrition-related national guidelines that are relevant to this discussion, including the 2006 AHA Diet and Lifestyle Recommendations[49]; both the 2005 and 2010 U.S. Dietary Guidelines for Americans[5,6]; and the recent introduction of MyPlate as the 2011 successor to the 2005 MyPyramid, which was the successor to the original Food Guide Pyramid.[99] All of these recommendations and guidelines are readily accessible, but it is beyond the scope of this chapter to provide an extensive overview of their specifics.

American Heart Association 2006 Recommendations

The 2006 AHA recommendations[49] confirmed the general recommendations of 2000[100,101] (table 4.1) and extended them in cases in which sufficient evidence had become available. Increased fish intake, especially oily fish high in marine omega-3 fats (twice a week), was a stronger recommendation in the 2006 AHA guidelines. Limited consumption of food items made with added sugar was an additional recommendation in those guidelines (note that there is now a separate AHA position statement devoted to this topic[50]). Emphasis on monitoring and maintaining normal blood glucose levels was added to the 2006 guidelines. In addition, the AHA recommendations addressed the importance of making sensible food choices when eating away from home and pointed out the importance of the availability of heart-healthy food choices in the food environment.

Egg Consumption

Historically, the AHA has advised the general public to limit dietary cholesterol intake to <300 mg/day, and especially to limit consumption of egg yolks and organ meats to control dietary consumption intake. However, studies have shown that there is much variation in individual responses to dietary cholesterol.[102]

The Nurses' Health Study, which followed 80,082 nurses for 14 years, determined that there was no evidence of a significant relationship between egg consumption and risk of CVD or stroke among healthy individuals when the equivalent of one egg per day was ingested.[103] However, this study noted an increased risk of CVD in study participants with diabetes with higher egg consumption. The Physicians' Health Study[104] also suggested that consumption of up to six eggs a week had no major effect on the risk of CVD and mortality. However, the consumption of greater than seven eggs per week was associated with a modest increase in total mortality. Similar to the Nurses' Health Study, this study did find that consumption of any eggs in study participants with diabetes was positively associated with an increase in stroke, MI, and all-cause mortality.

The National Cholesterol Education Program recommends that individuals with diabetes and heart disease limit their intake of egg yolks to two per week.[101] This coincides with the 2010 Dietary Recommendations as well as the AHA recommendations suggesting that healthy adults limit their intake of dietary cholesterol to <300 mg/day and that those with high risk factors for CVD (e.g., diabetes) limit their intake to <200 mg/day.

2010 U.S. Dietary Guidelines

The U.S. Dietary Guidelines are updated every 5 years. The 2010 Guidelines place stronger emphasis on reducing calorie consumption and increasing physical activity (these were also goals of the 2005 and previous guidelines).[5] There is nothing particularly new in these guidelines and there

Table 4.1 The Therapeutic Lifestyle Changes Diet

	Prevention	Coronary disease present
Total fat	≤30% of total daily calories	≤25% to 35% of total daily calories[a]
Saturated fat Trans fat	≤10% of total daily calories	≤7% of total daily calories
Monounsaturated fatty acids Cholesterol	10% of total daily calories <300 mg/day	≥13% of total daily calories <200 mg/day

[a]Based on lipid panel (triglycerides)

continues to be a particularly disturbing continuity with the guidelines of past editions: When it comes to recommending what to eat more of, the guidelines suggest food categories, but when it comes to recommending what to reduce, limit, or avoid in the diet, they emphasize nutrients. However, these guidelines do recommend limiting foods higher in fats; this list includes whole milk, fatty meats, and so on.

Despite the fact that many individuals somewhat limit carbohydrates in their meal plans for either weight management or blood glucose control, carbohydrates can and should be incorporated into most meal plans. The 2010 Dietary Guidelines remind us that one-fourth of each meal should be derived from a grain or starch. The guidelines specifically recommend that half of our total carbohydrates come from whole grains. In addition, they recommend that Americans aim to replace most refined grains with whole-grain foods.

Besides limiting refined carbohydrates, the 2010 Dietary Guidelines state that individuals should limit intake of carbohydrates in the form of "added sugars."[5] The physiological response to sugars that are naturally present in foods (e.g., fruits and milk) and those that are added to foods during preparation or processing ("added sugars") is similar. However, sugars naturally present in foods are considered "part of the food's total package of nutrients and contain other healthful components." In comparison, foods containing added sugars may provide few essential nutrients and little dietary fiber. Moreover, added sugars have implications for weight gain without contributing to overall nutritional adequacy of the diet. Added sugars and fats together contribute a significant portion to the total calories consumed by Americans.

The major sources of added sugars in the American diet are soda, energy drinks, and sport drinks (representing 36% of added sugars); grain-based desserts (representing 13% of added sugars); sugar-sweetened fruit drinks (10% of added sugars); dairy-based desserts such as ice cream (6% of added sugars); and candy (6% of added sugars). The Dietary Guidelines recommend that foods and beverages sweetened with any form of added sugars be replaced with choices that have no or minimal added sugars. Foods and beverages containing nonnutritive sweeteners such as sucralose, aspartame, or saccharin may replace beverages or foods that otherwise contain added sugars in moderation. For example, sweetened soda can be replaced with either unsweetened soda or water.

In addition to limiting added sugars and increasing whole grains, the AHA suggests that the carbohydrates we consume should include sources of soluble fibers.[50] It has been demonstrated that for every 1 to 2 g of soluble fiber ingested, LDL-C may be decreased by 1%. Sources of soluble fiber include fruits, vegetables, legumes, oats, barley, and psyllium. To maximize the soluble fiber intake while limiting added sugars, they suggest that people select whole fruits rather than fruit juices or fruits canned in syrup.

Introduction of MyPlate

Even more recent than the release of the 2010 Dietary Guidelines is the introduction of MyPlate, which replaces MyPyramid.[99] The MyPlate graphic is a plate divided into four sections; the two largest sections are vegetables and fruits, and the two smaller sections are grains and protein (see "The New Focus of the AHA's MyPlate and Accompanying Recommendations"). To the side of the plate is a smaller circle suggesting a beverage and representing dairy. The plate is certainly more intuitive than the pyramid and has fewer categories (omitting fats) than the old pyramids.

Summary

In summary, these nutrition recommendations suggest that an optimal diet is a plant-based diet composed of high nutrient density and low energy density foods. These recommendations are not a significant departure from past nutrition knowledge, just refinements and shifts in emphasis and priority. Obesity is the biggest nutrition-related health problem of the past and the coming decade. Weight control and energy intake restriction remain daunting challenges,

The New Focus of the AHA's MyPlate and Accompanying Recommendations

Balancing Calories

- Enjoy your food, but eat less.
- Avoid oversized portions.

Foods to Increase

- Make half your plate vegetables and fruits.
- Make at least half your grains whole grains.
- Switch to fat-free or low-fat (1%) milk.

Foods to Reduce

- Reduce foods high in sodium. Compare sodium in foods like soup, bread, and frozen meals, and choose the foods with lower numbers.
- Reduce added sugars. Drink water instead of sugary drinks.
- Reduce foods high in fats.

---

and recent efforts have fallen dismally short of expectations and needs. Many of us need to eat less. In particular, the advice really should be to eat fewer *sugars* (emphasis on the plural). Corn sweetener, corn syrup, dextrose, lactose, maltose, and levulose are sugars. Honey, molasses, maple sugar, and turbinado are primarily sugar, as are "concentrated fruit juices" and "organic, whole, unbleached, unrefined, evaporated, sugar cane juice." These can be found in thousands of packaged, processed convenience foods (including many foods labeled "low fat").

The reality is we really do not need more studies to determine what the healthiest diet is, or what the healthiest components of that healthy diet are. What we really need is to change the food environment and social norms that surround eating. We need to prepare more of our own food and diminish the demand for sugar-, fat-, and salt-laden processed convenience foods. We need

to at least put more effort into finding out about and appreciating the sources of the foods we buy.

Although perhaps not yet well defined or easy to substantiate, there is currently a grassroots groundswell of interest around food and a growing social movement around sustainable food. Individuals who make the most substantial, lasting, and healthiest modifications to their diet may do so for reasons that go beyond personal health. Clearly health is one reason, but there are other compelling reasons that include cultural and environmental issues. Research has begun to explore the possibility of social responsibility as a motivator for making successful and healthful dietary changes among college students, with some encouraging preliminary findings.[105] Perhaps by the time the next revision of nutrition guidelines comes out there will be more substantial information on this topic and more practical advice to share.

Cardiac Rehabilitation in the Inpatient and Transitional Settings

The first line of rehabilitation after an acute cardiac event begins in the acute-care inpatient setting. This chapter provides recommendations regarding the structure and process of inpatient and transitional cardiac rehabilitation while recognizing emerging trends in the field and ongoing changes in health care.

Decreasing length of stay (LOS) following the acute event remains the largest challenge to providing proper rehabilitation in the acute setting. The usual LOS has decreased to approximately 3 to 5 days following an uncomplicated cardiac event, including acute coronary syndrome (ACS), ST-elevation myocardial infarction (STEMI) or non-STEMI, and heart surgery (coronary artery bypass grafting [CABG] or valve repair, replacement, or both). The task of the inpatient health care professional has become increasingly challenging because of the decreased LOS. In addition to mobilization, vital components include assessment, readiness for discharge, recommendations for home care, and referral to outpatient cardiac rehabilitation/secondary prevention (CR/SP) programming. Since the initiation of inpatient CR (IPCR), a variety of postacute or transitional settings have been developed to bridge acute IPCR and discharge to home. These have become increasingly important due to the shortened LOS following a cardiac event. This chapter addresses the continuum of care from the acute event to successful discharge to home.

OBJECTIVES

This chapter addresses programming considerations for

- the inpatient setting, including clinical pathways and staffing considerations;
- transitional facilities; and
- home programming.

Assessment, Mobilization, and Risk-Factor Management

Patient assessment, mobilization, identification of cardiovascular disease risk factors, and discharge requirements (including basic education regard-ing self-care and management and facilitating entry into outpatient CR/SP) are cornerstones of CR in the acute-care setting. IPCR commences once a referral (either directly or via standing orders) is made (guideline 5.1).

Guideline 5.1   Cardiac Rehabilitation Within the Inpatient and Transitional Settings

Following a physician referral or by standing order, patients hospitalized for an event or procedure associated with cardiovascular disease should be provided with a program of IPCR consisting of

- initial or daily (or both) clinical status assessment and mobilization;
- identification of and information regarding modification of cardiovascular disease risk factors and self-care; and

- a comprehensive discharge plan that includes a discussion of follow-up options for transitional care, home programming, and formal outpatient CR.

Assessment of each patient referred for IPCR services is accomplished via a thorough chart review and a patient interview (guideline 5.2).

Guideline 5.2   Initial Patient Assessment

The initial interview of patients referred to IPCR should consist of

- assessment for admitting diagnosis, present illness and clinical status, current signs and symptoms, past medical history, social history, employment status, risk factors for coronary artery disease and other chronic diseases, comorbidities, and alcohol or substance abuse; and identification of support systems for future health behavior change and medical issues.

The purpose of the chart review and assessment is to

- verify diagnosis and current medical status,
- identify cardiovascular disease risk factors (figure 5.1) in order to begin planning education and interventions, and
- determine the existence of any comorbidities or complications that may increase the risk of a recurrent cardiac event.

The patient interview is essential to supplement the medical information in the chart for personal, family, and social history; home and food management needs; and availability of resources after discharge. Management of a variety of parameters not limited to cardiovascular disease risk factors is critical to the success of the CR program. Emphasis during this initial encounter, however, should be on assessing the patient for

- readiness for activity (figure 5.2),
- readiness to learn (figure 5.3), and
- discharge requirements.

The CR professional should assess whether patient goals are reasonable and realistic (guideline 5.3). Early recognition of unrealistic goals (e.g., return to work or unrealistic expectations for physical activity [PA]) allows staff to determine the need for intervention.

Guideline 5.3 **Assessment of Patient Goals for Cardiac Rehabilitation**

Patient-set, individualized goals for rehabilitation should be assessed to facilitate compliance and postevent adaptation. As appropriate, goals should be developed for such areas as

- physical function and return to work,

- risk factor reduction through health behavior change,
- psychological well-being and quality of life, and
- family and social support.

Figure 5.1 Cardiovascular Disease Risk Factor Checklist

Smoking	Dyslipidemia	Hypertension
__ Current smoker or quit at time of hospitalization Number of packs per day _____ Years smoked _____ Total pack-years _____ __ Former smoker, quit smoking <6 months before admission Total pack-year history _____ __ Never smoked or quit ≥6 months before admission Total pack-year history _____ __ Uses other tobacco products Identify: _____ _____	__ Abnormal lipid levels diagnosed before admission __ Pt reports compliance with prescribed lipid-lowering medication __ Previous lipid values or lipids drawn within 24 h of admission Chol _____ LDL _____ HDL _____ Trig _____ __ Unknown __ History of normal lipid levels	__ Diagnosed before hospitalization BP _____ __ Pt reports compliance with anti-HTN medication __ Pt reports discontinuing current medication __ Unknown __ History of normal blood pressure
Physical inactivity	**Stress or psychological concerns**	**Body composition**
__ Pt did not exercise three or more times per week or ≥150 min per week in 3 months before hospitalization __ Pt reports regular exercise	__ Pt reports history of high stress levels __ History of prior psychological or psychiatric treatment __ No history of perceived high stress or prior problem Appears, acts, or reports being __ angry __ depressed __ hostile __ lonely	Current height _____ Current weight _____ BMI _____ __ Healthy weight, BMI <25 __ Overweight, BMI 25 to 29.9 __ Obese, BMI 30 to 40 __ Very obese, BMI >40 __ Waist Circumference _____ At risk: __ Males >102 cm (>40 in.) __ Females >88 cm (>35 in.)
Diabetes	**Alcohol or substance abuse**	**Other**
__ Elevated blood glucose levels on admission or diagnosed __ Fasting BS or __ HbA1c __ Normal blood glucose levels __ Metabolic syndrome	__ History of alcohol or substance abuse at time of admission __ Pt denies history but initial presentation suggestive __ No evidence of alcohol or substance abuse	_____ _____ _____ _____ _____ _____

Response is required in each category. Abbreviations: Pt, patient; BP, blood pressure; Chol, cholesterol; LDL, low density lipoprotein; HDL, high density lipoprotein; Trig, triglycerides; HTN, hypertension; BMI , body mass index; BS, blood sugar; HbA1c, glycosylated hemoglobin

Assessment Parameters for Inpatient Cardiac Rehabilitation (and Transitional) Activity Program

The patient is considered appropriate for daily ambulation and mobilization if

- there has been no new or recurrent chest pain during previous 8 h period;
- neither CK nor troponin levels are rising;
- there are no new signs of decompensated failure (e.g., dyspnea at rest with bibasilar rales); and
- no new significant, abnormal rhythm, or electrocardiogram changes occurred during the previous 8 h period.

Progression of Activity

Progression of activity depends on the initial assessment as well as the daily physical assessment, documented in patient's chart (appendix B). Patient may be considered for progression of activity when response to previous activity includes

- appropriate heart rate increase (≤30 bpm, absence of chronotropic incompetence)
- appropriate systolic blood pressure (SBP) response to activity (increasing with activity, 10-40 mm Hg from resting SBP);
- no new rhythm or ST changes identified by telemetry with previous activity; and
- no new cardiovascular symptoms such as palpitations, dyspnea, excessive fatigue, or chest pain with previous activity.

Patients reporting any of these out of normal range or limits must be assessed by a physician and approved for resumption of activity.

Figure 5.2 Assessment parameters for inpatient education program

If assessment indicates that patient is "not ready to learn," *do not proceed with teaching;* document assessment, and defer teaching due to lack of readiness.

1. **Before proceeding with any teaching encounter,** confirm readiness to learn.

Is the patient physically able to learn now?	Is the patient psychologically willing to learn now?
• Stable physical condition • Adequate energy level and alertness (may be limited by fatigue, medication) • Absence of brain injury with event (anoxia or hypoxia not present)	• Appropriate emotional state (may be limited by anxiety or depression) • Awareness of cardiac problem (informed of diagnosis; not in denial)

2. **To determine teaching sequence,** ask patient to complete a learning assessment tool (see Example of a Learning Assessment Tool); proceed to teach topics identified by patient as priorities.

Generally, activity performance progresses from supine through sitting and standing to ambulation. Assessment may include activities of daily living (ADLs), such as grooming, dressing, and bathing (showering). In some instances the patient may require medical intervention before resuming upright or other PA. Abnormal responses must be documented and should be brought to the attention of the clinician. If no contraindications are noted (see "Abnormal Responses to Inpatient Exercise Indicating Discontinuation of Exercise Until Physician Assessment and Reapproval for Activity"), patients may proceed with ambulation as tolerated.

Abnormal Responses to Inpatient Exercise Indicating Discontinuation of Exercise Until Physician Assessment and Reapproval for Activity

Abnormal blood pressure changes including decrease in systolic blood pressure (SBP) of ≥10 mm Hg; and increase in SBP of >40 mm Hg

Significant ventricular or atrial arrhythmias

Second- or third-degree heart block

Signs or symptoms of exercise intolerance, including angina pectoris, marked dyspnea, or electrocardiogram changes suggestive of ischemia

Progression of activity depends on the initial and daily assessment. Patients should be assessed on a daily basis by the physician or the physician's designate before ambulation or activity within IPCR. Daily chart review and assessment by IPCR professionals before activity should include review of progress notes as well as assessment of rhythm, heart rate (HR), and blood pressure (BP) as they relate to ambulation and exercise (guideline 5.4).

Progression may vary from a more rapid increase in PA tolerance in the low-risk patient (patient with uncomplicated ACS or a patient without left ventricular dysfunction) to a slower progression in higher-risk or more debilitated patients, such as those with congestive heart failure (CHF). Table 5.1 lists common PAs used in IPCR as well as approximate MET (metabolic equivalent) values for those activities. Tolerance to activity always overrides other considerations for progression of PA during the mobilization phase of IPCR.

Management of risk factors begins immediately with the assessment of patient readiness to learn and capacity to understand the disease

Table 5.1 Types of Activities Commonly Used in Early Cardiac Rehabilitation

Activity	Method	METs
Toileting	Bedpan Commode Urinal (in bed) Urinal (standing)	1.5-2.5
Bathing	Bed bath Tub bath Shower	1.5-2.0
Walking	Flat surface 2 mph 2.5 mph 3 mph	 2-2.5 2.5-2.9 3-3.3
Upper body exercise (low to moderate effort; no resistance)	While standing Arms Trunk	 2.5-3.0
Stair climbing	One flight = 12 steps Down one flight Up one or two flights	 3.0-4.0

Based on B.E. Ainsworth et al., 2011, "2011 compendium of physical activity: A second update of codes and met values," *Medicine and Science in Sports and Exercise* 43(8): 1575-1581.

Med Sci Sports Exerc. 2011;43:1575-1581. Retrieved [01/25/2012] from the World Wide Web. https://sites.google.com/site/compendiumofphysicalactivities/

Guideline 5.4 Physical Assessment and Initial Physical Activity Mobilization by Inpatient Cardiac Rehabilitation

- Before beginning the activity portion of IPCR, a physician, nurse, physical therapist, or CR staff member with appropriate skills and competencies should perform a baseline physical assessment (see section on staffing), including heart and lung sounds, palpation of peripheral pulses, and self-care skills and ability. Results of the assessment must be documented along with baseline heart rate, blood pressure, and cardiac rhythm.

- Daily assessments must include chart review (after physician or nursing rounds, if possible), cardiac rhythm, heart rate, and blood pressure data, along with current clinical status.

process. Providing the patient and family with information and resources for risk factor intervention is critical. However, the reduced LOS and time constraints often restrict the IPCR staff to addressing only the most important concerns, such as survival skills and smoking cessation (guideline 5.5).

Adult learning theory provides the foundation for effective in-hospital patient education. "Example of a Learning Assessment Tool" illustrates a tool to assess readiness and priorities for learning. A growing body of evidence supports the idea that patients can identify what is important for them to know, and that teaching to those patient

Guideline 5.5 Smoking Cessation Intervention

- The smoking status of each acute-care cardiac patient must be assessed and documented.
- All current smokers must be offered intervention.
- Educational and behavioral intervention should assist patients through the period when they are

not smoking in the hospital, assess readiness to continue smoking cessation after discharge, and provide information on maintenance of smoking cessation if patients are ready and willing.

Example of a Learning Assessment Tool

Dear Patient:

Like most people with heart problems, you probably have many questions. During the next few days we want to address those concerns that are uppermost in your mind. So, to help plan our discussions, please check all topics for which you would like more information:

____ treatments and related equipment

____ heart structure and function

____ heart arteries, normal/abnormal

____ activity progression during hospital stay

____ what to do for chest pain

____ emergency planning for home*

____ heart attack and healing

____ your risk factors

____ how to take your pulse

____ high blood pressure

____ high blood cholesterol

____ your medications

____ fitness and health

____ eating for a healthy heart

____ sexual activity and your heart

____ emotional changes after heart problems

____ development of heart disease

____ stress and your heart

____ smoking and your heart*

____ alcohol and your heart

____ guidelines for activities at home*

____ activity/exercise precautions*

____ heart catheter procedure

____ bypass graft surgery

____ heart balloon procedure

____ stent placement

____ heart failure

____ internal cardiac defibrillator

____ CR/SP program*

____ treadmill exercise test

____ effects of heart problems on families

____ return-to-work questions*

____ heart rhythms

Other questions you would like to have answered:

_____

*These topics will be discussed by the cardiac rehabilitation staff before you go home.

Adapted from *Critical Care Nursing*, P.M. Comoss, Optimizing patient recovery—inpatient cardiac rehabilitation, edited by J.M. Clochese et al. pg. 1413, copyright 1993, with permission of Elsevier.

priorities results in the most effective education, especially during short LOS.[1,2]

IPCR education programs are based on individually selected learning priorities, with only one exception, the universal need for safety-related information. Materials such as handouts, pamphlets, and videos can be used to supplement the learning experience. Staff must choose those materials that best reinforce topics of importance, giving special attention to the reading level of selected teaching aids. Materials appropriate to a 6th to 8th grade reading level are recommended to help ensure that the majority of patients can understand them. Resources for many appropriate IPCR topics can be found readily on the Internet.[3-5]

Management of cardiac risk factors requires behavior counseling along with patient education. Chapter 8 discusses risk factor management in greater detail. Reduced LOS often precludes interventions for modifying specific risk factors. Consequently, the role of IPCR staff is to identify risk factors (where possible, inform patients of their implications, and provide information about how they may obtain additional assistance for risk

factor intervention following hospital discharge). In addition, clear, concise documentation about when and with whom the patient should follow up with about these issues within the first weeks after discharge will ensure the continuum of care and increase compliance (see figure 5.3). Early family involvement in the management of risk factors and continued care is critical to the success of the interventions and must be encouraged.

Discharge Planning

Discharge planning has taken on greater significance with decreased LOS. An IPCR can no longer be viewed as a phase that the patient will finish before being discharged; thus, discharge planning should focus on making appropriate connections for continued CR/SP, for example, referral to an outpatient CR/SP program before hospital discharge. The American Association of Cardiovascular and Pulmonary Rehabilitation (AACVPR) performance measures related to referral to outpatient CR/SP indicate that programs consider implementing an automatic referral process to CR/SP in the discharge orders.[6-9]

Figure 5.3   Example of discharge instructions and intervention follow-up checklist

Item	Provider of service	Responsible for follow-up	Date of appointment
Transitional care or home health			
Physician follow-up • Cardiologist • Surgeon • Primary care physician			
Outpatient cardiac rehabilitation/ secondary prevention program			
Risk factor follow-up • Smoking cessation program • Lipid management • Hypertension management • Stress management, psychosocial counseling, or both • Weight management • Diabetes management • Medication management			
Insurance and reimbursement issues			
Transportation			
Additional therapies • Physical therapy • Occupational therapy			

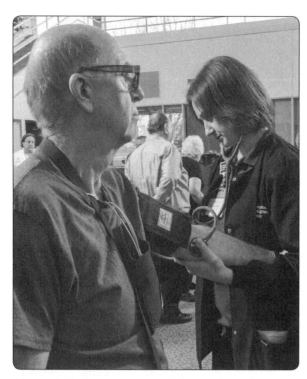

Abnormal responses to activity, such as decrease in SBP, must be documented and should be brought to the attention of the clinician.

For example, the referral process could include a prescription for CR/SP in the discharge packet, along with a list of CR/SP programs close to the patient's home (with contact information). The performance measures for referral to outpatient CR/SP stipulate that information about the inpatient stay should be sent to the outpatient facility and that the patient should be provided with sufficient information about how to enroll. They also include a sample script for inpatient practitioners to use to endorse the benefits of outpatient CR/SP to patients.

Enrollment in CR/SP is more likely if patients are strongly encouraged to attend by their health care practitioners. A science advisory of the American Heart Association (endorsed by AACVPR) encourages consistent communication about the importance of CR/SP from all health care professionals who interact with a hospitalized patient, including nurses, physical therapists, registered dietitians, clinical exercise physiologists, and physicians.[10] This advisory also recommends that an "inpatient CR director" be identified and empowered to direct the IPCR process, including working with administrators and other health care professionals to facilitate enrollment in CR/SP after discharge.

The following are discharge planning issues that should be addressed by health care providers, including the CR/SP staff, during the first month after discharge:

- Return to work
- Driving
- Household activity
- Stair climbing
- Lifting
- Sexual activity
- Walking
- Recreational and social activities

Transition to Outpatient CR/SP

All patients hospitalized with a primary diagnosis of ACS, chronic stable angina (CSA), CABG, a percutaneous coronary intervention (PCI), cardiac valve surgery, or cardiac transplantation should be referred to an outpatient CR/SP. However, regardless of where (or whether) the patient continues outpatient CR/SP, addressing safety is the highest priority for discharge planning. Survival skills (recognition of signs and symptoms, nitroglycerin use, when to call the doctor, and emergency assistance) and recommendations specifically with respect to ADLs, activity, and basic self-care are essential to patient safety. IPCR professionals should be active participants in the discharge planning team, especially by providing the patient assistance in evaluating options for both formal and informal continuation of CR/SP. Formal program options (transitional programs) that precede entrance into a more typical outpatient program are discussed in the next section of this chapter.

Implementation Strategies

Checkpoints and criteria for discharge readiness assessment[11] include

- physiological and symptom stability,
- functional ability,
- cognitive and psychomotor competency to perform adequate self-care,
- perceived self-efficacy,

- availability of social support, and
- access to health care resources.

Functional level and tolerance for PA should be documented by CR staff on a daily basis; this can provide exercise tolerance data that may be useful for home activity guidelines and CR/SP.

Clinical Pathways

Exercise and PA, education, and behavior counseling have traditionally been provided to patients within the construct of a structured and sequenced IPCR program. Historically, such programs were separate from routine daily patient care, but the current health care environment requires increased interdepartmental cooperation for quality improvement and cost containment.[12] The use of a clinical pathway provides a framework for the overall care of cardiac patients and integrates IPCR services into a comprehensive care plan.[13]

Clinical pathways provide a description of the typical course of treatment for patients with a particular diagnosis such as ACS, PCI, or CABG. The purpose of a clinical pathway as a case management tool is to standardize care so that LOS is predictable for the majority of patients in the respective diagnostic groups. As clinical guides, the pathways provide a protocol for progressing patients through the hospital stay. Furthermore, they serve as tools for evaluating both the process and the outcomes of patient care. Clinical pathways are intended to be comprehensive and multidisciplinary and are generally specific to each facility. Categories of patient care typically mapped out on the path include the following:

- Physical activity
- Consultations
- Diagnostics
- Discharge planning
- Education
- Medications
- Nutrition
- Treatments

Table 5.2 Sample Grid for Clinical Pathway

	Day 1	Day 2	Day 3	Day 4
Consults		CR to assess: • Readiness for activity • Readiness to learn		
Activity	Bed rest until stable, then OOB in chair Bedside commode	Routine CCU activities Sitting warm-up, walk in room	Up in room; standing warm-up Walk 5 to 10 min in hall two or three times a day (first time with supervision)	Up in room; standing warm-up Walk 5 to 10 min in hall three or four times a day Walk down and up flight of stairs with supervision
Education	Orient to CCU Give basic explanation of event and treatment plan	Assess readiness to learn; when patient is ready, teach survival lesson, for example, signs and symptoms recognition, preventive medications, nitroglycerine use, emergency plan	Assess readiness to learn Discuss safety, self-care, precautions for home	Review survival lesson Discuss postdischarge plans: • Provide phone number to call with questions • Discuss CR/SP follow-up: where, when • Discuss MD and specialist follow-up
Discharge planning				Provide CR/SP predischarge visit Evaluate for follow-up CR/SP services: home, transitional, outpatient

MI length of stay = 4 days. Abbreviations: OOB, out of bed; CCU, coronary care unit; CR/SP, cardiac rehabilitation/secondary prevention.

Variations in the Pathway

Preexisting conditions	Cardiovascular complications
General frailty	Postoperative bleeding
Chronic renal insufficiency	Arrhythmia
Cerebrovascular accident	Pulmonary infections
Orthopedic problems	Perioperative myocardial infarction
Cognitive impairment	Reduced left ventricular function
	Cerebrovascular accident
	Postoperative wound infections

Table 5.2 provides a simplified, basic sample of a clinical pathway. Clinical pathways allow visualization of the overall plan of care by outlining the sequence of intended care. Because activity progression and education are core elements of the IPCR program, these services are listed under the "Activity" and "Education" headings. **Note that this pathway is only an example of the activity progression and that both activity progression and teaching must be individualized.** Additionally, special visits by the IPCR staff for the initial assessment or predischarge instructions may be included under "Consults." To ensure optimal integration of IPCR services as well as to clarify roles and responsibilities, staff members, including those from IPCR, should participate in the multidisciplinary committee that designs each cardiac-related clinical pathway.

Once clinical pathways for cardiac patients are developed and implemented, usual patients progress accordingly. Variations in a clinical pathway secondary to comorbidities or complications such as those listed in "Variations in the Pathway" may occur. Although such problems may disrupt the treatment timeline, they usually do not eliminate the need for IPCR services. The IPCR specialist may make case-by-case adjustments, documenting those adjustments so that other members of the rehabilitation team are aware of the variance and can implement associated changes accordingly. Variance tracking is a part of the data collection requirements of clinical pathways.

Staffing

Considerations for staffing have been previously described and they include defining responsibility, competency, and productivity (guideline 5.6).[14] CR specialists, including exercise specialists, physical therapists, occupational therapists, nurses, and other staff, are traditional providers of IPCR services. The integration of the IPCR team and services into clinical pathways often involves a reallocation of staff resources. Table 5.3 provides an example of such role delineations. The particular role assigned depends on the needs, expectations, and resources of each facility.

CR Specialist

Even within the dedicated CR specialist role, variations in practice patterns exist. Responsibilities range from daily delivery of exercise and education services to a single, focused predischarge visit. Figure 5.4 contrasts the various roles. Again, the AACVPR Core Competencies adequately outline and detail these competencies for CR professionals.[14]

 Guideline 5.6   Staff Responsibilities

- Competencies for each member of the IPCR team should be defined as specified in the AACPR Core Competencies document.[14]

Table 5.3 Clinical Pathways and Staff Allocation

Role	Focus	Function
Cardiac or diabetic educator (RN, clinical exercise specialist, PT, dietitian, other allied health staff)	All cardiac patients in hospital	Responsible for teaching preventive strategies for risk factor modification and recovery from medical or surgical interventions
Rehabilitation specialist (RN, clinical exercise specialist, PT, OT, other allied health staff)	Postacute recovery	Responsible for evaluation, ambulation and exercise, and education of patients eligible for IPCR
RN or LPN	Postacute, postsurgery recovery and nursing care	Responsible for assisting with daily care (e.g., getting patients OOB, inspecting incision sites, doing medication teaching, assisting with transfer) as well as exercise and education where appropriate and necessary
Cardiovascular clinical nurse specialist, NP, PA, or case manager	Selected or all cardiac patients	Role defined by institution; may include implementation of teaching, activity progression, and discharge planning, or may include the coordination of the bedside RN staff for purposes of IPCR

Abbreviations: RN, registered nurse; PT, physical therapist; OT, occupational therapist; LPN, licensed practical nurse; IPCR, inpatient cardiac rehabilitation; NP, nurse practitioner; PA, physician assistant; OOB, out of bed.

Figure 5.4 **Inpatient cardiac rehabilitation specialist role variations**

Minimum	Moderate	Maximum
Predischarge visit for: • Education—emergency plan, precautions for home • Exercise—activity evaluation (e.g., stair climbing, 6-minute walk test), treadmill demonstration, and home program • Discussion of need for CR/SP or transitional follow-up; seek referral to the outpatient program	Shared responsibility with unit nursing staff for daily services: • Responsible for education, exercise, or both • Responsible for a selected combination of risk factor topics and exercise • Discuss need for CR/SP or transitional follow-up; seek referral and provide patient with information to facilitate enrollment	All day-to-day rehabilitation services: • Education—daily sessions based on individual priorities • Exercise—daily assessment and activity advancement based on protocol or clinical pathways • Discuss need for CR/SP or transitional care follow-up; provide referral

Abbreviation: CR/SP, cardiac rehabilitation/secondary prevention

Other Health Professionals

Clinical pathways encourage multidisciplinary involvement in the CR process. To optimize results, staff nurses or other qualified health care professionals may share responsibility with the CR specialists for activity progression, patient teaching, and other aspects of the CR process as long as they meet the specific core competency. Once the extent of the involvement of CR specialists and other staff has been clarified, respective job descriptions must be revised to reflect roles and responsibilities. CR specialists are expected to meet the AACVPR Core Competencies and

to be working toward appropriate specialty certification.[14]

All staff members require ongoing in-service education to maintain CR program excellence. Programs combining classroom instruction with supervised clinical practice are recommended. Such training not only improves the quality of inpatient care and therefore the CR program, but also helps fulfill the expectation for specialty training that ensures competence.[15] Continuing education modules via conferences and webinars are offered by various organizations, including AACVPR. Productivity and staffing standards must be consistent with the volume of IPCR patients.

Space and Equipment

The most common physical site for the delivery of IPCR services is the patient room and care unit where the patient is housed, usually the intensive care unit, coronary care unit, or intermediate-care unit or nonmonitored medical–surgical bed. Bedside activity and patient and family education can take place in the room or in another facility, while progressive ambulation can be carried out in adjacent hallways. It is prudent to use telemetry for patients on monitored units.

Ideally, facilities have dedicated space for evaluations, mobility exercises, or both. An inpatient exercise room specially equipped with treadmills and bicycle ergometers to limit hallway traffic and further advance functional capacity before discharge can be useful. Alternatively, patients may be transported to the CR/SP center (time and space permitting) for an introductory visit or even brief activity before discharge. An outpatient center visit may encourage early entry into the CR/SP.

Educational equipment and supplies, including an audiovisual system with a collection of educational programs, along with pamphlets and other handouts designed for use in patient edu-cation sessions, are recommended. Office space that serves as a work area and contact point for IPCR staff, as well as for storage of supplies is also recommended. Access to a conference room or small classroom is useful for group teaching.

Transitional Programming

Patients must leave the hospital with a clear plan for follow-up. They must be advised and instructed about progression of activity begun in the hospital. Unfortunately, shortened LOS and limitations in patient readiness to learn often reduce opportunities for effective patient teaching in the hospital; this is particularly true in complicated or elderly patients and in patients with significant preexisting comorbidities. When patients do not move directly from the inpatient to the outpatient setting, the immediate postdischarge (transition) period may provide an opportunity for participation in a transitional program, depending on the needs and capabilities of the individual patient as well as the options available in the area. Figure 5.5 illustrates admission criteria for three of the most current transitional tracks.

Because of cardiac complications, comorbidities, or age-related frailty, some patients are

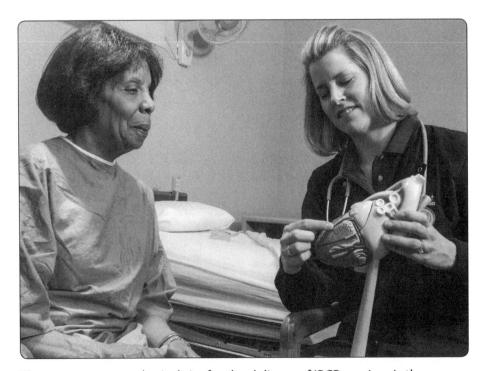

The most common physical site for the delivery of IPCR services is the patient room and care unit where the patient is housed.

Figure 5.5 Admission criteria for transitional programs

Skilled nursing facility	Inpatient rehabilitation facility	Home health care
Patients are temporarily unable to carry out some activities of daily living. They do not need 24 h rehabilitation nursing or evaluation and management by a rehabilitation physician as many as three times per week.	Patients require specific rehabilitation therapies; patients should be capable of participating in at least 3 h of combined rehabilitation per day; they should require 24 h rehabilitation nursing and evaluation and management by a physician with expertise in rehabilitation at least three times per week.	Patients are limited in their ability to provide for themselves independently at home and are in need of skilled nursing care or home physical or occupational therapy or social work services.

medically ready for discharge from acute-care facilities without the ability to perform ADLs or to ambulate household distances, while others may require physical therapy or other services in addition to CR in order to return to home safely. These types of patients benefit from referral to an alternative level of care such as subacute rehabilitation in a skilled nursing facility (SNF), acute inpatient rehabilitation in a hospital unit, or an inpatient rehabilitation facility (IRF).

Skilled Nursing Facility

Skilled nursing units may be available within the acute-care hospital or as independent centers. Such facilities have specific admission criteria based on patient ability to carry out ADLs. Patients who require assistance with basic ADLs such as feeding, toileting, dressing, grooming, bathing, transferring, and walking after a cardiac event may qualify for admission to a skilled nursing facility.

Inpatient Rehabilitation Facility

Over the past several decades, inpatient rehabilitation facilities have been developed as a bridge between the acute-care facility and independent home living.[16,17] These programs prepare patients for a safe and independent return to home using a multidisciplinary approach that includes physical, occupational, vocational, and recreational therapy; speech pathology; nutrition; psychology and psychiatry; and continued medical and nursing management. Such a team approach should reduce fragmentation of care; improve patient outcomes; and enhance patient, family, staff, and physician satisfaction.

Admission criteria to inpatient rehabilitation programs generally include a greater need for skilled nursing, physician, and rehabilitation care compared to subacute or skilled nursing facili-

ties. This can include management of medical issues such as fluid status; dysrhythmia; tracheotomy care; oxygen and bronchodilator therapy; wound care; intravenous therapy; and adjustments of medications for comorbidities such as depression, postoperative confusion, diabetes, and hypertension. The frequency and intensity of therapy sessions are greater. Sessions include individual and group education; gait retraining; strength, endurance, and range of motion exercise; ADL evaluation and retraining; cognitive evaluation and retraining; and therapy specific to any preexisting or postoperative neurological or musculoskeletal disabilities that may interfere with recovery. Patients with permanent disabilities (e.g., paraplegia, amputation, neuromuscular disorders) who have had acute cardiac problems may also benefit from the multidisciplinary assistance that an inpatient rehabilitation hospital can provide. Rehabilitation goals are set by the patient, family, and the multidisciplinary team and generally include return to independent community function, with referral to home care or CR/SP programming as appropriate.

Inpatient rehabilitation facilities use standardized, objective, and valid tools to measure outcomes. Evaluations such as the Functional Independence Measure, among others, are used to measure improvement from admission to discharge.[17] Longstanding national registries track outcomes for these patients related to functional improvement, discharge destination, and readmissions. Published data demonstrate the efficacy of such programs with respect to functional outcomes.[18-20]

Home Health Care

Many patients who leave the hospital after short stays are in need of follow-up care that until recently would have been provided in the hospital.

Nursing care such as wound care, medication instruction and administration, BP or blood sugar surveillance, and anticoagulation may be more than the patient or the home caregiver can manage, prompting referral to home health care. In addition, some patients may need physical or occupational therapy, or both, to assess their safety at home, including their ability to climb stairs and care for themselves safely. The availability of home health nursing services, especially for the postsurgical and CHF populations, provides an alternative for managing recovery that is attractive to patients, physicians, and payers alike.

Under Medicare standards, patients must be "homebound," which means that they are unable to leave their homes unassisted, to receive home health services. A number of cardiac patients may qualify for several weeks of home care due to either physical limitations, lack of mobility, or temporary restrictions imposed by the medical team (i.e., driving restrictions). A patient who is being transported by another person to day care for any reason other than medical appointments is not considered homebound. The maximum length of time for insurance coverage is determined individually. Payers may cover follow-up home care for a fixed number of visits or weeks as a routine component of total case management.

Specific Considerations for Transitional Care

Two major issues must be addressed when patient options for transitional care programs are being explored: (1) who provides care and (2) the level of reimbursement. Nurses, physical therapists, and others who typically staff skilled nursing facilities and home care agencies are trained to provide services designed to meet specific functional and medical goals to enable a patient to return to (or stay) at home. Therefore they may not have received specific training regarding CR issues. However, these individuals can develop competencies through in-service training provided by CR professionals; or, alternatively, CR specialists may be hired to staff these programs. Staff physical assessment skills should include electrocardiogram telemetry monitoring, which is not typically available in skilled nursing facility or home settings. Although transitional settings may provide CR exercise and education services, CR services alone in these settings are usually not reimbursable by Medicare. Medicare reimburses only for skilled nursing or specific therapy such as physical or occupational therapy, based on medical necessity criteria for these services. This emphasizes the need for specialized training and experience related to CR for these providers if the delivery of postacute care for cardiac patients in these transitional settings is to be maximally effective.

The clinical pathway can also be a primary tool for service delivery in transitional settings. Transitional clinical pathways can build on the inpatient programming results by gradually increasing ambulation and PA and by introducing upper body exercises. Performance parameters similar to those used with inpatient programs apply; and the same education assessments, curriculums, and teaching aids can be used to address individual priorities.

In an attempt to provide continuity of CR service from one setting to the next, some programs have developed pathways that span the entire CR continuum: inpatient, transitional, outpatient, and maintenance. Two major advantages have been documented with this approach: (1) downtime between CR settings is minimized, and (2) referrals from tertiary treatment centers to community CR/SP programming are maximized.[21]

This continuity of care is as beneficial to the uncomplicated patient who is discharged quickly as it is to the more complicated patient who requires transitional care. Ironically, patients considered "uncomplicated" may have the fewest options for posthospitalization or transitional care, since it tends to be provided most often to patients at higher levels of acuity and dysfunction. Additionally, because uncomplicated patients often have shortened LOS, less time in the hospital is available for education and activity. Unfortunately, some uncomplicated patients may not be able to enter an outpatient program immediately. Therefore, traditional outpatient CR program staff should consider developing transitional programs.

Summary

Current AACVPR (see chapter 2) guidelines recommend early initiation of outpatient CR/SP, that is, within 1 to 3 weeks postevent. The innovative transitional programs discussed here and summarized in "Summary of Cardiac Rehabilitation Structure Recommendations Within the Inpatient and Transitional Settings" and "Summary of Process Recommendations for Cardiac Rehabilitation (CR) in the Inpatient and Transitional Settings," including subacute facilities, rehabilitation hospitals, home care, and specifically designed transitional programs within traditional outpatient settings, meet the expectation of a quality continuum of rehabilitation care.

Summary of Cardiac Rehabilitation Structure Recommendations Within the Inpatient and Transitional Settings

Exercise

1. Design and implementation should be based on physiological principles that can be used by a variety of health professionals within either an inpatient or a transitional setting, and should be integrated into a cooperative clinical pathway.

2. Flexibility in the PA plan is critical to individualization; alternatively, an individualized plan may be developed for patients who do not fit the clinical pathway.

3. Specific criteria for beginning and advancing inpatient activities are required.

Education

1. A standardized collection of cardiac teaching plans that outline the content area topics (see figures 5.3 and 5.5) should be available.

2. Appropriate and readable teaching aids are required to reinforce patient education content.

3. Patients must be involved in identifying their own high-priority learning needs.

4. Patient readiness to learn should be assessed before every potential teaching encounter.

5. Each teaching encounter should be evaluated; this evaluation includes patient comprehension.

Discharge planning

1. At a minimum, one predischarge visit for every CR patient must

   - address survival skills and postdischarge "dos and don'ts,"
   - evaluate and estimate predischarge functional ability, and
   - provide information about outpatient programming.

Summary of Process Recommendations for Cardiac Rehabilitation (CR) in the Inpatient and Transitional Settings

Mechanism

1. Define the purpose and goals of the inpatient or transitional CR program.

2. Clarify CR expectations between rehabilitation specialists and other health care professionals.

Resources

1. Specify the extent of responsibility each rehabilitation specialist has (minimum, shared, maximum).

2. Document the time required for delivery of rehabilitation services.

3. Complete the scope of practice statement for all professionals involved in CR service delivery and insert into job descriptions.

(continued)

(continued)

4. Develop and present in-service training for health care professionals outside the immediate inpatient team who will assume some rehabilitation responsibilities.

5. Develop standards clarifying the criteria for educational and exercise therapy within the IPCR program.

Continuity

1. CR staff must participate in discharge planning to facilitate CR/SP follow-up.

2. Identify potential transitional resources and respective patient qualifications, including
   - subacute facilities,
   - acute rehabilitation hospitals, and
   - home care follow-up.

3. Advisory or educational assistance (or both) should be available to transitional programs.

4. Continuation to CR/SP programming after transition is complete is strongly recommended.

Medical Evaluation and Exercise Testing

Data gathered from the initial medical evaluation of patients before entry into cardiac reha-bilitation are used to design and implement an effective program in which specific outcomes are defined and targeted. The American Heart Association (AHA) guidelines for comprehensive secondary prevention provide a useful framework for evaluation and management prevention guidelines.[1] This information is most useful for stratifying the patient in two ways:

- It establishes patient risk for progression of atherosclerosis and the likelihood of future cardiac events.

- It establishes patient risk for adverse cardiac events during prescribed exercise training, as well as whether exercise is contraindicated and, if not, the level of supervision and monitoring recommended during the initial training period. (Stratification of these factors is discussed separately in chapter 7.)

OBJECTIVES

This chapter discusses
- the components of the history and physical examination,
- the methods and protocols for exercise testing,
- interpretation of results,
- additional imaging modalities, and
- alternative methods for evaluating physical activity status.

Information from the medical evaluation and exercise testing may be provided by the primary care physician, cardiologist, or surgeon before initiation of cardiac rehabilitation/secondary prevention (CR/SP) or through direct evaluation by the medical director of the CR/SP program during the initial session (guideline 6.1). A medical history, with particular attention to cardiovascular status, and a detailed review of risk factors and their management are essential components of the initial assessment and will serve to target and individualize the program (see "Components of the Medical History"). The CR/SP specialist should determine whether patients are experiencing symp-

Guideline 6.1 Medical Evaluation and Exercise Testing

- To establish a safe and effective program of comprehensive cardiovascular disease risk reduction and rehabilitation, each patient should undergo a careful medical evaluation and exercise test before participating in an outpatient cardiac rehabilitation/secondary prevention program.

- The 6-minute walk test (see later subsection on this test) can be used as a surrogate measure of exercise capacity when standard treadmill or cycle testing is not available. It is not useful in the objective deter-

mination of myocardial ischemia, and is best used in a serial manner to evaluate changes in exercise capacity with training over time.

- The specific components of the medical evaluation should include a medical history, physical examination, and resting electrocardiogram.

- The exercise test should be repeated any time that symptoms or clinical changes warrant, as well as in the follow-up assessment of the exercise training outcome.

Components of the Medical History

1. **Medical diagnoses:** A variety of diagnoses should be reviewed, including, but not limited to, cardiovascular disease including existing coronary artery disease; previous MI, angioplasty, cardiac surgery, angina, and hypertension; pulmonary disease, including asthma, emphysema, and bronchitis; cerebrovascular disease, including stroke; diabetes; peripheral arterial disease; anemia, phlebitis, or emboli; cancer; pregnancy; musculoskeletal imbalances and neuromuscular and joint disease; osteoporosis; emotional disorders and eating disorders.

2. **Symptoms:** Angina; discomfort (pressure, tingling, pain, heaviness, burning, numbness) in the chest, jaw, neck, or arms; atypical angina, such as light-headedness, dizziness, or fainting; shortness of breath; rapid heartbeats or palpitations, especially if associated with physical activity, eating a large meal, emotional upset, or exposure to cold.

3. **Risk factors for atherosclerotic disease progression:** Hypertension, diabetes, obesity, dyslipidemia, smoking, and physical inactivity.

4. **Recent illness, hospitalization, or surgical procedure.**

5. **Medication dose and schedule, drug allergies.**

6. **Other habits:** Including alcohol or illicit drug use.

7. **Exercise history:** Information on habitual level of activity, such as frequency, duration, intensity, and type of exercise.

8. **Work history:** With an emphasis on current or expected physical and mental demands, noting upper and lower extremity requirements; estimated time to return to work.

9. **Psychosocial history:** Including living conditions and housemates; marital and family status; transportation needs; family needs; domestic and emotional problems; depression, anxiety, or other psychological disorders.

Based on Fletcher et al. 2001.

toms of angina, dyspnea, palpitations, or syncope and should ask patients about previous occurrence of myocardial infarction (MI), percutaneous coronary intervention, or bypass surgery. Ideally, measurements of cardiac function via echocardiography and coronary anatomy should be available and noted. A complete list of medications, dosing intervals, and compliance with the drug regimen should be reviewed, because these may affect the response to exercise. Comorbid conditions such as pulmonary, endocrine, and neurological illnesses and behavioral and musculoskeletal conditions should be evaluated.

Detailed social and occupational histories yield valuable information and allow the tailoring of exercise training and goals to meet individual needs. When developing the patient assessment protocol for all patients, CR/SP staff should seek consultation, as needed, from social services and vocational rehabilitation specialists who are familiar with the array of medical, psychological, economic, and legal factors that influence return-to-work issues. Family and community resources that can assist patients with family concerns and returning to work should also be considered.

Physical Examination

The initial physical examination should be performed by a physician or other appropriately trained and qualified health care provider under the direction of a physician who is actively involved in the routine care of patients with cardiovascular disease (CVD) (see guideline 6.2 and "Components of the Physical Examination"). A current resting standard 12-lead electrocardiogram (ECG) is useful in assessing heart rate (HR), rhythm, conduction abnormalities, and evidence of prior MI. The resting ECG serves as an important reference for future comparison, particularly if the patient develops new signs or symptoms suggestive of ischemia, infarction, or dysrhythmias.

Musculoskeletal complaints and injury are not uncommon, especially when a patient is beginning an exercise program. Therefore,

 Guideline 6.2   Physical Examination

- The physical examination, at a minimum, should focus on the resting HR; blood pressure; and pulmonary, cardiac, vascular, and musculoskeletal areas (see "Components of the Physical Examination").

Components of the Physical Examination

1. Body weight, height, body mass index, waist-to-hip ratio, waist circumference at the level of the umbilicus
2. Pulse rate and regularity
3. Resting blood pressure
4. Auscultation of the lungs, with specific attention to uniformity of breath sounds in all areas (absence of rales, wheezes, and other abnormal breath sounds)
5. Auscultation of the heart, with specific attention to murmurs, gallops, clicks, and rubs
6. Palpation and auscultation of carotid, abdominal, and femoral arteries
7. Palpation and inspection of lower extremities for edema and presence of arterial pulses and skin integrity (particularly in those with diabetes)
8. Absence or presence of xanthoma and xanthelasma
9. Examination related to orthopedic, neurologic, or other medical conditions that might limit exercise testing or training
10. Examination of the chest and leg wounds and vascular access areas in patients after coronary bypass surgery or percutaneous coronary revascularization

Based on Fletcher et al. 2001.

musculoskeletal function should be assessed before exercise training begins. Assessment of lower extremity strength, flexibility, and balance should be performed with hopes of preventing injuries related to weight-bearing exercise. CR/SP staff should assess posture and alignment and determine whether there is a history of musculoskeletal injury.

In patients who have undergone coronary artery bypass surgery via median sternotomy, it is important to evaluate for sternal stability by identifying any movement in the sternum, pain, clicking, or popping. Sternal bone healing to attain adequate sternal stability is usually achieved by 8 weeks.[2] Infection, nonunion, and instability occur in about 2% to 5% of cases and are often predisposed by clinical factors such as diabetes mellitus, obesity, immunosuppression, advanced age, and osteoporosis.[3]

Risk Stratification and Identification of Contraindications for Exercise Training

Recommendations for risk stratifying patients as they enter outpatient CR/SP are outlined in chapter 7. The classifications are presented as a means of classifying patients with respect to risk of event during exercise and risk of progression of atherosclerosis. They do not consider accompanying morbidities (for example, insulin-dependent diabetes mellitus, morbid obesity, severe pulmonary disease, complicated pregnancy, or debilitating neurological or orthopedic conditions) that may constitute a contraindication to exercise or necessitate closer supervision during exercise

Absolute and Relative Contraindications to Exercise Training

Absolute
- Recent change in the resting ECG suggesting significant ischemia, recent MI, or other acute cardiac event
- Unstable angina
- Uncontrolled cardiac arrhythmias
- Symptomatic severe aortic stenosis or other valvular disease
- Decompensated symptomatic heart failure
- Acute pulmonary embolus or pulmonary infarction
- Acute noncardiac disorder that may affect exercise performance or may be aggravated by exercise (e.g., infection, thyrotoxicosis)
- Acute myocarditis or pericarditis
- Acute thrombophlebitis
- Physical disability that would preclude safe and adequate exercise performance

Relative*
- Electrolyte abnormalities
- Tachyarrhythmias or bradyarrhythmias
- High-degree atrioventricular block
- Atrial fibrillation with uncontrolled ventricular rate
- Hypertrophic obstructive cardiomyopathy with peak resting left ventricular outflow gradient of >25 mmHg
- Known aortic dissection
- Severe resting arterial hypertension (systolic blood pressure [BP] >200 mmHg and diastolic BP >110 mmHg)
- Mental impairment leading to inability to cooperate with testing

*Contraindications can be superseded if benefits outweigh risks of exercise.

Adapted from J. Gibbons et al., 2002, ACC/AHA 2002 guideline update for exercise testing. A report of the American College of Cardiology/American Heart Association Task Force on practice guidelines (Committee on Exercise Testing) (Bethesda, MD: American College of Cardiology), 5. Available: http://my.americanheart.org/idc/groups/ahaecc-internal/@wcm/@sop/documents/downloadable/ucm_423807.pdf training sessions. Patients with conditions as outlined in "Absolute and Relative Contraindications to Exercise Training" should be considered for exclusion from exercise training.

Exercise Testing

An exercise test is a key component of the initial assessment made before a patient begins an exercise program. Graded exercise tests are used to assess the ability to tolerate increased physical activity; ECG, hemodynamic, and symptomatic responses are monitored for manifestations of myocardial ischemia, dysrhythmias, or other exertion-related abnormalities. The exercise test may be used for diagnostic, prognostic, and therapeutic applications.[4] The test may also be a motivational tool for patients as well as verification to the family of patient improvement. Various published position statements present additional in-depth information regarding applications of exercise testing, methods of conducting exercise tests, and guidelines for managing exercise testing laboratories.[4-7] Apart from their use as a diagnostic tool, exercise tests are equally useful to staff as a functional tool. The test is quite useful in assessing cardiorespiratory fitness and for developing an exercise prescription. It can also be used to measure functional changes over time to assess exercise training outcomes. Exercise tests and simulated work tests also help determine an individual's ability to return to work.[8] Not all patients referred for CR/SP services are necessarily candidates for exercise testing or exercise participation, and patients should not be denied participation simply on the basis of not having

Absolute and Relative Contraindications to Exercise Testing

Absolute

- Acute MI (within 2 days)
- High-risk unstable angina
- Uncontrolled cardiac dysrhythmias causing symptoms or hemodynamic compromise
- Active endocarditis
- Severe symptomatic aortic stenosis
- Decompensated symptomatic heart failure
- Acute pulmonary embolus or pulmonary infarction
- Acute noncardiac disorder that may affect exercise performance or be aggravated by exercise (e.g., infection, renal failure, thyrotoxicosis)
- Acute myocarditis or pericarditis
- Physical disability that would preclude safe and adequate test performance
- Inability to obtain consent

Relative*

- Left main coronary stenosis or equivalent
- Moderate stenotic valvular heart disease
- Electrolyte abnormalities
- Tachyarrhythmias or bradyarrhythmias
- Atrial fibrillation with rapid ventricular rate, for example >150 bpm
- Hypertrophic cardiomyopathy
- Mental impairment leading to inability to cooperate with testing
- High-degree atrioventricular block
- Severe resting arterial hypertension (systolic BP >200 mmHg and diastolic BP >110 mmHg)

*Contraindications can be superseded if benefits outweigh risks of exercise.

Adapted from J. Gibbons et al., 2002, ACC/AHA 2002 guideline update for exercise testing. A report of the American College of Cardiology/American Heart Association Task Force on practice guidelines (Committee on Exercise Testing) (Bethesda, MD: American College of Cardiology), 5. Available: http://my.americanheart.org/idc/groups/ahaecc-internal/@wcm/@sop/documents/downloadable/ucm_423807.pdf undergone preentry exercise testing. Information regarding exercise prescription for patients without exercise testing is presented in chapter 7. "Absolute and Relative Contraindications to Exercise Testing" outlines the contraindications to exercise testing.

Safety and Personnel

Exercise is associated with an increased risk for a cardiovascular event. However, the safety of exercise testing is well documented, and the overall risk of adverse events is quite low. Among several large series of subjects with and without known CVD, the rate of major complications (including MI and other events requiring hospitalization) is <1 to as many as 5 per 10,000 tests, and the rate of death is <0.5 per 10,000 tests; however, the incidence of adverse events varies depending on the study population.[10] Among more than 2,000 subjects who completed exercise testing in the HF-ACTION study (Heart Failure: A Controlled Trial Investigating Outcomes of Exercise Training), there were no deaths, and the rate of nonfatal major cardiovascular events was <0.5 per 1,000 tests.[11] Patients with recent MI, reduced left ventricular systolic function, exertion-induced myocardial ischemia, and serious ventricular arrhythmias are at highest risk.[7]

Central to the prevention of exercise-induced complications are appropriate screening and risk stratification of patients before beginning an exercise program. Although the risk of an event is greater in patients with coronary artery disease (CAD), several clinical characteristics are associated with those patients at highest risk. Matching of patient medical history and clinical status to established contraindications to exercise should be incorporated into the assessment protocol before the patient gives informed consent and prepares for testing.[12]

Before preparation for the exercise test, the patient must give informed consent. An example of a consent form is presented in appendix C. The patient should have ample time to read the form before testing, and a staff person should ask whether the patient has any questions about the consent form or the test procedures and provide satisfactory explanations before proceeding.

Maintenance of appropriate emergency equipment, establishment of a workable emergency plan, and regular practice of the plan (with critiques) are fundamental to ensuring the safety of a CR/SP program. Chapter 12 discusses the important considerations for managing emergency situations.

The AHA has described the degree of required supervision for exercise testing.[5] The level of supervision depends primarily on the type of patients being tested. For patients who are at higher risk, for example those with recent MI, heart failure, or arrhythmia, the supervising physician should determine the necessity for direct physician monitoring of the test.[13] In other cases, properly trained nonphysician health care professionals may conduct the test and directly monitor patient status throughout testing and recovery, provided that they have been deemed competent by the physician supervisor per established guidelines.[14] In all cases, the supervising physician must be immediately available to respond. For nonphysicians, certification in the clinical track by the American College of Sports Medicine (ACSM) provides evidence of competencies to supervise exercise testing.[6] In addition, the credentialing body for cardiovascular technology provides a cardiographic technician certification that encompasses not only exercise testing but also Holter monitoring and pacemaker evaluation.[15] Successful completion of an advanced cardiac life support (ACLS) course is also recommended. The program medical director must be responsible for ensuring the availability of the proper equipment and the staffing of the exercise testing laboratory, including establishing laboratory policies and procedures. The physician is also responsible for final data interpretation and approval and delivery of emergency care (including ACLS) according to established standards.[5,14]

Medications

Although diagnostic exercise tests typically are performed with medications withheld to better assess any underlying ischemic response, functional testing performed before entrance into a CR/SP program should occur with the patient taking medications as prescribed. For example, withholding beta-blockers before exercise testing will interfere with HR prescription for exercise training. Under ideal conditions, the functional exercise test should be administered at a time when the patient normally exercises and following normal medication ingestion time.

Exercise Test Modality and Protocols

The appropriate testing modality and protocol should be selected after patient assessment.

Restrictions, limitations, or both can affect individual performance and therefore the usefulness of the exercise test. Exercise tests may be submaximal or maximal with respect to the effort required. In addition to common indications for stopping the exercise test (see "Indications for Terminating Exercise Testing"), submaximal exercise testing often has a predetermined end point: a specific peak HR such as 120 bpm, a percentage of predicted maximum HR such as 70%, an arbitrary metabolic equivalent (MET) level such as 5 METs, or a submaximal rating of perceived exertion (RPE) such as 13 to 15. Submaximal tests may be used before hospital discharge at 4 to 6 days after acute MI.[16] This low-level test can provide sufficient data for evaluating the ability to engage in activities of daily living or other physical activity, and serves as a baseline for early ambulatory exercise prescription.

Symptom-limited tests are designed to continue until the patient demonstrates signs and symptoms that require termination of exercise.[4]

Symptom-limited tests are usually selected when testing is performed more than 14 days after acute MI. Minimum required physiological and perceptual measurements to be collected before, during, and following exercise testing are listed in "Minimum Requirements for Measures Assessed During Exercise Testing."

Although several exercise testing protocols are available for both treadmill and stationary cycle ergometers, it is most important that the protocol be selected according to the individual patient-estimated physical fitness based on age, underlying disease, and current activity level. Patients who are deemed to be higher risk (e.g., recent history of dysrhythmia or symptoms during low levels of effort) or who are clearly deconditioned should be tested using a less aggressive exercise protocol. Validated questionnaires, which estimate an individual's exercise capacity and assist in appropriate protocol selection, are available.[17,18] A wide variety of treadmill and cycle ergometer testing protocols are well summarized by the ACSM.[6] Treadmill and

Indications for Terminating Exercise Testing

Absolute indications

- ST elevation (>1.0 mm) in leads without Q waves (other than V1 or aV$_R$)
- Drop in systolic blood pressure (SBP) of >10 mmHg (persistently below baseline) despite an increase in workload, when accompanied by any other evidence of ischemia
- Moderate to severe angina (grade 3 to 4; "Frequently used Angina and Dyspnea Rating Scales" presents descriptions and grades for angina scale)
- Central nervous system symptoms (e.g., ataxia, dizziness, or near-syncope)
- Signs of poor perfusion (cyanosis or pallor)
- Sustained ventricular tachycardia
- Technical difficulties monitoring the ECG or SBP
- Patient request to stop
- Development of bundle branch block that cannot be distinguished from ventricular tachycardia

Relative indications

- ST or QRS changes such as excessive ST displacement (horizontal or downsloping of >2 mm), or marked axis shift
- Drop in SBP of >10 mmHg (persistently below baseline) despite an increase in workload, in the absence of other evidence of ischemia
- Increasing chest pain
- Fatigue, shortness of breath, wheezing, leg cramps, or severe claudication
- Dysrhythmias other than sustained ventricular tachycardia, including frequent multifocal ectopic beats including ventricular pairs, supraventricular tachycardia, heart block, or bradyarrhythmias

Adapted, by permission, from J. Gibbons et al., 2002, *ACC/AHA 2002 guideline update for exercise testing. A report of the American College of Cardiology/American Heart Association Task Force on practice guidelines* (Committee on Exercise Testing) (Bethesda, MD: American College of Cardiology), 5. Available: http://my.americanheart.org/idc/groups/ahaecc-internal/@wcm/@sop/documents/downloadable/ucm_423807.pdf

Minimum Requirements for Measures Assessed During Exercise Testing

Pretest procedures and assessments

- Minimum of 5 min of rest before initial measures are taken
- Informed consent
- Demonstration of equipment use (as required)
- Explanation of maximal effort or desired end point(s)
- Explanation of rating scales (use standardized instructions where available)
- 12-lead ECG in supine and in position of exercise
- Blood pressure in supine and in position of exercise
- Assessment of medications, when last taken
- Current symptom status

Exercise assessments

- 12-lead ECG during last minute of each stage, or at least every 3 min if single stage test is administered
- Blood pressure and perceived exertion during last minute of each stage, or at least every 3 min if single stage test is administered
- Other rating scales as appropriate

Posttest procedures and assessments

- Minimum of 6 min in sitting or supine position, or until near-baseline measures are reached. A period of active cool-down may be included in the 6 min recovery period; for functional (nondiagnostic) exercise tests, a 1 to 3 min cool-down is recommended, depending on the level of exertion (additional time for heavier exertion), to minimize postexercise effects of venous pooling in the lower extremities.
- 12-lead ECG every minute.
- Blood pressure immediately after exercise, then every 1 or 2 min until normotensive or near-baseline measures are reached.
- Rating of symptoms each minute as long as they persist after exercise. Patients should be observed until all symptoms have subsided and the ECG is within acceptable limits as determined by the supervising clinician.

---

cycle ergometers may employ staged or continuous ramp protocols. Work rate increments during staged protocols can vary from 1 to 2.5 METs (1 MET = 3.5 mL · kg^{-1} · min^{-1} oxygen uptake), whereas those of ramp protocols are designed to use less abrupt increments. Treadmill testing provides a more common form of physiological stress (i.e., walking), with subjects more likely to attain a higher oxygen uptake and peak HR. Cycling may be preferable when orthopedic or other specific patient characteristics limit ability to walk or bear weight during exercise. The most frequently used stepped treadmill protocols are the Bruce (table 6.1), the modified Bruce, and the Naughton.[6] Ramp protocols are designed to have stages no longer than 1 min and for the patient to

Table 6.1 Bruce Protocol for Treadmill Testing

Stage	Time	Speed (mph)	Grade (%)	METs
Rest	00.00	0.0	0.0	1.0
Modified Bruce protocol	3.00	1.7	0.0	2.2
	3.00	1.7	5	3.4
1	3.00	1.7	10.0	4.6
2	3.00	2.5	12.0	7.0
3	3.00	3.4	14.0	10.1
4	3.00	4.2	16.0	12.9
5	3.00	5.0	18.0	15.1
6	3.00	5.5	20.0	16.9
7	3.00	6.0	22.0	19.2

attain peak effort within 8 to 12 min. Thus, ramp protocols must be individualized to patient effort (table 6.2).

The cycle ergometer is smaller, quieter, and less expensive than a treadmill. Because the cycle ergometer requires less movement of the arms and thorax, quality ECG recordings and BP measurements are easier to obtain. Stationary cycling may be unfamiliar to many patients, and its success as a testing tool is highly dependent on patient motivation. Thus, the test may end before the patient reaches a true cardiopulmonary end point. However, unlike treadmill testing, which is fully weight bearing, cycle testing protocols are independent of weight because the seat supports the body weight. As shown in table 6.2, the MET level attained varies with patient body weight. The energy requirement (oxygen uptake) of non–weight-bearing activity is inversely proportional to body weight. That is, at the same workload, the higher the body weight, the lower the oxygen uptake.

The following recommendations may assist in selecting an appropriate cycling protocol:

- Select a protocol appropriate to level of fitness.
- When using a mechanically braked ergometer, keep pedal rpm constant, for example at 50 rpm.
- After a zero-load warm-up of 1 to 2 min, use 25 W or less (150 kilopond-meter [kgm]) increments for patients who are deconditioned or weigh less than 150 lb (68 kg). Use 50 W (300 kgm) increments for more fit or heavier patients.

- Set stages at a minimum of 2 min in duration, increasing the load by 25 W or less as clinical judgment indicates.
- When ramping protocols are used, electronically braked cycle ergometers are preferred since they generally allow programming of incremental workloads at stages <1 min. Similar to treadmill ramp protocols, customized cycle ergometer ramp protocols that accommodate a wide range of fitness levels need to be established by individual exercise testing laboratories.

Once the appropriate test equipment and protocol are selected, the exercise component of a symptom-limited exercise test should last approximately 8 to 12 min.[19] Low-level ramps or protocols that increase metabolic demand by 1 MET per stage are appropriate for high-risk patients with functional capacities less than 7 METs; metabolic demands greater than or equal to 2 METs per stage may be appropriate for low- to intermediate-risk patients with functional capacities equal to or greater than 7 METs. Similar considerations are necessary when one is adjusting ramp rates. Smaller increments in MET requirements for each stage permit a more specific determination of the ischemic or anginal threshold and result in a more accurate estimation of oxygen uptake at the corresponding work rate. The widely used Bruce treadmill protocol (2 to 3 METs per stage) is less accurate in this regard.[20]

During treadmill exercise, encourage patients to walk freely, using the handrails for balance only when necessary. Excessive gripping alters the BP response and decreases the oxygen requirement

Table 6.2 Approximate Metabolic Equivalent (MET) Loads During Cycle Ergometer Assessments

BODY WEIGHT		EXECISE RATE (KG · M · MIN⁻¹/WATTS						
kg	lb	300/50 METs	450/75	600/100	750/125	900/150	1050/175	1200/200
50	110	5.1	6.6	8.2	9.7	11.3	12.8	14.3
60	132	4.6	5.9	7.1	8.4	9.7	11.0	12.3
70	154	4.2	5.3	6.4	7.5	8.6	9.7	10.8
80	176	3.9	4.9	5.9	6.8	7.8	8.8	9.7
90	198	3.7	4.6	5.4	6.3	7.1	8.0	8.9
100	220	3.5	4.3	5.1	5.9	6.6	7.4	8.2

Based on American College of Sports Medicine 2006.

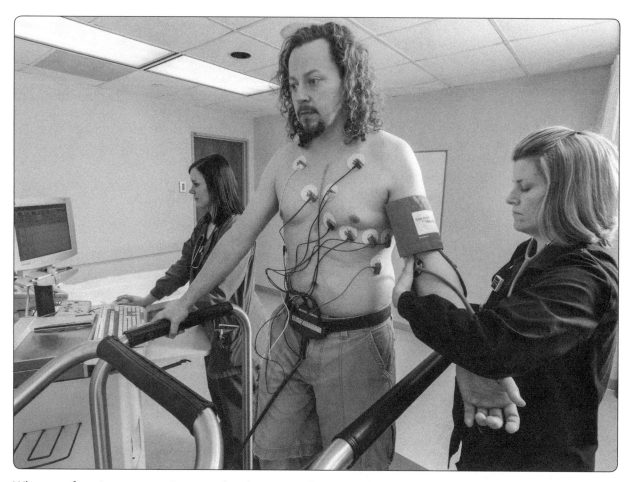

When performing an exercise test, closely monitor heart rate and blood pressure.

(METs) for each workload, resulting in an overestimation of exercise capacity and inaccurate HR- and BP-to-workload equivalents. Most patients adapt quickly if instructed to lightly rest a finger or two from one or both hands on the handrail. Exercise capacity can be reasonably estimated for functional purposes from both treadmill and cycle workloads provided that the equipment is calibrated regularly and accurately. When precise determination of oxygen uptake is necessary, as in assessing patients for heart transplant, evaluation by expired gas analysis is preferred.

Symptom Rating Scales

Before exercising, patients should be familiarized with the symptom rating scales. Rating of perceived exertion and scales for angina, dyspnea, and claudication are shown in "Frequently Used Angina and Dyspnea Rating Scales" and "Intermittent Claudication Rating Scale."

Cardiopulmonary Exercise Testing

Cardiopulmonary exercise testing (CPX) uses ventilatory gas exchange analysis during exercise and is a useful tool for assessment of patients with CVD.[9] Measures of gas exchange primarily include oxygen uptake ($\dot{V}O_2$), carbon dioxide output ($\dot{V}CO_2$), minute ventilation, and ventilatory threshold. Oxygen uptake at peak exercise is considered the most reliable measure of aerobic capacity and cardiorespiratory function. The technical aspects and clinical applications of CPX are discussed in detail elsewhere.[10] Such testing is appropriate for

- evaluation of exercise capacity in selected patients with heart failure to assist in the estimation of prognosis and assess the need for cardiac transplantation;
- assistance in the differentiation of cardiac versus pulmonary limitations as a cause of

Frequently Used Angina and Dyspnea Rating Scales

5-grade angina scale

0	No angina
1	Light, barely noticeable
2	Moderate, bothersome
3	Severe, very uncomfortable
4	Most pain ever experienced

5-grade dyspnea scale

0	No dyspnea
1	Mild, noticeable
2	Mild, some difficulty
3	Moderate difficulty, but can continue
4	Severe difficulty, cannot continue

10-grade angina/dyspnea scale

0	Nothing
0.5	Very, very slight
1	Very slight
2	Slight
3	Moderate
4	Somewhat severe
5	Severe
6	
7	Very severe
8	
9	
10	Very, very severe

Intermittent Claudication Rating Scale

0	No claudication pain
1	Initial, minimal pain
2	Moderate, bothersome pain
3	Intense pain
4	Maximal pain, cannot continue

exercise-induced dyspnea or impaired exercise capacity, when the etiology is uncertain;

• evaluation of the patient response to specific therapeutic interventions in which the improvement of exercise tolerance is an important goal or end point; and

• a more precise determination of the appropriate intensity for exercise training through identification of the ventilatory threshold.

Normal values for maximal oxygen uptake among healthy adults at different ages are available and may serve as a useful reference in the evaluation of exercise capacity.[21-24] Exercise training intensities to maintain or improve health and fitness among individuals with or without heart disease can be derived from direct measurements of peak oxygen uptake.[19] This may be most useful when the HR response to exercise is not a reliable indicator of exercise intensity (e.g., in patients with atrial fibrillation).

Contemporary exercise testing systems have simplified techniques of CPX testing. However, these systems require meticulous maintenance and calibration for optimal use. Personnel involved with both test administration and interpretation must be trained and proficient in these techniques. Finally, the test requires additional time as well as patient cooperation.[10]

Diagnostic Utility

Exercise tests are very useful in the detection of ischemia for diagnostic and management purposes. Abnormalities in exercise capacity, HR, BP, and exercise ECG are important findings. Cardiac events are more likely to occur in patients with lower exercise capacities and those who exhibit exercise-induced hypotension. Other markers of adverse prognosis are abnormal HR recovery (HR drop of <12 bpm within the first minute of recovery),[25] inability to attain 85% maximal predicted HR,[26] and frequent ventricular ectopy in recovery (ventricular couplets or runs of ventricular tachycardia).[27]

The most common and useful ECG definition of a positive test is a horizontal or downsloping ST depression that is greater than or equal to 1 mm for at least 60 to 80 ms after the end of the QRS complex.[4] Stress test ECG findings must be interpreted in the context of clinical information regarding the baseline ECG, the patient's cardiovascular history, and the presence or absence of symptoms. Clearly, exercise testing in persons with documented CVD (prior MI or coronary angiogram demonstrating significant coronary stenosis) is not used for diagnosis, but rather for the detection of inducible ischemia, disease management, and estimation of prognosis. With patients for whom the diagnosis is in question, the description of symptoms can be most helpful. Typical angina can be defined as substernal chest discomfort (it may also begin in, or radiate into, the arms or jaw) that is provoked by exertion or emotional stress and is relieved by rest and nitroglycerin. Typical or definite angina, particularly in men older than 50 years and women older than 60 years, makes the pretest probability of disease so high that the test result does not dramatically change the probability of the presence of coronary disease. Atypical angina is defined as chest discomfort that lacks one of the earlier-mentioned characteristics. It may also include discomfort other than in the chest, arms, or jaw and other symptoms such as shortness of breath, all of which serve to complicate the diagnosis. Symptoms of atypical angina generally indicate an intermediate pretest likelihood of coronary disease, particularly in men older than 30 years and women older than 50 years.[4]

Sensitivity is the percentage of patients with disease (e.g., ≤50% lesion of at least one major coronary artery) who will have an abnormal test. *Specificity* is the percentage of patients free of disease who will have a normal test. The sensitivity and specificity of exercise ECG are each approximately 70%. However, those levels are affected based on the subgroup of patients being evaluated.[4] *Positive predictive value* of an abnormal test result is the percentage of persons with an abnormal test who have the disease, whereas the *negative predictive value* of a normal test result is the percentage of persons with a normal test who do not have the disease. It is important to understand that the positive and negative predictive values of the test are dependent on the prevalence of disease within the population being tested. Thus, evaluation of the pretest likelihood of disease allows for the most appropriate interpretation of the test results. For example, an abnormal test result is more likely to be a true positive (high positive predictive value) in a 60-year-old man with typical angina, and more likely to be a false positive (low positive predictive value) in a 25-year-old woman with atypical symptoms.

Several other factors influence test interpretation. Failure to achieve 85% maximum predicted HR limits the estimation of posttest probability if no abnormalities are detected, because the patient has not reached a diagnostic level of stress from which sensitivity estimates have been derived.[9] The presence of left bundle branch block, left ventricular hypertrophy with repolarization abnormalities, or resting ST-segment depression (≥1 mm) and the use of digoxin therapy confound the interpretation of the exercise ECG.[29] In such patients, exercise testing with either nuclear or echocardiographic imaging offers the advantage of greater sensitivity and specificity for the detection of CAD. In severely debilitated patients who are unable to perform an exercise test, pharmacologic testing has been used to evaluate ischemia. Unfortunately, the data from pharmacologic tests are not particularly useful in exercise prescription because hemodynamic and ischemic responses during such tests are not directly related to exercise effort. These tests are discussed later in this section.

Exercise Testing With Imaging Modalities

Cardiac imaging modalities are indicated when potential ECG changes are likely to be nondiagnostic, or when it is important to determine the extent and distribution of ischemic myocardium or to exclude or confirm a positive or negative exercise ECG. Cardiac imaging with echocardiography before and after exercise can diagnose and localize the extent of myocardial ischemia. Radioactive agents are used to obtain nuclear myocardial perfusion scans at rest and with exercise.

Exercise Echocardiography

Echocardiography can be combined with exercise ECG in an attempt to increase the sensitivity and specificity of stress testing, as well as to determine the extent of myocardium at risk for ischemia. Echocardiographic images at rest are compared with those obtained while the patient bicycles or immediately after treadmill exercise. Images must be obtained within 1 to 2 min after exercise, because abnormal wall motion begins to normalize after this point.

Myocardial contractility normally increases with exercise, whereas ischemia causes hypokinesis, akinesis, or dyskinesis of the affected segments. Therefore, a test is considered positive when wall-motion abnormalities develop in previously normal areas with exercise or worsen in an already abnormal segment. Exercise echocardiography has a weighted mean sensitivity of 86%, specificity of 81%, and overall accuracy of 85% for the detection of CAD.[30] Patients with a normal exercise echocardiogram have a low risk of future cardiac events, including revascularization procedures, MI, or cardiac death. Exercise echocardiography has been shown to be highly accurate in diagnosing CAD in patients in whom there may be an increased incidence of false-positive exercise ECG (e.g., women).[30,31]

Exercise Nuclear Imaging

Exercise tests with nuclear imaging are also performed with ECG monitoring. There are several different imaging protocols using only technetium (Tc)-99m or thallous (thallium) chloride-201. These agents are usually injected about 1 min before the end of exercise, and images are obtained. Rest images are compared to exercise images to determine the areas of myocardial ischemia. Perfusion defects that are present during exercise but not seen at rest suggest ischemia. Perfusion defects that are present during exercise and persist at rest suggest previous MI or scar. In this manner, the extent and distribution of ischemic myocardium can be identified. Exercise nuclear single photon emission computed tomography (SPECT) imaging has a sensitivity of 87% and specificity of 73% for detecting CAD with ≥50% coronary stenosis.[32]

Pharmacologic Stress Testing

Patients unable to undergo exercise stress testing for reasons such as deconditioning, peripheral arterial disease, orthopedic disability, neurological disease, or concomitant illness can often benefit from pharmacologic stress testing. Two of the most common tests are dobutamine stress echocardiography (DSE) and nuclear scintigraphy with dipyridamole, adenosine, or regadenoson. Indications for these tests include establishing a diagnosis of CAD, determining myocardial viability before revascularization, assessing prognosis after MI or in chronic angina, and evaluating cardiac risk preoperatively. Little information can be gained from these tests to aid in the exercise prescription, since the HR and BP response at the ischemic threshold cannot be directly compared to that during exercise. Pharmacologic studies can, however, provide information regarding ventricular function and the extent of myocardium that may become ischemic; thus they are useful in risk stratification, particularly as it relates to the exercise program.

Dobutamine is a synthetic catecholamine and acts predominantly as a beta-1 agonist but also has some beta-2 and alpha-1 stimulatory effects. At lower doses, it increases cardiac output by causing an increase in contractility and HR. At higher doses, its principal effect is to bring about an increase in HR. Patients who have inadequate HR response to dobutamine may also receive an additional infusion of atropine to further stimulate HR response. As a result of the increased cardiac work, myocardial oxygen demand increases. If significant coronary artery stenoses are present, an oxygen supply-and-demand mismatch may occur, resulting in ischemia and abnormal wall motion.[30]

Dipyridamole, adenosine, and regadenoson cause coronary vasodilation in normal epicardial arteries, but not in stenotic segments. As a result, a coronary steal phenomenon occurs with a relatively increased flow to normal arteries and a relatively decreased flow to stenotic arteries. Nuclear perfusion imaging under resting conditions is then compared with imaging obtained after coronary vasodilation. Interpretation of the test is similar to that for exercise nuclear scans.[32]

Alternative Opportunities for Evaluating Physical Activity Status

Several opportunities exist for the evaluation of physical activity status in addition to symptom-limited exercise testing. These include the 6-minute walk test; estimation of exercise tolerance from the clinician–patient interview, questionnaires, or both; and controlled job simulation.

Six-Minute Walk Test

The 6-minute walk test (6MWT)[33] can be used as a surrogate measure of exercise capacity when standard treadmill or cycle testing is not available. It is not useful in the objective determination of myocardial ischemia, and is best used in a serial manner to evaluate changes in exercise capacity with training over time. The 6MWT protocol is presented in appendix D.

Clinician–Patient Interview and Questionnaires

Although interviews and surveys are not a substitute for exercise testing, clinicians may obtain rough estimations of exercise tolerance by using MET activity tables and questioning patients about those activities that induce fatigue or symptoms.[34,35] In addition, a number of physical activity surveys have been used to quantify activity.[36] The Duke Activity Status Index and the Specific Activity Scale are examples of such scales.[37,38]

Controlled Job Simulation

Data from an exercise test can be compared to readily available MET tables to assist in making recommendations for safe vocational and avocational activities.[24] However, mechanical efficiency, specific job-task requirements, and environmental and psychological stressors can substantially alter the responses measured in the laboratory. While not usually performed in CR/SP programs, controlled simulation of physical tasks can aid physicians and employers in determining whether a patient can safely return to work.[8]

Summary

A careful evaluation of patient medical status and exercise testing results before participation in an outpatient cardiac rehabilitation/secondary prevention (CR/SP) is essential to identifying limitations to exercise participation, describing patient CVD progression risk factor profile, and facilitating the development of patient and staff goals as they relate to expected outcomes. Recognizing the appropriate methodologies for accomplishing these objectives and understanding potential alternatives to the evaluation of physical activity status are integral to the process, and ultimately to the success of the individual patient in CR/SP.

Outpatient Cardiovascular Rehabilitation and Secondary Prevention

M edical therapies, interventional techniques, and research on the effects of lifestyle intervention for coronary heart disease (CHD) continue to proliferate. The importance of comprehensive health behavior change in the efficacious management and prevention of CHD has been increasingly validated and is an established component of chronic disease management. The structure of outpatient cardiac rehabilitation/secondary prevention (CR/SP) must account for and address the risk of disease progression and the risk of a recurrent cardiac event. It is critical not only to expand the number of participating and eligible patient populations, but also to implement and deliver innovative models for secondary prevention through a variety of programming techniques. Integrating the rapidly growing knowledge base of the etiology and progression of atherosclerosis, as well as the efficacy of healthy behaviors as agents for primary and secondary prevention in CR/SP, is necessary to positively affect patient outcomes.

OBJECTIVES

This chapter focuses on

- assessment and management of risk factors for cardiovascular disease (CVD) progression,
- stratification of risk for events during exercise and appropriate supervision, and
- implementation of models for secondary prevention.

Primary and secondary prevention have been subjects of epidemiological and experimental research for decades. Many prominent groups have issued practice guidelines for primary and secondary prevention (see table 7.1 for these statements), including the American Association of Cardiovascular and Pulmonary Rehabilitation (AACVPR), the American College of Cardiology (ACC), and the American Heart Association (AHA). These documents present the basis for the utilization and efficacy of a CR/SP model to provide a multifaceted program for secondary prevention of CHD. The notion that secondary prevention is not only possible, but also feasible and effective, is well established.[1] An aggressive therapeutic regimen, using optimal targets for intervention that addresses all modifiable CHD risk factors, has become the basis for managing persons with CHD in CR/SP. A broad array of assessments, therapeutic modalities, and follow-up

Table 7.1

STATEMENTS ON SMOKING AND TOBACCO	
Office of the Surgeon General	**2007** **Children and Secondhand Smoke Exposure-Excerpts From The Health Consequences of Involuntary Exposure to Tobacco Smoke: A Report of the Surgeon General** Office of the Surgeon General website. Available at: www.surgeongeneral.gov/library/smokeexposure/index.html.
	2006 **The Health Consequences of Involuntary Exposure to Tobacco Smoke: A Report of the Surgeon General** Office of the Surgeon General website. Available at: www.surgeongeneral.gov/library/secondhandsmoke/index.html.
	2004 **The Health Consequences of Smoking: A Report of the Surgeon General** Office of the Surgeon General website. Available at: www.cdc.gov/tobacco/data_statistics/sgr/2004/index.htm.
	2001 **Women and Smoking: A Report of the Surgeon General** Office of the Surgeon General website. Available at: www.surgeongeneral.gov/library/womenandtobacco/index.html.
	2000 **Reducing Tobacco Use: A Report of the Surgeon General** Office of the Surgeon General website. Available at: www.surgeongeneral.gov/library/tobacco_use/index.html.
	2010 **How Tobacco Smoke Causes Disease: The Biology and Behavioral Basis for Smoking-Attributable Disease** Office of the Surgeon General website. Available at: www.surgeongeneral.gov/library/tobaccosmoke/report/index.html.
American Heart Association/American College of Cardiology Statements	**2004** **Air Pollution and Cardiovascular Disease** American Heart Association website. Available at: http://circ.ahajournals.org/cgi/content/full/109/21/2655.
	2010 **Impact of Smokeless Tobacco Products on Cardiovascular Disease** American Heart Association website. Available at: http://circ.ahajournals.org/cgi/reprint/CIR.0b013e3181f432c3v1.
American Lung Association	**2009** **Helping Smokers Quit** American Lung Association website. Available at: www.lungusa.org/assets/documents/publications/other-reports/smoking-cessation-report-2009.pdf

STATEMENTS ON DYSLIPIDEMIA AND NUTRITION *(CONTINUED)*	
European Society of Cardiology/European Atherosclerosis Society	**2011** **ESC/EAS Guidelines for the Management of Dyslipidaemias** Eur Heart J. 2011;32:1769-1818. Available at: http://eurheartj.oxfordjournals.org/content/early/2011/06/27/eurheartj.ehr158.full.pdf+html.
United States Department of Agriculture	**2010** **Dietary Guidelines for Americans: 2010** USDA website. Available at: www.health.gov/dietaryguidelines/dga2010/DietaryGuidelines2010.pdf.
American Heart Association	**2010** **A Scientific Statement From the American Heart Association: Interventions to Promote Physical Activity and Dietary Lifestyle Changes for Cardiovascular Risk Factor Reduction in Adults: A Scientific Statement From the American Heart Association** American Heart Association website. Available at: http://circ.ahajournals.org/cgi/reprint/CIR.0b013e3181e8edf1. **2009** **Dietary Sugars Intake and Cardiovascular Health: A Scientific Statement From the American Heart Association** American Heart Association website. Available at: http://circ.ahajournals.org/cgi/reprint/CIRCULATIONAHA.109.192627. **2009** **Omega-6 Fatty Acids and Risk for Cardiovascular Disease: A Science Advisory From the American Heart Association Nutrition Subcommittee of the Council on Nutrition, Physical Activity, and Metabolism; Council on Cardiovascular Nursing; and Council on Epidemiology and Prevention** American Heart Association website. Available at: http://circ.ahajournals.org/cgi/reprint/CIRCULATIONAHA.108.191627. **2006** **Understanding the Complexity of Trans Fatty Acid Reduction in the American Diet: American Heart Association Trans Fat Conference 2006. Report of the Trans Fat Conference Planning Group** American Heart Association website. Available at: http://circ.ahajournals.org/cgi/reprint/CIRCULATIONAHA.106.181947. **2005** **Managing Abnormal Blood Lipids: A Collaborative Approach** American Heart Association website. Managing Abnormal Blood Lipids: A Collaborative Approach. Available at: http://circ.ahajournals.org/cgi/content/full/112/20/3184. **2004** **Implications of Recent Clinical Trials for the National Cholesterol Education Program Adult Treatment Panel III Guidelines** American Heart Association website. Available at: http://circ.ahajournals.org/cgi/content/full/110/2/227. **2004** **AHA Science Advisory: Antioxidant Vitamin Supplements and Cardiovascular Disease** American Heart Association website. Available at: http://circ.ahajournals.org/cgi/content/full/110/5/637. **2002** **Third Report of the National Cholesterol Education Program (NCEP) Expert Panel on Detection, Evaluation, and Treatment of High Blood Cholesterol in Adults (Adult Treatment Panel III) Final Report** American Heart Association website. Available at: http://circ.ahajournals.org/cgi/content/full/106/25/3143.

(continued)

STATEMENTS ON DYSLIPIDEMIA AND NUTRITION *(CONTINUED)*	
Institute of Medicine	2002 **Dietary Reference Intakes for Energy, Carbohydrate, Fiber, Fat, Fatty Acids, Cholesterol, Protein, and Amino Acids** Institute of Medicine website. Available at: http://books.nap.edu/openbook.php?record_id=10490.
World Cancer Research Fund and the American Institute for Cancer Research	2007 **Food, Nutrition, Physical Activity, and the Prevention of Cancer: A Global Perspective** World Cancer Research Fund and the American Institute for Cancer Research website. Available at: www.dietandcancerreport.org.
American Dietetic Association	2007 **Dietary Fatty Acids - Position of the American Dietetic Association and Dietitians of Canada** American Dietetic Association website. Available at: www.eatright.org/About/Content.aspx?id=8353. 2008 **Health Implications of Dietary Fiber** American Dietetic Association website. Available at: www.eatright.org/About/Content.aspx?id=8355.
STATEMENTS ON HYPERTENSION	
American College of Sports Medicine	2004 **Exercise and Hypertension** ACSM website. Available at: http://journals.lww.com/acsm-msse/Fulltext/2004/03000/Exercise_and_Hypertension.25.aspx.
National High Blood Pressure Education Program	2003 **The Seventh Report of the Joint Commission on Prevention, Detection, Evaluation and Treatment of High Blood Pressure.** http://www.nhlbi.nih.gov/guidelines/hypertension.
STATEMENT ON DIABETES	
American College of Sports Medicine and the American Diabetes Association	2011 **Exercise and Type 2 Diabetes: American College of Sports Medicine and the American Diabetes Association: Joint Position Statement** ACSM website. Available at: http://journals.lww.com/acsm-msse/Fulltext/2010/12000/Exercise_and_Type_2_Diabetes__American_College_of.18.aspx. Clinical Practice Recommendations. Diabetes Care website. Diabetes Care. 2011;34:S1-S2. Available at: http://care.diabetesjournals.org.
STATEMENTS ON PHYSICAL ACTIVITY	
American College of Sports Medicine	2009 **Exercise and Physical Activity for Older Adults** ACSM website. Available at: http://journals.lww.com/acsm-msse/Fulltext/2009/07000/Exercise_and_Physical_Activity_for_Older_Adults.20.aspx.
Centers for Disease Control and Prevention	2008 **Physical Activity Guidelines for Americans** Centers for Disease Control and Prevention website. Available at: www.health.gov/PAGuidelines/pdf/paguide.pdf.

STATEMENTS ON PHYSICAL ACTIVITY *(CONTINUED)*	
American Heart Association	2007 **Resistance Exercise in Individuals With and Without Cardiovascular Disease: 2007 Update** Williams MA, Haskell WL, Ades PA, et al. Circulation. 2007;116:572-584. 2007 **Physical Activity and Public Health: Updated Recommendation for Adults From the American College of Sports Medicine and the American Heart Association** Haskell WL, Lee IM, Pate RR, et al. *Circulation.* 2007;116:1081-1093. 2006 **Physical Activity Intervention Studies** What We Know and What We Need to Know: A Scientific Statement From the American Heart Association. Marcus BH, Williams DM, Dubbert P, et al. Circulation. 2006;114:2739-2752. 2006 **Physical Activity and Public Health** Updated Recommendation for Adults From the American College of Sports Medicine and the American Heart Association. Haskell WL, Lee IM, Pate RR, et al. *Circulation.* 2007;116:1081-1093. 2006 **AHA Scientific Statement: Physical Activity Intervention Studies.** Marcus BH, Williams DM, Dubbert PM, et al. *Circulation.* 2006;114:2739-2752.
STATEMENT ON WEIGHT LOSS AND BODY COMPOSITION	
American College of Sports Medicine	2009 **Appropriate Physical Activity Intervention Strategies for Weight Loss and Prevention of Weight Regain for Adults** ACSM website. Available at: http://journals.lww.com/acsm-msse/Fulltext/2009/02000/Appropriate_Physical_Activity_Intervention.26.aspx.
American Dietetic Association	2009 **Weight Management** American Dietetic Health Implications of Dietary Fiber. Available at: http://andevidencelibrary.com/files/Docs/WM%20Position%20Paper.pdf.

is required for comprehensive secondary prevention. Tracking and reporting outcomes to patients, physicians, and payers is essential to the ongoing reimbursement, success, and acceptance of secondary prevention programs.

Case management models for delivering preventive and rehabilitative services are effective methods for secondary prevention in CR/SP.[2-4] Inclusion of CR/SP in the clinical pathway beginning in the acute-care phase and continuing through the outpatient phase is necessary for comprehensive patient care.

Secondary prevention efforts within the health care setting remain limited, but have the potential to increase as health care reform progresses. Several reports indicate that primary risk factors are more prevalent after CVD events secondary to poor compliance with prescription medication or lifestyle change.[5] Utilization rates of CR/SP have experienced little change since earlier studies found that 11% to 37% of eligible patients were being referred to outpatient CR/SP. This is despite the evidence that outpatient CR/SP confers demonstrated reductions in mortality and morbidity (21-34%).[6,7] More recent investigations indicate that a mere 14% to 31% of eligible Medicare patients are referred to CR/SP.[8] Thus, despite widespread confirmation of the safety and efficacy of CR/SP, as well as an emphasis aimed at the medical community to aggressively implement this therapy and recommended lifestyle interventions, secondary prevention is neither widely used nor effectively employed. Accordingly, future efforts should focus on methods to increase referral rates for CHD patients with eligible diagnoses. It has been reported that specific strategies can increase the referral rates.[9,10] Following publication of those reports, AACVPR/ACCF/AHA updated a statement on performance measures to include specific referral guidelines.[11]

Structure of Secondary Prevention

AACVPR/ACCF/AHA statements regarding performance measures, core components, and secondary prevention guidelines provide standards that specify structure for CR/SP.[1,11,12] Assessment and management of all established risk factors for CHD as well as associated health behaviors are addressed in both documents. The European Society of Cardiology "Guidelines on Cardiovascular Disease Prevention," provide additional preventive strategies for CHD.[13] These guidelines and subsequent statements issued by national organizations can guide CR/SP structure and development and may be useful for maintaining and updating program design concurrent with a rapidly evolving body of literature.

The core components of CR/SP should be formulated with the primary goals of reducing CVD morbidity and mortality, improving physical and psychological function, and enhancing quality of life. This can be accomplished through changing health behaviors that lead to disease progression, specifically behaviors related to tobacco use; dyslipidemia; nutrition; exercise; stress; psychological health; and control of metabolic disorders such as diabetes, metabolic syndrome, and obesity. Optimal management of these lifestyle behaviors and metabolic disorders results in stabilization and, perhaps, regression of the atherosclerotic process.[4,14-16] So-called usual care has been demonstrated to be significantly less effective in preventing the progression of atherosclerosis and recurring events than optimal lifestyle interventions.[17] Thus, a paradigm focusing on aggressive health behavior change along with adjunctive medical therapy as required should receive increasing emphasis early in an ongoing outpatient CR/SP (see guideline 7.1).

Optimal secondary prevention requires a team of health care professionals to function in close partnership with physicians to assist and guide

---

Guideline 7.1 Structure of Cardiac Rehabilitation/Secondary Prevention Programming

- All patients should be assessed for the presence and extent of modifiable cardiovascular disease risk factors, including smoking, physical inactivity and sitting time, obesity, dietary pattern, psychosocial dysfunction including depression, exercise capacity, hypertension, dyslipidemia, impaired glucose tolerance, and diabetes.

- Depending on the medical history and physiological and psychological status, the majority of patients should begin aggressive, optimal SP while still in the hospital and should continue after discharge.

- Standard practice guidelines should be followed for preventive pharmacologic therapy. These should be implemented during hospitalization.

- Minimally, outcome assessment must include objective clinical measures of exercise performance and self-reported measures of exertion and behavior as required by the Centers for Medicare and Medicaid Services.[39]

- Automatic referral should be offered to all eligible patients to increase referral rates. The use of referral and transition from inpatient to outpatient CR/SP is a critical point in the referral and admission process to outpatient CR/SP.

Early outpatient CR/SP should begin within 1 to 3 weeks of discharge from the hospital. Most patients, including those with uncomplicated percutaneous transluminal coronary angioplasty with or without stent, should begin within 1 week of hospital discharge. The evaluation, intervention, and expected outcomes are specified for all of these behaviors in the AACVPR performance measures document.[11,55]

patients toward safe and efficacious therapy. Core competencies for CR/SP professionals are specified in an AACVPR/AHA position statement.[18] It is critical that secondary prevention programs foster close partnerships with primary care and specialty physicians to maximize medical management for patients enrolled in CR/SP.

Coaching and Case Management

The usual-care therapeutic approach to health behavior change in which a knowledgeable "expert" provides goals consistent with national practice standards is not an effective means to foster behavior change.[3,19] Individualized case management is an integrated disease-management process that provides specific risk factor intervention strategies. The patient is the center of the process and takes an active role, particularly in goal setting to accomplish mutually agreed-upon short-term and long-term goals and outcomes that reduce risk. Therapeutic approaches should be coordinated with primary care and specialty physicians, as well as other selected health care professionals as necessary. Case management techniques are especially efficient in outpatient CR/SP using a team approach consisting of three primary steps:

1. Assess all risk factors for disease progression and recurrent CVD events and subsequently coach each patient to make positive changes in health behaviors associated with those risk factors.
2. Establish rapport and maintain communication with patients by using face-to-face communication, as well as other methods such as electronic communication and reminder techniques as appropriate.
3. Provide ongoing follow-up to assess progress and reset goals as appropriate.

Finally, continued support for health behavior change is essential for addressing lapses and for promoting successful change. This model allows for individualized therapeutic modalities as well as implementation of algorithms for each risk factor with full patient agreement and understanding.

Contemporary CR/SP provides the tangible patient support necessary for successful behavior change. Consistent contact gives CR/SP staff the opportunity to provide feedback and reinforce

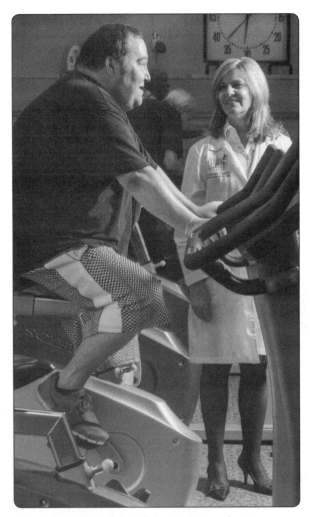

Consistent contact with patients, such as personal discussion during exercise, provides CR/SP staff opportunities to reinforce positive health behavior changes.

positive health behavior changes. Contact can take many forms, including personal discussion during exercise and education sessions, telephone calls, e-mails, letters or other written correspondence, or visits to the facility for follow-up counseling and testing.

Assessment and Management of Risk Factors for Disease Progression

The progression and vulnerability of established plaque and the development of new plaque are partially dependent on the presence of proinflammatory and other atherogenic risk factors.[20,21]

Thus ongoing tracking and management of cardiovascular risk factors through the behavior change process is one of the most important spheres of influence of CR/SP on positive patient outcomes.

Risk factor assessment should be performed at entry into and exit from the CR/SP. (See guideline 7.2.) Additionally, reassessing risk factors throughout participation in the program provides educational opportunities that may facilitate the behavior change that is critical to improved patient outcomes. This reinforcement is perhaps the most effective tool that CR/SP professionals can employ. CR/SP professionals should consider prioritizing and implementing all required variables for assessment included in the document on performance measures.[11]

The presence of multiple risk factors increases the risk of recurrent or new cardiovascular events.[22] Additionally, specific combinations of risk factors, such as high low-density lipoprotein (LDL) levels, high triglycerides, and impaired glucose metabolism (insulin resistance syndrome or diabetes), are associated with significantly increased risk in patients with CHD.[23] Screening and assessment requirements for entry into SP are outlined in guideline 7.2.

Assessment of risk for progression of CHD helps to establish the appropriate length and intensity of CR/SP and to prioritize risk factor intervention in CR/SP. After the initial assessment, assisting the establishment of "patient-centered" goals according to readiness and self-efficacy is indicated as the next step in setting up comprehensive SP. (See chapter 3 for a more detailed discussion of the basic principles of health behavior change.) Establishing patient-owned, short-term and long-term goals with the assistance (coaching) of CR/SP professionals is one of the most effective ways to facilitate positive health behavior change.[24,25] Putting goals in writing, often in contractual form, can be an effective method for promoting health behavior change.[26] Table 7.2 shows the therapeutic goals and recommended lifestyle interventions for optimal secondary prevention in patients with CVD.[1]

 Guideline 7.2   Screening and Assessments*

At the time of program entrance and exit, all patients should undergo or have the following current screening and assessments:

Current medical history—medical or surgical profile (or both), including complications, comorbidities, and other pertinent medical history

- Physical examination—cardiopulmonary systems assessment and musculoskeletal assessment, particularly upper and lower extremities and lower back
- Resting 12-lead electrocardiogram
- Current medications, including dose and frequency
- CVD risk profile, including the following:
  - Identification of age and gender and menopausal status if female
  - Use of tobacco products
  - History and level of control of hypertension
  - History and level of control of dyslipidemia including lipid profile (total cholesterol, low-density lipoproteins, high-density lipoproteins, and triglycerides); lipid profile before event or 6 to 8 weeks postevent; dietary pattern, specifically macronutrient content including dietary fat, saturated fat, cholesterol, and caloric intake
- Body composition (weight; height; body mass index; waist circumference, waist-to-hip ratio preferred, relative body fatness [percent fat] acceptable)
- Fasting blood glucose or hemoglobin A1c and history of diabetes mellitus
- Physical activity status including exercise capacity (entry exercise test preferred), leisure time physical activity, daily sitting or sedentary time
- Psychosocial history including evidence of depression, level of anger and hostility; family history
- Level of anger and hostility
- Other identified questionnaire data

*See chapter 6 for a complete discussion of evaluation and assessment.

Table 7.2 Practice Standards and Statements Regarding Secondary Prevention of Atherosclerotic Disease and Risk Factor Modification

Risk factor	Therapeutic goal	Practice standard or guideline
Smoking	No exposure to firsthand or secondhand tobacco or other smoke	1. Surgeon General's reports: 2010, 2007 2. AHA/ACC statements: 2010, 2004 3. American Lung Association: 2009
Dyslipidemia	LDL-C <100 mg/dL or LDL <70 mg/dL (AHA, 2004) If triglycerides are >200 mg/dL, non-HDL-C should be <130 mg/dL	1. EAS guidelines: 2011 2. ADA: 2010 3. AHA: 2010, 2009 4. WCRR, AICR: 2007 5. USDA: 2002 6. IOM: 2002
Hypertension	Normal: <120/<80 mmHg Risk increases linearly with: • SBP >115 mmHg • DBP >75 mmHg	1. ACSM: 2007 2. JNC7: 2003
Physical inactivity	• Adults should do at least 150 min (2 h and 30 min) a week of moderate-intensity, or 75 min (1 h and 15 min) a week of vigorous-intensity aerobic physical activity performed in bouts of at least 10 min. • For additional and more extensive health benefits, adults should increase their aerobic physical activity to 300 min (5 h) a week of moderate-intensity, or 150 min a week of vigorous-intensity aerobic physical activity. • Adults should also do muscle strengthening activities that are moderate or high intensity and involve all major muscle groups on 2 or more days per week. • All adults should avoid inactivity. • All adults should avoid prolonged sitting time.	1. ACSM: 2009 2. CDC: 2008 3. AHA: 2007
Overweight and obesity	**Body mass index (BMI)** • Normal weight = 18.5 to 24.9 • Overweight ≥25.0 to 29.9 • Obesity ≥30.0 **Waist circumference** • Men: <40 in. (<101 cm) • Women: <35 in (<89 cm) **Waist-to-hip ratio (WHR)** *Men:* • Low risk ≤0.95 • Moderate risk ≥0.96 to 1.0 • High risk ≥1.0 *Women:* • Low risk ≤0.80 • Moderate risk ≥0.81 to 0.85 • High risk >0.85	1. ACSM: 2009 2. ADA: 2009
Diabetes and insulin resistance	**Categories of increased risk (prediabetes)** • Impaired fasting glucose: 100 to 125 mg/dL • Impaired glucose tolerance: 140 to 199 mg/dL • Glycated hemoglobin: 5.7% to 6.4% **Criteria for the diagnosis of type 2 diabetes** • Glycated hemoglobin: ≥6.5% • Fasting plasma glucose: ≥126 mg/dL (7.0 mmol/L) • 2 h plasma glucose: ≥200 mg/dL (11.1 mmol/L) during an oral glucose tolerance test	1. ADA: 2011 2. ACSM: 2010
Secondary prevention guidelines		1. AHA/ACC: 2011, 2010 2. EACVRP: 2010

Abbreviations: AHA, American Heart Association; ACC, American College of Cardiology; EAS, European Atherosclerosis Society; WCRF-AICR, World Cancer Research Fund-American Institute for Cancer Research; USDA, United States Department of Agriculture; IOM, Institutes of Medicine; ADA, American Diabetes Association; JNC7, The Seventh Report of the Joint National Committee on Prevention, Detection, Evaluation, and Treatment of High Blood Pressure; ACSM, American College of Sports Medicine; CDC, Centers for Disease Control and Prevention; EACVRP, European Association of Cardiovascular Rehabilitation and Prevention.

Guidelines for Risk Factor Intervention

If present, each of the risk factors listed in table 7.2 is appropriate for intervention. Modifying CHD risk factors has been shown to be efficacious for reducing risk of subsequent CVD events and progression of CAD.[27] The national guidelines, practice standards, and scientific statements cited in table 7.1 provide significant support and documentation for the efficacy of risk factor modification.

Stratification of Risk for Events During Exercise

As just noted, the presence of multiple risk factors increases the risk for progression of disease, as well as for CVD events. It is prudent to assess for the risk of progression of disease and for the risk of events. "Stratification of Risk for Cardiac Events During Exercise Participation" provides information relative to the level of risk for each risk factor mentioned. "Optimal" should be considered the outcome goal for patients, but current clinical status and extent of behavior change required must be considered when setting goals with patients. Research indicates that patient-set (self-set) goals and goal ownership are significantly related to achieving the desired outcomes.[24]

The goal of an exercise program is for patients to achieve physiological, symptomatic, psychological, and vocational benefits of physical activity using exercise training implemented at an acceptable (low) level of risk. A key element of safety is stratification of patients according to risk for acute CVD complications during exercise (guideline 7.3). Risk stratification criteria for events during exercise or activity are not well established or differentiated from those related to general mortality. It is less clear whether risk for an exercise-related event is related to the exercise or to the overall risk of morbidity and mortality.[28] Despite these potential limitations, stratification of patients for risk of an event during exercise is a clinical tool that can help determine the appropriate level of supervision for individual patients.

For those diagnosed with CHD, the risk of CVD events during exercise is low.[29-31] It has also been reported that the risk of an event for patients with congestive heart failure (CHF) during exercise is minimal.[32,33] Physical activity (especially "unaccustomed" activity) can trigger CVD events, but increased habitual physical activity and higher levels of cardiovascular fitness significantly lower risk during exercise.[34,35] More recently, it has been shown that events are more common during the early sessions of CR/SP.[36] Additionally, it has been demonstrated that the size of the program, the level of experience of the professional supervision, and presence or absence of electrocardiogram (ECG) monitoring are not related to event rate.[37] Finally, noncompliance with the exercise prescription increases risk of mortality.[38]

CR/SP can minimize risk through appropriate assessment at program entry, conservative implementation of the exercise prescription (especially during the early stages of CR/SP), frequent and high-quality training of CR/SP professionals in emergency response, and ongoing clinical and symptomatic assessment of patients during each exercise session. This does not diminish the potential importance of ECG monitoring. However, CR/SP professionals should understand that monitoring, in itself, does not necessarily prevent or reduce complications during CR/SP.

The risk stratification model presented in the sidebar "Stratification of Risk for Cardiac Events During Exercise Participation" uses variables common to established models and allows categorization into a single risk category. This model is helpful for identifying the lowest-risk, moderate-risk, and highest-risk patients. Lowest-risk patients have all of the characteristics listed, whereas the highest-risk patients have any one of the characteristics listed. Those who do not fit either classification are considered to be moderate risk.

Patients who have not undergone exercise testing before entering CR/SP and those with nondiagnostic exercise tests may be inadequately categorized using criteria from "Stratification of Risk for Cardiac Events During Exercise Participation". For such patients the approach to risk stratification should be more cautious, and the initial exercise prescription at program entry should be conservative. Patients with non-diagnostic exercise tests or tests that may not be useful for exercise prescription include the following:

Stratification of Risk for Cardiac Events During Exercise Participation

Characteristics of patients at lowest risk for exercise participation (all characteristics listed must be present for patient to remain at lowest risk)

- Absence of complex ventricular dysrhythmia during exercise testing and recovery
- Absence of angina or other significant symptoms (e.g., unusual shortness of breath, light-headedness, or dizziness during exercise testing and recovery)
- Presence of normal hemodynamics during exercise testing and recovery (i.e., appropriate increases and decreases in heart rate and systolic blood pressure with increasing workloads and recovery)
- Functional capacity ≥7 metabolic equivalents (METs)

Nonexercise testing findings:

- Rest ejection fraction ≥50%
- Uncomplicated myocardial infarction (MI) or revascularization procedure
- Absence of complicated ventricular arrhythmias at rest
- Absence of congestive heart failure (CHF)
- Absence of signs or symptoms of postevent or postprocedure ischemia
- Absence of clinical depression

Characteristics of patients at moderate risk for exercise participation (any one or combination of these findings places a patient at moderate risk)

- Presence of angina or other significant symptoms (e.g., unusual shortness of breath, light-headedness, or dizziness occurring only at high levels of exertion [≥7 METs])
- Mild to moderate level of silent ischemia during exercise testing or recovery (ST-segment depression <2 mm from baseline)
- Functional capacity <5 METs

Nonexercise testing findings:

- Rest ejection fraction = 40% to 49%

Characteristics of patients at high risk for exercise participation (any one or combination of these findings places a patient at high risk)

- Presence of complex ventricular arrhythmias during exercise testing or recovery
- Presence of angina or other significant symptoms (e.g., unusual shortness of breath, light-headedness, or dizziness at low levels of exertion [<5 METs] or during recovery)
- High level of silent ischemia (ST-segment depression ≥2 mm from baseline) during exercise testing or recovery
- Presence of abnormal hemodynamics with exercise testing (i.e., chronotropic incompetence or flat or decreasing systolic BP with increasing workloads) or recovery (i.e., severe postexercise hypotension)

Nonexercise testing findings:

- Rest ejection fraction <40%
- History of cardiac arrest, or sudden death
- Complex dysrhythmias at rest
- Complicated MI or revascularization procedure
- Presence of CHF
- Presence of signs or symptoms of postevent or postprocedure ischemia
- Presence of clinical depression

Reproduced from *Cardiology Clinics*, Vol. 19, M.A. Williams, "Exercise testing in cardiac rehabilitation: Exercise prescription and beyond," Copyright 2001, with permission from Elsevier.

> ### Guideline 7.3 Stratification of Risk for Exercise Events
>
> All patients diagnosed with cardiovascular disease (CVD) entering outpatient CR/SP programming should be stratified according to risk for the occurrence of CVD events during exercise and for risk of progression of atherosclerotic disease.

- Those with abnormal resting ECG, including left bundle branch block, left ventricular hypertrophy with or without resting ST-T wave changes, nonspecific intraventricular conduction delays, Wolff-Parkinson-White ECG pattern, and ventricular-paced rhythms
- Those on digitalis therapy
- Those who test negative for ischemia but who fail to achieve 85% of predicted maximal heart rate, and those with significant additional medical problems (comorbidities) that limit exercise capacity. Stress testing using pharmacologic challenge that is not symptom limited is less likely to be useful for exercise prescription. (See chapter 6 for a more detailed discussion.)

Clinical Supervision During Exercise

Guidelines concerning clinical supervision, perhaps the most important safety feature, in CR/SP remain an area of discussion. Decisions regarding the intensity of clinical supervision, including necessary personnel and the type and duration of the supervision and frequency of ECG monitoring (continuous vs. intermittent), should be established by the CR/SP program medical director and staff with input from the referring physician as appropriate.

The following sidebar, "Reducing Cardiovascular Disease Complications During Exercise Within Cardiac Rehabilitation/Secondary Prevention Programs (CR/SPPs)" suggests various programming methods to assist program staff with safety. More intense clinical supervision is required for patients who are at a higher level of acuity, who exhibit new or recurring cardiovascular or other symptoms, or who experience a change in health status. Additionally, enhanced awareness of patient status during exercise is prudent when the intensity of the exercise prescription is increased. The monitoring of clinical parameters before, during, and following exercise provides further safeguards (see guideline 7.4). As part of clinical supervision, staff members must provide thorough instruction regarding patient self-assessment and reporting responsibilities about symptoms and feelings of well-being to CR/SP staff. The safety and efficacy of the exercise program can be maximized through communicating with patients and conducting and implementing frequent clinical and symptomatic assessment for well-being and clinical status, as well as for compliance with the exercise prescription.

Early Outpatient Exercise Program

Early outpatient CR/SP may begin within 1 to 3 weeks postdischarge from the hospital if clinical status allows and may last up to 36 sessions (or longer based on medical necessity). Sessions are most commonly scheduled for 3 days per week, although numbers of sessions per week may vary from one to five and may include more than one session per day, if indicated. The intensity of clinical supervision is usually highest during this phase and may include ECG monitoring. The following sidebar, "Physician Roles in Cardiac Rehabilitation and Secondary Prevention (CR/SP)" outlines the physician roles in the provision of clinical supervision. Professionally qualified staff members such as registered nurses and registered or certified clinical exercise physiologists or specialists should provide physicians with documented evidence of unusual or abnormal responses. In each instance, this documentation should prompt the attention of a physician, with additional documentation of such review and plan of action.

Intensive Cardiac Rehabilitation

A novel format for outpatient cardiac rehabilitation, termed intensive cardiac rehabilitation (ICR), has been approved for reimbursement by

Reducing Cardiovascular Disease Complications During Exercise Within Cardiac Rehabilitation/Secondary Prevention Programs (CR/SPPs)

Program policies

- Ensure that all patients have physician referral and have appropriate assessment before entry into the program and at periodic follow-up intervals.
- Ensure that all patients receive ongoing assessment before, during, and after each exercise session.
- Maintain an emergency plan for adverse events and provide for frequent mock emergency practice and critique sessions for all staff members.
- Maintain physician standing orders for potential emergent and nonemergent medical events.
- Ensure on-site availability of medical supervision; monitoring and resuscitation equipment, including a defibrillator (as well as maintenance of such equipment); and appropriate medications.
- Emphasize duration of activity over intensity of effort, particularly in higher-risk patients and during early sessions (first month) in the program.

Patient education

- Emphasize to patients that they must be knowledgeable about and alert for warning signs and changes in their condition, both at home and within the CR/SP program, including chest discomfort or other angina-like symptoms, light-headedness or dizziness, irregular pulse, weight gain, and shortness of breath.
- Instruct patients about the appropriate responses to such changes in their condition.
- Stress the importance of adhering to the exercise prescription (i.e., target heart rate or perceived exertion, exercise workloads, duration of effort, and choices of exercise equipment).
- Emphasize the importance of warm-up and cool-down as they relate to the safety of exercise.
- Remind patients to adjust exercise levels according to various environmental conditions such as heat, humidity, cold, and elevation.

During the exercise session

- Evaluate each patient before exercise for recent changes in condition, body weight, BP, medication adherence, and electrocardiogram (ECG) if used.
- Use ECG monitoring as appropriate.
- If necessary, adjust the intensity and duration of the daily exercise prescription based on the clinical status before exercise and upon response to activity.
- Maintain supervision during and following exercise, including periodic checks of shower or locker room facilities, until the patient has left the facility.
- Modify recreational activities as appropriate and minimize competition.

Reproduced from *Cardiology Clinics*, Vol. 19, M.A. Williams, "Exercise testing in cardiac rehabilitation: Exercise prescription and beyond," Copyright 2001, with permission from Elsevier.

Medicare. Centers for Medicare and Medicaid Services (CMS) Publication 100-03 defines this ICR as "a physician-supervised program that furnishes CR services more frequently and often in a more rigorous manner."[39] Simply stated, an ICR program may offer up to six sessions per day and twice the total number of sessions (72 vs. 36) allowed in a traditional CR/SP program. A CR/SP program is limited to two sessions per day for up to 36 sessions (over 18 weeks). There is no restriction on the number of days per week on which either ICR or a traditional CR/SP program may offer sessions. There are additional requirements for ICR services to demonstrate "efficacy," mandating that very specific outcomes be assessed and that the program demonstrate

Guideline 7.4   Recommended Methods and Tools for Daily Assessment of Risk for Exercise

The preexercise assessment should include interviewing the patient about recent signs and symptoms, adherence to the medication schedule, and subjective feelings of well-being. Risk may also be assessed with the following clinical measures:

- Signs or symptoms of effort intolerance
- Continuous or intermittent electrocardiogram (ECG) monitoring
  - Telemetry or hardwire monitoring
    - "Quick-look" using the defibrillator paddles
    - Periodic rhythm strips
- Blood pressure
- Pulse, heart rate, or both (by palpation, ECG monitor, or both)
- Rating of perceived exertion
- Exercise tolerance

Physician Roles in Cardiac Rehabilitation and Secondary Prevention (CR/SP)

- ***Supervising physician*** means a physician who is immediately available and accessible for medical consultations and medical emergencies at all times during which services are being provided to individuals within CR/SP and intensive cardiac rehabilitation programs.

- ***Standards for supervising physicians.*** Physicians acting as the supervising physician must possess all of the following:

  1. Expertise in the management of individuals with cardiac pathophysiology
  2. Cardiopulmonary training in basic life support or advanced cardiac life support
  3. A license to practice medicine in the state in which the CR/SP program is offered

- CR/SP services are prescribed and supervised by a physician pursuant to a written individualized treatment plan established, reviewed, and signed by a physician every 30 days (in consultation with appropriate staff participating in the program). The plan sets forth the diagnoses; the type, amount, frequency, and duration of the items and services provided under the plan; and the goals under the plan.

- ***Medical director*** means a physician who oversees or supervises a CR/SP or intensive cardiac rehabilitation program at a particular site.

- ***Standards for the physician responsible for CR/SP program.*** A physician responsible for a CR/SP program or intensive cardiac rehabilitation programs is identified as the ***medical director.*** The medical director, in consultation with staff, is involved in directing the progress of individuals in the program and must possess all of the following:

  1. Expertise in the management of individuals with cardiac pathophysiology
  2. Cardiopulmonary training in basic life support or advanced cardiac life support
  3. A license to practice medicine in the state in which the CR/SP program is offered

- The medical director and the supervising physician are not required to be, and most often are not, the same person.

Reprinted from http://edocket.access.gpo.gov/cfr_2010/octqtr/pdf/42cfr410.49.pdf

"significant reduction" in five of those outcome variables. These are summarized in the following CMS statement: "The ICR program must also demonstrate through peer-reviewed published research that it accomplished a statistically significant reduction in five or more of the following measures for patients from their levels before CR services to after CR services: (1) LDL; (2) triglycerides; (3) body mass index; (4) systolic blood pressure (BP); (5) diastolic BP; and, (6) the need for cholesterol, BP, and diabetes medication."[39] It is noteworthy that these requirements are descriptive of a comprehensive program. That is, in order to provide "significant reduction in five or more" of the measures, an ICR program must address multiple CHD risk factors and health behaviors. All programs that offer ICR must be approved by CMS under the national determination process. The application process is described and contact information provided in the CMS publication referred to here.

ECG Monitoring in Early Outpatient CR/SP

As previously stated, ECG monitoring does not necessarily ensure either efficacy or safety. It is not, by itself, a valid or reliable measure of the clinical value of exercise or secondary prevention services or of the duration of an exercise program. Rather, ECG monitoring is one of several available methods and techniques that can be used for clinical supervision of patients. ECG monitoring during exercise sessions is frequently required for insurance reimbursement, often with the delineation of a "maximum" number of "allowable" sessions. There is less specific information available regarding program exit criteria other than the maximal number of sessions. Program staff should ensure familiarity with the insurance requirements of each patient. Ideally, the length of the supervised CR/SP should be determined on an individual basis according to outcomes and individual needs. Further recommendations for the use of ECG monitoring and duration of CR/SP based on risk of exercise events are presented in the following sidebar, "Recommendations for Intensity of Supervision and Monitoring Related to Risk of Exercise Participation."

ECG monitoring seems to be linked inversely with risk, but no firm predictors exist to help identify patients for whom it may not be necessary.[40] Continuous ECG monitoring is intended to

- detect dangerous dysrhythmias or other significant ECG changes that are amenable to treatment before complications arise;
- monitor compliance with the exercise prescription, especially with respect to heart rate; and
- increase patient self-confidence for independent activity.

Given the variable occurrence of dysrhythmias, however, and given that the safety of exercise regimens has been determined only by means of aggregate data, the use of continuous versus intermittent ECG monitoring remains a matter of clinical judgment. The type and frequency of ECG monitoring depend on the overall clinical status of the patient and the response to the exercise session. Intermittent ECG monitoring enables observation when indicated, such as at the time of a suspected change in clinical status as assessed by observation, measurement, or symptomatology, but does not afford detection of silent or sudden-onset dysrhythmias and thus should be used judiciously. Accordingly, the optimal approach balances patient benefit with safety.

Innovation in CR/SP

CMS, through updated guidelines and regulations, has opened the door to innovation in CR/SP programs. ICR is one route to innovation but is perhaps more complicated than is practical for many programs to implement. The ICR requirement for peer-reviewed, published research, which is (apparently) specific to each program that wishes to implement ICR, may be burdensome. Additionally, the method of enforcement is at this point uncertain. New regulations allow CR/SP, either traditional or ICR, the potential of multiple sessions per day with no upper limit on number of days per week. The result is a more intensive approach to CR/SP services. It has been demonstrated that a format using increased exercise duration and daily caloric expenditure in a CR/SP program can effectively modify several CVD risk factors and the risk for metabolic syndrome.[41]

Thus a more intensive approach to exercise within CR/SP, along with innovation in the process of risk factor modification (e.g., use of coaching), is indicated as a potential avenue to improve services for many patients. Offering sessions lasting 90 to 120 min, up to 5 days per week, is within these revised regulations. Additionally, modifications to the exercise prescription such as increased duration and intensity (on some days) may be indicated and allowable.

Maintenance CR/SP

CHD patients who have completed early outpatient CR/SP or who have CVD risk factors can benefit from attending a maintenance CR/SP to

Recommendations for Intensity of Supervision and Monitoring Related to Risk of Exercise Participation

Patients at lowest risk for exercise-related event

- Direct medical supervision of exercise should occur for a minimum of 6 to 18 exercise sessions or 30 days postevent or postprocedure, beginning with continuous electrocardiogram (ECG) monitoring and decreasing as appropriate (e.g., at 6-12 sessions).

- For the patient to remain at lowest risk, the ECG and hemodynamic findings must remain normal; there should be no development or progression of abnormal signs and symptoms or intolerance to exercise within or outside the supervised program. Progression of the exercise regimen should be appropriate.

Patients at moderate risk for exercise-related event

- Direct staff supervision of exercise should occur for a minimum of 12 to 24 exercise sessions or 60 days postevent or postprocedure; begin with continuous ECG monitoring and decrease to intermittent or no ECG monitoring as appropriate (e.g., at 12-18 sessions).

- To move the patient to the lowest risk category, ECG and hemodynamic findings during exercise must be normal; there should be no development or progression of abnormal signs and symptoms or intolerance to exercise within or outside the supervised program. Progression of the exercise regimen should be appropriate.

- Abnormal ECG or hemodynamic findings during exercise or the development or progression of abnormal signs and symptoms or intolerance to exercise within or outside the supervised program, or the need to severely decrease exercise levels, may result in the patient's remaining in the moderate risk category or even moving to the high risk category.

Patients at highest risk for exercise-related event

- Direct staff supervision of exercise should occur for a minimum of 18 to 36 exercise sessions or 90 days postevent or postprocedure, beginning with continuous ECG monitoring and decreasing to intermittent ECG monitoring as appropriate.

- For a patient to move to the moderate risk category, ECG and hemodynamic findings during exercise should be normal; there should be no development or progression of abnormal signs and symptoms or intolerance to exercise within or outside the supervised program. Progression of the exercise regimen should be appropriate.

- Findings of the development or progression of abnormal ECG or hemodynamic findings during exercise including intolerance to exercise within or outside the supervised program should be evaluated immediately. Significant limitations in the ability to participate may result in discontinuation of the exercise program until appropriate evaluation, and intervention where necessary, can take place.

facilitate ongoing and additional health behavior change associated with reductions in recurrent CVD events.[42] Indeed, maintenance CR/SP and the accompanying healthy lifestyle behaviors encouraged through continued secondary (and primary, if applicable) prevention are integral to decreasing morbidity and mortality and enhancing health-related quality of life in patients with CHD.[43]

Maintenance CR/SP can take many forms and is often structured around an individualized exercise prescription tailored to clinical status and comorbidities, orthopedic considerations, and cardiorespiratory fitness. Patients are monitored less intensively than in early outpatient CR/SP; thus, specific guidelines for clinical supervision should be implemented by the program director in consultation with the medical director. Patients may receive periodic heart rate and blood pressure assessment; intermittent or "quick-look" ECG monitoring; and counseling and support regarding health behavior change and risk factors, cardiovascular symptoms, and exercise prescription. Qualified staff (i.e., registered nurse, American College of Sports Medicine [ACSM] Registered Clinical Exercise Physiologist, ACSM Certified Clinical Exercise Specialist, and other certified clinical professionals) should be immediately available and properly trained to administer emergency support. Exercise progression and cardiovascular indicators should be closely monitored for changes in clinical status that may warrant further evaluation. Moreover, professional staff can determine whether ancillary programming, such as diabetes education, psychosocial evaluation, or nutrition counseling, may be beneficial to patients and make referrals as indicated.

In addition to basic exercise instruction and monitoring, maintenance CR/SP provides the ideal setting for continued risk factor modification and behavior change. Education can take many forms, including group lectures, individualized chart reviews, and newsletters or other written material, as well as verbal interaction during exercise sessions. A group education format also provides opportunities for social interaction among patients that should not be undervalued. Settings such as these facilitate support networks that may enhance health outcomes and participation in CR/SP.[44,45] Varied educational opportunities can provide patients with more than simply "supervised exercise"; patients receive comprehensive care aimed at positively influencing myriad CHD risk factors related to cardiovascular health, which may reduce the risk for future CVD events.[1]

As with many other lifestyle behaviors, the success of maintenance CR/SP depends on adherence. Beyond basic exercise sessions using standard equipment, supplementary programming such as group resistance training sessions, fitness classes (e.g., yoga, tai chi), aquatic exercise, aerobics, team sports (as appropriate), and other

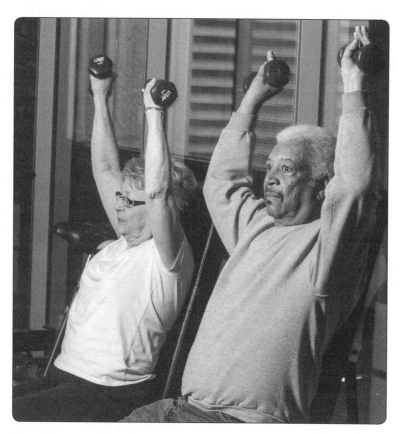

Beyond basic exercise sessions using standard equipment, supplementary programming such as group resistance training sessions may increase program adherence.

exercise modalities may augment CR/SP offerings for selected coronary patients and increase adherence. Techniques that improve compliance with healthy lifestyle behaviors, such as motivational interviewing[46-50] and goal setting,[51] are useful and valid strategies as well. Finally, identifying barriers to maintenance CR/SP, such as financial considerations, transportation issues, time constraints, and orthopedic limitations, allows patients and staff to work cohesively toward developing an action plan to circumvent factors limiting compliance. Honest and confidential communication among all parties influencing patient care is critical to maintaining adherence for those who experience such barriers to exercise.

Implementation of Secondary Prevention

The implementation of secondary prevention as described here can be challenging. Attempting to reduce the cost of health care has become the trend and a necessity in the current economic environment. CR/SP has been demonstrated to be cost-effective in both supervised, institutional settings and home-based settings.[52-54] Offering multidisciplinary programming to address the myriad issues facing patients with CHD can be challenging in the face of limited financial resources; creativity is essential. Identifying available programs offered outside CR/SP is one solution. In the hospital setting and in many communities, a variety of programs address general lifestyle issues such as managing stress, dietary change, and smoking cessation. Program staff may establish links with other in-house programs or outside agencies to offer access to these programs that extend services and provide potential discounts, ongoing support, and even periodic reassessment. Through use of resources such as these and others, programs may extend services.

Following patient progress through periodic assessment of cardiovascular risk factors and planned follow-up programming helps to ensure that outcomes are optimized; thus, accurate and detailed record keeping and continued patient contact are critical to long-term success. This process requires attention to detail, orderly record keeping, and established flags to alert staff to timely follow-up. Computer software specific to this task, particularly systems that allow careful tracking of outcomes, is helpful but not an absolute necessity. Chapter 11 presents a more detailed discussion of outcomes assessment.

Summary

Implementation of multifaceted CR/SP is prudent and necessary, since CR/SP has been shown to reduce CVD morbidity and mortality as well as to improve function and quality of life. Entry assessment for safety and disease progression helps program staff establish priorities for therapeutic modalities, helps patients understand the health behaviors that require change, and may identify the most efficacious therapy. Clinical supervision, which may include ECG-monitored exercise, is necessary; the intensity of clinical supervision required depends on individual patient status. In addition, home programming for patients, with or without supervised CR/SP, is an excellent adjunct to any patient-centered program of CVD risk reduction and is recommended here. Home programming can take many forms and is amenable to the use of technological innovations such as phone, e-mail, and Skype connection with professional staff. However, CR/SP must be more than an exercise program. The treatment of risk for progression of CVD disease requires a multifactorial effort by CR/SP staff, physicians, and other health care professionals and programs as indicated, including outcome assessment to validate the efficacy of services.

Modifiable Cardiovascular Disease Risk Factors

Cardiac rehabilitation/secondary prevention (CR/SP) programs are, in fact, risk factor intervention programs. The American Heart Association in the latest set of secondary prevention guidelines provides practitioners with specific recommendations for each risk factor.[1] Risk factor intervention and management is effective for both primary and secondary prevention. Additionally, in a set of Core Competencies published by the American Association of Cardiovascular and Pulmonary Rehabilitation (AACVPR), the authors state that, "Effective lifestyle management of CVD and associated risk factors" is a basic core competency for all cardiac rehabilitation professionals.

Lastly, cardiac rehabilitation programs have been shown to be effective in decreasing morbidity and mortality of participating patients by delivering secondary prevention programs within the service.[3]

OBJECTIVES

This chapter describes the basic assessment and intervention strategies for the following modifiable cardiovascular disease (CVD) risk factors:

- Tobacco use
- Dyslipidemia
- Hypertension
- Physical inactivity
- Diabetes
- Psychosocial concerns
- Obesity
- Emerging risk factors

Tobacco Use

Tobacco smoking continues to be the leading cause of preventable deaths in the United States today.[1] One in five deaths from CVD is attributable to smoking. Moreover, the global mortality from tobacco use is expected to climb from 3 million deaths in 1990 to 10 million in 2025.[1] Smoking is associated with an increased risk of CVD events in patients with established disease, including recurrent myocardial infarction (MI), sudden death, and restenosis after percutaneous coronary intervention (PCI). In individuals with coronary heart disease (CHD), smoking cessation is associated with a 36% reduction in the risk of all-cause mortality, making it an important secondary prevention intervention.[2] As a result of the high rates of relapse upon cessation even weeks, months, and years after quitting, the U.S. Public Health Service Clinical Practice Guideline on Treating Tobacco Use and Dependence, first published in 2000 and updated in 2008, suggests that tobacco dependence must now be considered a chronic condition that requires repeated intervention.[3]

Smoking causes numerous problems within the CV system and is associated with increased risk in those with vascular disease including CHD, peripheral arterial disease, abdominal aortic aneurysm, and stroke. Nicotine, the most important by-product of smoking, promotes catecholamine release, increasing heart rate and blood pressure and thus increasing myocardial oxygen demand. In addition, nicotine constricts peripheral arteries, interfering with blood flow to tissues; lowers the threshold for ventricular fibrillation; and increases platelet activation. Finally, nicotine has adverse effects on the lipoprotein panel, decreasing high-density lipoprotein cholesterol and increasing the oxygenation of low-density lipoprotein cholesterol, promoting atherogenesis. Carbon monoxide, another by-product of smoking, injures vascular endothelium and interferes with the ability of red blood cells to carry oxygen, thus reducing the amount of oxygen delivered to the heart muscle. Many other constituents in tobacco smoke augment platelet aggregability, promoting adherence of platelets to damaged endothelium.[4,5]

The improved outcome associated with smoking cessation in those with CVD is apparent soon after quitting and in people of all age groups, including the elderly. For example, the risk of MI decreases by 50% within 2 years of cessation, and the rate of restenosis following PCI and deaths following bypass surgery are decreased after cessation.[5]

Assessment of Tobacco Use

The U.S. Tobacco and Dependence Treatment clinical practice guideline suggests that health care professionals take every opportunity to identify and document tobacco use in all practice settings.[3] Because numerous patients are identified for CR/SP programs at the time of hospitalization, this setting serves as an important entryway for smoking cessation intervention. Moreover, at the time of hospitalization, patients are focused on their health; they experience the worst of withdrawal in the first 48 to 72 h of quitting and are forced to follow hospital smoking bans. Thus, a mechanism for identifying all smokers at the time of hospitalization, such as including smoking status as a vital sign and applying the mandated smoking status code on electronic records to identify smokers, is critically important for patient outcomes (guideline 8.1).

In outpatient CR/SP programs, smokers can be identified through intake forms that collect information about risk factors, or through interviews that are often part of taking a medical history. This

---

 Guideline 8.1   Evaluation of Tobacco Use

To reduce the risk associated with tobacco use, all health care professionals must take every opportunity to

- identify smokers and those who use other types of tobacco in all practical settings,

- document these encounters in the patient health record, and

- provide an environment that facilitates repeated interventions.

information should be electronically stored, with efforts directed at cessation. With the enforcement of hospital smoking bans, many smokers view themselves as having stopped smoking once they have entered the hospital. Therefore, it is critical that interviewers ask the appropriate question to identify smokers. The question "Have you smoked or used oral tobacco products in the past 30 days?" is more specific than "Do you smoke or use oral tobacco products?"

Once screening is completed, the next step in intervening is to determine willingness to quit smoking. Staff members may simply ask, "Are you willing to quit smoking now?" or "Are you willing to make an attempt to quit smoking now?" The clinical practice guideline indicates that those patients who are willing to quit tobacco should be provided appropriate treatments.[3] In addition, those who are unwilling to make an attempt to quit smoking should be offered a brief intervention designed to enhance their motivation. Ways to enhance motivation include

- encouraging patients to indicate why quitting smoking is personally relevant to them, being as specific as possible;
- helping patients to identify the acute, long-term, and environmental risks associated with continued smoking;
- helping patients determine potential benefits of quitting by selecting personal rewards;
- identifying barriers or roadblocks to quitting; and
- repeating the intervention (motivational interview) every time an unmotivated patient

visits a clinic setting (see "Motivational Interview").

A key to remembering the structure of such an intervention is to focus on the 5 Rs:

- Relevance
- Risks
- Rewards
- Roadblocks
- Repetition

For patients who are ready to make an attempt to quit smoking, additional information about their smoking status is helpful and allows individualized counseling. However, the clinical practice guideline also notes that smoking cessation interventions should not depend solely on formal assessments such as questionnaires, the clinical interview, or physiological measures such as carbon monoxide or pulmonary function measures to guide them.[3] These assessments do not consistently produce higher long-term quit rates than nontailored interventions of equal intensity. Thus, time allotted to undertake these assessments must be weighed against the time available for counseling and intervention.

A smoking history (see appendix K) may provide additional information that is useful for individualizing counseling about smoking. Documenting whether other household members smoke may help determine the patient level of support and whether family members may also benefit from counseling. Determining past experience with serious attempts to quit and

Motivational Interview

Relevance	Personalize why quitting is relevant (i.e., wishes of family members, health).
Risks	Ask patient to identify negative consequences of tobacco use:
	• Acute risks: Shortness of breath, chest discomfort
	• Long-term risks: MI, stroke, chronic obstructive pulmonary disease (COPD)
	• Environmental: Respiratory infections in children, heart disease in spouses
Rewards	Ask patient to identify benefits of stopping smoking (e.g., improving symptoms, saving money, setting a good example for children).
Roadblocks	Ask patient to identify barriers to quitting (e.g., weight gain, depression, withdrawal symptoms).
Repetition	Repeat this intervention at every clinic visit or within any other setting.

length of cessation, success with previous smoking interventions, and previous use of pharmacologic therapies can be helpful in planning an appropriate intervention. People with a history of depression have more difficulty quitting than those without such a history. Therefore, using standardized tools to measure depression as part of an evaluation of the psychosocial status, or incorporating single-item measures such as the scale depicted in the "Example of a Single-Item Measure of Psychological Status" sidebar, which has been shown to correlate with other clinical measures of depression, can be useful in counseling.[6] Moreover, patients who are depressed are appropriate candidates for the use of buproprion SR to help them quit smoking.

Alcohol use is another important question to address when individualizing counseling for people attempting to quit smoking. Smokers who consume large amounts of alcohol or abuse alcohol find it difficult to quit. Success with quitting is extremely low, and little research has been conducted showing the efficacy of smoking interventions in this population. Confronting patients about inappropriate alcohol use may be necessary when intervening with them. Determining the frequency of use and weekly consumption, as well as screening for alcohol abuse, provides important insights useful for counseling. The CAGE Questionnaire (see appendix L) is the most common screening tool for potential alcohol abuse.[7] A "yes" response to any of the questions may indicate potential alcohol abuse, and two or more positive responses increases the probability of past or present abuse. Questions in the smoking history (appendix K) related to alcohol consumption are also useful in this regard. The frequent underreporting of alcohol use, and the cardiotoxic effects of high consumption in patients with CVD, require health care professionals to assess and openly discuss this issue.[8,9] Referral to an alcoholism treatment program may be warranted.

Intervention

The clinical practice guideline highlights evidence from randomized controlled trials suggesting several key findings that are important when intervening with smokers:

- The more intense the treatment, the greater the rate of cessation. Intensive interventions are more effective and should be used whenever possible.

- Treatment can be maximized by increasing the length of individual sessions to greater than 10 min and the number of treatment sessions to four or more sessions (>30 min contact time).

- Use of multiple types of providers (e.g., physicians, nurses, pharmacists) enhances cessation rates.

- Proactive telephone calls and individual and group counseling are effective cessation formats. State quit lines and 1-800-Quit-Now, the national quit line, are effective compared to no or minimal interventions.

- Practical counseling (problem solving and skills training) and use of social support significantly improve cessation outcomes.

- Pharmacologic therapies increase cessation rates and should be encouraged for all quitters except where contraindications exist. In some cases, combination therapies have been shown to be more effective than single drugs.

- The combination of counseling and medications is more effective for smoking cessation than either one alone; both should be provided.[3]

Example of a Single-Item Measure of Psychological Status

How troubled are you now by feeling miserable or depressed?

0	1	2	3	4	5	6	7	8	9
Not	Hardly		Slightly		Moderately		Markedly		Severely

Patients scoring 5 or greater may have problems with depression, and further clinical evaluation should be suggested.

Many of these recommendations have been applied in helping cardiac patients to quit smoking.[6,10] In general, exercise training alone as part of CR/SP has not been shown to improve smoking cessation rates in this population. However, nurse case management with more intensive interventions has been shown to improve cessation rates in those with established CHD.[6,10,11] Although relapse rates continue to be greater than 50% in cardiac patients, smoking cessation is still the single most important intervention proven to reduce morbidity and mortality in these individuals, making it a high priority for all clinicians. Finally, because most smokers do not attend formal cessation programs, which often provide behavioral skills training over 10 to 12 weeks, offering education and reinforcement for quitting is important on an ongoing basis.

Because smokers move along a continuum from contemplation to preparation to action to quitting (maintenance), numerous health care providers must strongly reinforce the message to quit, keeping in mind that "readiness to quit" is critical in determining when a patient may take action.[12] Physician advice to quit is extremely powerful, and CR/SP specialists should not only encourage patients to quit but also cue physicians to provide the same strong message. Personalizing the message to include information about the smoking hazards related to the disease offers patients a greater understanding of the risks associated with continuing to smoke.

At a minimum, all health care professionals involved in secondary prevention can help people to quit smoking by

- identifying smokers at every encounter;
- asking if they are willing to make an attempt to quit smoking (see the "Assessment of Tobacco Use" section);
- aiding the smoker in using interventions, including providing strong advice about the need to quit and offering self-help materials such as videotapes and pamphlets for those willing to quit and community resources for those unwilling to quit; and
- arranging for follow-up, either in person or via telephone.

In addition, CR/SP specialists should provide behavioral counseling and monitor the effects of pharmacologic therapies for patients interested in quitting. An algorithm for patients who are smoking at the time of an encounter with a secondary prevention program is presented in appendix M. Due to the high risk of recurrent events, all patients who choose not to quit should also be offered follow-up. Contracting with them to limit the number of cigarettes they smoke each day, aggressively modifying other CVD risk factors, and ensuring that patients are well protected with other interventions known to affect prognosis (such as angiotensin-converting enzyme [ACE] inhibitors, antiplatelet agents, beta-blockers, statins, and antihypertensive medications) may improve overall survival and in time alter their perspective on quitting smoking.

A person who has not quit smoking but is interested in doing so will need help with cessation. Patients should set a quit date within 1 to 2 weeks of the encounter so that their commitment to cessation does not wane. They must also decide whether to quit "cold turkey" or use other methods, such as switching brands or decreasing the number of cigarettes smoked in the days before they quit. Pharmacotherapy may be needed before quitting. Health care professionals can use this opportunity to review the smoking history, highlighting the most relevant items, such as success with previous attempts, availability of social support, use of alcohol, and problems that may have hindered past success. In addition, CR/SP specialists should prepare individuals for their "quit day" by asking them to remove all ashtrays and tobacco products, inform family members of their intent to quit, and obtain pharmacologic therapies if they have not done so already.

For patients who have quit smoking during hospitalization, relapse prevention counseling and other behavioral interventions such as contracting increase their chances of success. Relapse prevention training has been used with great success for those with addictive behaviors such as those related to excessive gambling, obesity, alcoholism, and smoking. Slips or lapses into the old behavior are common when a person gives up smoking, and they often relate to emotional states such as frustration, boredom, or depression; interpersonal conflict with family members, friends, or colleagues; or social pressure. Relapse prevention interventions to help people cope involve

- identifying high-risk situations likely to cause relapse;
- determining both behavioral and cognitive coping skills and practicing them through role rehearsal;
- using lifestyle changes such as relaxation, imagery, and exercise to support the quitting effort; and
- knowing what to do if a slip occurs.

In addition to the preceding, as noted in the algorithm, people also need counseling about

- potential weight gain,
- common withdrawal symptoms that may pose an important need for pharmacologic therapy,
- the difficulty in quitting associated with alcohol use,
- integrating social support networks such as family members and friends to aid in quitting,
- the psychological craving associated with quitting that occurs through urges, and
- the psychological sense of loss associated with giving up cigarettes.[13]

Exercise through CR/SP also helps individuals as they quit smoking by improving psychological well-being and minimizing weight gain and withdrawal symptoms. Thus, CR/SP professionals should encourage active participation in the exercise component of a cardiac rehabilitation/secondary prevention (CR/SP) program. Self-help materials such as pamphlets, videotapes, and audiotapes developed by the American Heart Association, the American Lung Association, and the American Cancer Society should also be used to supplement counseling and to reinforce information provided by program specialists. An abundance of reputable Internet sites offer resources to help smokers through the early stages of quitting to complement in-person counseling. Individuals may also want to avail themselves of a state-sponsored quit line or the national quit line. One of the advantages of using the quit lines is the lack of cost associated with this type of intervention and ready access to well-trained smoking cessation counselors. Unfortunately, only about 1% of all smokers avail themselves of these services.[11]

Pharmacologic Therapy

The clinical practice guideline indicates that all patients should be encouraged to use pharmacologic therapies for smoking cessation except in special circumstances.[3] Numerous studies indicate a lack of association between the use of nicotine replacement products and acute cardiovascular events.[14-16] Precautions with the use of nicotine replacement products continue to exist for patients who are within 2 weeks of an MI, those with serious arrhythmias, and those with serious or worsening angina. However, with some patients, one must also weigh the risks associated with continued smoking, noting that the amount of nicotine is far greater in cigarettes than in nicotine replacement products.

Presently, seven first-line medications are indicated to help smokers in their attempts to quit. These include buproprion SR, varenicline, and five nicotine replacement therapies: nicotine gum, nicotine inhaler, nicotine lozenge, nicotine nasal spray, and the nicotine patch. Personal preference and previous use can often guide the choice of an agent. Recent data have shown the benefit of varenicline as an effective agent in patients with CVD.[3] The following are important facts about the use of these pharmacologic agents: (1) 4 mg nicotine gum is more useful for highly dependent smokers than 2 mg gum; (2) buproprion SR has been especially helpful for those with a history of depression; and (3) pharmacologic therapies (nicotine patch or gum and buproprion) have not been shown to prevent weight gain but simply to delay it. Most patients benefit from the use of an agent for 8 to 12 weeks, with a small proportion needing therapy for 24 weeks. In addition, recent evidence suggests the benefit of combining pharmacotherapies such as varenicline, the nicotine patch, and buproprion.[3] It should be noted that the U.S. Food and Drug Administration (FDA) published a safety announcement in mid-2011, notifying the public that the smoking cessation aid varenicline may be associated with a small, increased risk of certain cardiovascular adverse events in patients who have CVD.[17]

CR/SP specialists should offer appropriate education and counseling regarding the administration of all pharmacologic agents. Education can be reinforced through written instructions developed to support these pharmacologic aids. Follow-up carried out through visits, telephone contacts, and e-mail increases the success of smoking cessation interventions. Studies suggest an increase in smoking cessation rates when four or more contacts are used to follow up with CHD patients.[18,19] Telephone contacts may be a convenient, effective method to provide positive reinforcement, to problem solve difficulties the patient encounters in quitting, and to help patients set another quit date if relapse has occurred. These telephone contacts are especially helpful in the early stages of quitting.

Abnormal Lipids

Approximately 44% of American adults have dyslipidemia.[1] These findings do represent, however, a decrease for non-Hispanic whites, non-Hispanic blacks, and Hispanics, the biggest decrease since 2003-2004 to 2007-2008 according to the National Health and Nutrition Examination Survey (NHANES) data. Specifically, decreases among these groups have resulted from changes in white males, black males, and Mexican American women. Strong evidence supports the benefits of lowering serum cholesterol levels and LDL-C in patients with CHD, particularly among those who have suffered a MI. Reductions in cardiovascular mortality, recurrent cardiac events, hospitalizations, and angiographic progression of atherosclerotic disease have been demonstrated with LDL-C lowering, including in women and the elderly.[1-9] Unfortunately, evidence suggests that despite the measurable benefit associated with lowering cholesterol levels, many patients who have been identified as having CHD continue to exhibit elevated cholesterol, which may also be due to poor adherence to the medication(s).[10-13] The results of these studies justify aggressive cholesterol evaluation and management as early

as possible in patients with known CHD (guideline 8.2).

Cholesterol is a fatlike substance (lipid) that is present in cell membranes and is a precursor of bile acids and steroid hormones. Cholesterol travels in the blood in distinct particles containing both lipid and proteins. These particles are called lipoproteins. The cholesterol level in the blood is determined partly by genetics; partly by environmental factors; and partly by health behaviors such as diet, calorie balance, and level of physical activity. Three major classes of lipoproteins are found in the blood: LDL-C, HDL-C, and very low-density lipoprotein cholesterol (VLDL-C). VLDL-C is a precursor of LDL-C; and some forms of VLDL-C, particularly VLDL-C remnants, appear to be atherogenic.[14]

LDL-C is estimated from measurements of total cholesterol, total fasting triglycerides, and HDL-C. If the triglyceride value is below 400 mg/dL, then its value can be divided by 5 to estimate the VLDL-C level. Because the level of total cholesterol is the sum of LDL-C, HDL-C, and VLDL-C, LDL-C can be calculated as follows (all quantities are in mg/dL):

$$\text{LDL-C} = \text{Total cholesterol} - \text{HDL-C} - (\text{Triglycerides}/5)$$

Because the LDL-C value is estimated from measurements that include triglycerides, blood samples should be collected from patients who have fasted for 9 to 12 h, having taken nothing by mouth except water and medications. For patients with triglyceride values over 400 mg/dL, estimation of LDL-C as just described is not accurate. In such cases, direct measurement of LDL by ultracentrifugation in a specialized laboratory is recommended if available. It is recommended that measurement of cholesterol occur within the first 24 h following the event or that it wait until 4 to 6 weeks after the event or procedure

Guideline 8.2   **Evaluation of Lipids**

All patients with established CHD should have a lipoprotein analysis for LDL-C determination after an overnight fast at 4 to 6 weeks postevent or postprocedure.[14-17]

to establish a true baseline on which therapeutic decisions can be made.[14-17] This is not to suggest, however, that therapeutic management and education should not begin immediately, especially in those patients whose lipids were previously found to be abnormal.[1] In all adults over the age of 20, a fasting lipoprotein profile should be obtained every 5 years.[14]

Clinical evaluation in patients with abnormal lipids should include a detailed history to determine potential contributors to elevated lipid levels such as various disease states, inappropriate diet, or, in some instances, medications. Secondary causes of abnormal lipids include the following:

- Diabetes mellitus
- Hypothyroidism
- Nephrotic syndrome
- Obstructive liver disease
- Drugs that may raise LDL-C levels or lower HDL-C, particularly progestins, anabolic steroids, corticosteroids, and certain antihypertensive agents; thiazide diuretics and loop diuretics can cause an elevation of total cholesterol, LDL-C, and triglycerides

Although limited in their impact, beta-adrenergic blocking agents without intrinsic sympathomimetic activity (ISA) or alpha-blocking properties increase serum triglycerides and lower HDL-C. However, it should be noted that these drugs are not contraindicated in the presence of abnormal lipids. Their use must be considered in the context of their benefit in treating other disorders versus their potential adverse effect on the lipid profile.

Because abnormal lipids sometimes are caused by familial genetic disorders, a careful family history can help to determine the etiology and management of LDL-C elevations in affected patients, as well as potentially identifying family members who need therapy for high cholesterol levels. Increasing evidence shows that additional factors such as lipoprotein(a), fibrinogen levels, and immune responses interact with lipids in ways that can also increase coronary risk. Homocysteine is no longer considered an additional factor to measure or treat for CVD.[18] Therefore population-wide screening for elevated homocysteine levels is not recommended. In selected patients with personal or family history of premature CVD,

especially without other known risk factors, evaluation of homocysteine levels may be prudent.

Specific areas of the physical examination relevant to abnormal lipids include a careful examination of the eyes to document corneal arcus, a funduscopic examination to detect retinal changes due to abnormal lipids, and an examination of the skin to detect xanthoma and xanthelasma. Specific laboratory assessment in the hyperlipidemic patient should include thyroid-stimulating hormone, fasting blood glucose, serum creatinine, and liver function tests—the latter to assess for hepatotoxicity from statin therapy. Lipids and liver function should be measured regularly to make sure that the patient is achieving and maintaining goals and has no medication-related side effects.

LDL-C, Traditional Risk Factors, and CHD Risk

The National Cholesterol Education Program (NCEP) was developed after evidence from epidemiological studies revealed a significant relationship between elevated cholesterol and CHD. Studies were then undertaken to determine whether lowering cholesterol would result in a decrease in CHD.[14] The NCEP Expert Panel on Detection, Evaluation, and Treatment of High Blood Cholesterol in Adults (Adult Treatment Panel III, ATP III) provides clinical guidelines for cholesterol testing and management. ATP III targets decreasing (treating) LDL-C while also emphasizing primary prevention in persons with multiple risk factors. The ATP III classifications are shown in "ATP III Classification of Cholesterol, HDL, and LDL" and "Traditional CVD Risk Factors." In 2004, after five major randomized trials had been completed, an update to the ATP III guidelines was written.[1] This update acknowledged the benefit of obtaining a lower LDL-C than had been specified in the ATP III guidelines for specific high-risk patients. Therefore, secondary prevention LDL goals were changed for high-risk patients (see table 8.1). HMG Co-A reductase inhibitors (statins) continue to be listed as the drug of choice for patients with CAD. The LDL-C treatment goal is <70 mg/dL.

In addition to using risk factors in the determination of overall treatment goals and interven-

ATP III Classification of Cholesterol, HDL, and LDL

Total cholesterol (mg/dL)

<200	Desirable
200-239	Borderline high
≥240	High

LDL-C (mg/dL)

<100	Optimal
100-129	Near optimal to above optimal
130-159	Borderline high
160-189	High
≥190	Very high

HDL-C (mg/dL)

<40	Low
≥60	High

Reprinted from National Institute of Health. Available: http://www.nhlbi.nih.gov/guidelines/cholesterol/atglance.pdf

Traditional CVD Risk Factors

Positive risk factors[a]

- Age: Men ≥45 years, women ≥55 years
- Family history of premature CHD
  - CHD in male first-degree relative <55 years
  - CHD in female first-degree relative <65 years
- Cigarette smoking
- Hypertension ≥140/90 mmHg or on antihypertensive medication
- Low HDL-C, <40 mg/dL

Negative risk factor

- High HDL-C, ≥60 mg/dL (presence of this negative risk factor removes one positive risk factor from the total number of risk factors)

[a]Diabetes is regarded as a CHD risk equivalent.

Abbreviations: CVD, cardiovascular disease; CHD, coronary heart disease; HDL-C, high-density lipoprotein cholesterol.

Reprinted from National Institute of Health, 2001, *National Cholesterol Education Program*.

tion strategies, ATP III emphasizes the need to assess 10-year CHD risk (MI or coronary death) as a part of this process in primary prevention.[20] Risk of development of CHD over a 10-year period using Framingham risk scoring for men and women is grouped into three categories (see "Risk Categories for Development of CHD in 10 Years" sidebar). A subset of moderately high-risk patients will have the option to reduce LDL-C to <100 mg/dL (see table 8.1). Risk factors used in the estimation of 10-year risk for a cardiac event include age, total cholesterol (an average of two readings), systolic blood pressure (BP) on the day of assessment, HDL, and smoking (yes/no, any amount or type) (see "Estimate of 10-Year Risk for Men and Women" sidebar and figure 8.1).[1,14]

Risk Categories for Development of CHD in 10 Years

High risk

Individuals in this category have a >20% risk for a new or recurring cardiac event (MI or coronary death) in a 10-year period and should be treated the most aggressively:

- Those with documented CHD
- Those at high CHD risk equivalent, including patients with symptomatic carotid artery disease, peripheral artery disease, abdominal aortic aneurysm, or diabetes

Moderate risk

Individuals in this category have a 10% to 20% risk for a cardiac event (MI or coronary death) in a 10-year period:

- Those with two or more traditional risk factors for CHD

Lowest risk

Individuals in this category have a <10% risk for a cardiac event (MI or coronary death) in a 10-year period:

- Those with no or one other traditional risk factor

Abbreviations: CHD, coronary heart disease; MI, myocardial infarction.

Based on National Institute of Health, 2001, *National Cholesterol Education Program*.

Estimate of 10-Year Risk for Men and Women

Risk factors used in the estimation of 10-year risk for a cardiac event include age, total cholesterol (an average of two readings), systolic blood pressure on the day of assessment, high-density lipoprotein cholesterol (HDL-C), and smoking (yes/no, any amount or type). Each risk factor is given points depending on the age group. Points are totaled to determine 10-year risk as a percentage.[14] The risk can be recalculated as the patient makes lifestyle changes to demonstrate reductions in coronary heart disease (CHD) risk (see figure 8.1).

Therapeutic Lifestyle Changes

It is important to recognize that the recommendations for target LDL-C levels, as well as levels for the initiation of nonpharmacologic (therapeutic lifestyle changes [TLC]) and pharmacologic therapies, are based on stratification of 10-year risk.[14] Table 8.1 identifies the risk categories and associated goals.

Treatment of dyslipidemia must include therapeutic lifestyle changes, including dietary intervention, physical activity, and weight loss, as a part of any risk reduction program. The most recent guidelines have condensed previous recommendations of the American Heart Association Step 1 and Step 2 diets, which gradually lowered cholesterol and saturated fat intake, to one diet that represents most of what was a part of the Step 2 diet (see "Therapeutic Lifestyle Changes"

sidebar). These dietary guidelines provide a range of 25% to 35% of total calories derived from total fat (which is especially helpful for people who have diabetes or are insulin resistant) but still recommend that intake of calories from saturated fat be kept <7% of total calories.[19] If the patient does not reach the LDL-C goal, other options include increasing or adding plant stanols and sterols and viscous fiber.

Dietary evaluation and counseling should serve as the foundation of treatment for patients with abnormal lipids. A registered dietitian or other appropriately trained individual specializing in dietary lipid management should perform a careful assessment of current eating habits and dietary composition. This assessment should include an estimation of total daily caloric requirements to achieve and maintain desirable body weight; total caloric intake; and dietary

Figure 8.1 Estimate of 10-Year Risk For Men And Women

Estimate of 10-year risk for men
(Framingham point scores)

Age (years)	Points
20-34	-9
35-39	-4
40-44	0
45-49	3
50-54	6
55-59	8
60-64	10
65-69	11
70-74	12
75-79	13

Total cholesterol, mg/dL	Points				
	Age 20-39	Age 40-49	Age 50-59	Age 60-69	Age 70-79
<160	0	0	0	0	0
160-199	4	3	2	1	0
200-239	7	5	3	1	0
240-279	9	6	4	2	1
≤280	11	8	5	3	1

	Points				
	Age 20-39	Age 40-49	Age 50-59	Age 60-69	Age 70-79
Nonsmoker	0	0	0	0	0
Smoker	8	5	3	1	1

HDL, mg/dL	Points
≥60	-1
50-59	0
40-49	1
<40	2

Systolic BP, mmHg	If untreated	If treated
<120	0	0
120-129	0	1
130-139	1	2
140-159	1	2
≥160	2	3

Point total	10-yr Risk, %
0	<1
1	1
2	1
3	1
4	1
5	2
6	2
7	3
8	4
9	5
10	6
11	8
12	10
13	12
14	16
15	20
16	25
≥17	≥30

Estimate of 10-year risk for women
(Framingham point scores)

Age (years)	Points
20-34	-7
35-39	-3
40-44	0
45-49	3
50-54	6
55-59	8
60-64	10
65-69	12
70-74	14
75-79	16

Total cholesterol, mg/dL	Points				
	Age 20-39	Age 40-49	Age 50-59	Age 60-69	Age 70-79
<160	0	0	0	0	0
160-199	4	3	2	1	1
200-239	8	6	4	2	1
240-279	11	8	5	3	2
≤280	13	10	7	4	2

	Points				
	Age 20-39	Age 40-49	Age 50-59	Age 60-69	Age 70-79
Nonsmoker	0	0	0	0	0
Smoker	9	7	4	2	1

HDL, mg/dL	Points
≥60	-1
50-59	0
40-49	1
<40	2

Systolic BP, mmHg	If untreated	If treated
<120	0	0
120-129	1	3
130-139	2	4
140-159	3	5
≥160	4	6

Point total	10-yr Risk, %
<0	<1
9	1
10	1
11	1
12	1
13	2
14	2
15	3
16	4
17	5
18	6
19	8
20	11
21	14
22	17
23	22
24	27
≥25	≥30

Reprinted from National Institute of Health, 2001, *National Cholesterol Education Program*. Available: http://www.nhlbi.nih.gov/guidelines/cholesterol/risk_tbl.htm

Table 8.1 National Cholesterol Education Program Adult Treatment Panel III: LDL-C Treatment Guidelines (2004 Revision, Adapted[1])

Risk category	LDL-C goal	Initiate TLC	Consider drug therapy**
High risk: CHD* or CHD risk equivalents[†] (10-year risk >20%)	<100g/dL (optional goal: <70 mg/dL)	≥100 mg/dL	≥100 mg/dL (<100 mg/dL: consider drug options)
Moderately high risk: 2+ risk factors (10-year risk 10% to 20%)	<130 mg/dL	≥130 mg/dL	≥130 mg/dL (100–129 mg/dL; consider drug options)
Moderate risk: 2+ risk factors (10-year risk <10%)	<130 mg/dL	≥130 mg/dL	≥160 mg/dL
Lower risk: 0–1 risk factor[§]	<160 mg/dL	≥160 mg/dL	≥190 mg/dL (160–189 mg/dL: LDL-lowering drug optional)

*CHD includes history of myocardial infarction, unstable angina, stable angina, coronary artery procedures (angioplasty or bypass surgery), or evidence of clinically significant myocardial ischemia.

**When LDL-lowering drug therapy is employed, it is advised that intensity of therapy be sufficient to achieve at least a 30% to 40% reduction in LDL-C levels.

†CHD risk equivalents include clinical manifestations of noncoronary forms of atherosclerotic disease (peripheral arterial disease, abdominal aortic aneurysm, and carotid artery disease [transient ischemic attacks or stroke of carotid origin or >50% obstruction of a carotid artery]), diabetes, and 2+ risk factors with 10-year risk for hard CHD >20%.

§Almost all people with zero or 1 risk factor have a 10-year risk 10%, and 10-year risk assessment in people with zero or 1 risk factor is thus not necessary.

Reprinted, by permission, from S.M. Grundy et al., 2004, "Implications of recent clinical trials for the National Cholesterol Education Program Adult Treatment Panel III guidelines," *Circulation* 110: 227-239.

Therapeutic Lifestyle Changes

- Diet
  - Saturated fat <7% of total calories; cholesterol <200 mg/day
  - Consider increased viscous (soluble) fiber (10-25 g/day) and plant stanols and sterols (2 g/day) as therapeutic options to enhance low-density lipoprotein cholesterol lowering
- Weight management
- Increased physical activity

Based on National Institute of Health, 2001, *National Cholesterol Education Program*.

composition, including, at least, an estimate of the percentage of total calories from fat, percentage of total calories from saturated fat, and daily cholesterol intake. Dietary intervention should not preclude the immediate use of pharmacologic therapy to appropriately lower lipid levels to the desirable range as outlined by ATP III.[14]

Insulin Resistance and the Metabolic Syndrome

Substantial evidence now exists to suggest a correlation between insulin resistance and CHD.[1,22-25] Although the LDL goal is still the primary target of therapy, other lipid and nonlipid goals are also targeted. The first-line therapy for people who are insulin resistant includes weight loss and exercise, both of which can have a great impact on insulin

resistance and reduce CHD risk. Both weight loss and physical activity have been shown to decrease insulin resistance, lower triglycerides (and VLDL-C), increase HDL, and possibly decrease blood pressure.[26,27] In helping to identify patients at risk for insulin resistance, ATP III recommends evaluating the characteristics listed in table 8.2, which are associated with insulin resistance. If three of the five characteristics are present, a diagnosis of metabolic syndrome is established. Insulin resistance is related to both genetic and environmental factors.[23,28] Increasing weight and lack of physical activity both contribute to this syndrome. Upon recognition of those characteristics in table 8.2, starting a treatment plan as described in the "Treatment of Insulin Resistance–Metabolic Syndrome" sidebar is appropriate.

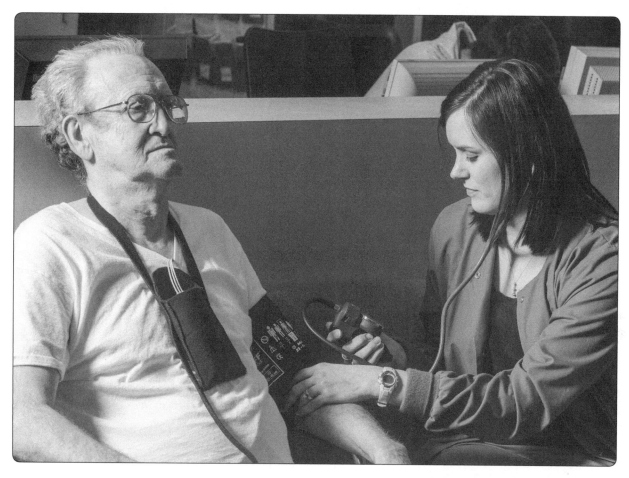

Systolic blood pressure on the day of assessment is one of the risk factors used in the estimation of 10-year risk for a cardiac event.

Table 8.2   Clinical Identification of the Metabolic Syndrome[a]

Risk factor	Defining level

Abdominal obesity[b]
    Men[c]
    Women
	Waist circumference[b]
	    >102 cm (>40 in.)
	    >88 cm (>35 in.)

Triglycerides	≥150 mg/dL

High-density lipoprotein cholesterol
    Men
    Women
	
	<40 mg/dL
	<50 mg/dL

Blood pressure	≥130/≥85 mmHg
Fasting glucose	≥110 mg/dL

[a]The presence of three or more of these characteristics identifies the metabolic syndrome.

[b]Both obesity and overweight are associated with insulin resistance and the metabolic syndrome. The presence of abdominal obesity, however, is more highly correlated with the metabolic risk factors than is an elevated body mass index. Therefore, the simple measure of waist circumference is recommended to identify the body weight component of the metabolic syndrome.

[c]Some male patients can develop multiple metabolic risk factors when the waist circumference is only marginally increased (e.g., 94-102 cm [37-39 in.]). Such patients may have a strong genetic contribution to insulin resistance. The benefit they gain from changes in lifestyle habits is similar to that of men with categorical increases in waist circumference.

Based on National Institute of Health, 2001, *National Cholesterol Education Program.*

Treatment of Insulin Resistance–Metabolic Syndrome

First-line therapies:

- Increasing physical activity
- Intensifying weight loss
- Treatment for lipid and nonlipid risk factors if they persist despite these lifestyle therapies
- Treatment for hypertension
- Use of aspirin for CHD patients to reduce prothrombotic state

Based on National Institute of Health, 2001, *National Cholesterol Education Program.*

Elevated Triglycerides

People who are insulin resistant often have elevated triglycerides, with or without elevated cholesterol levels, and are at further increased risk for CHD.[15,28,29] In these cases, other goals may be necessary after the LDL goal is obtained. Non-HDL-C is total cholesterol minus HDL-C.[31] Using non-HDL-C as a goal when elevated triglyceride levels are present is a new addition to the guidelines. Specific guidelines for levels of elevated triglycerides are listed in the "ATP III Classification of Serum Triglycerides" sidebar. Treatment goals and intervention recommendations for elevated triglycerides and low HDL are described in table 8.3, "Intervention Recommendations for Elevated Triglyceride Levels" sidebar, and "Treatment of Low HDL-C (<40 mg/dL)" sidebar. As mentioned earlier, intensifying weight management and increasing physical activity are always part of the treatment regimen.[14]

Table 8.3 Treatment Goals and Intervention Recommendations for Elevated Triglycerides and Low HDL-C[a]

Risk category	LDL goal (mg/dL)	Non-HDL goal (mg/dL)
CHD and CHD risk equivalent (10-year risk for CHD >20%)	<100	<130
Multiple (2+) risk factors and 10-year risk for CHD ≤20%	<130	<160
0 or 1 risk factor	<160	<190

[a]If triglyceride level is ≥200 mg/dL after LDL-C goal is reached, secondary goal for non-HDL-C (total cholesterol minus HDL-C) is 30 mg/dL higher than LDL-C goal.

Abbreviations: HDL-C, high-density lipoprotein cholesterol; LDL-C, low-density lipoprotein cholesterol; CHD, coronary heart disease.

Reprinted, by permission, from National Cholesterol Education Program, 2003, "Executive Summary of the third report of the Expert Panel on Detection, Evaluation and Treatment of High Blood Cholesterol in Adults (Adult Treatment Panel III)," *JAMA* 289(19): 2560-2572.

ATP III Classification of Serum Triglycerides

<150 mg/dL	Normal
150-199 mg/dL	Borderline high
200-499 mg/dL	High
≥500 mg/dL	Very high

Based on National Institute of Health, 2001, *National Cholesterol Education Program.*

Intervention Recommendations for Elevated Triglyceride Levels

If triglycerides are 200 to 499 mg/dL after LDL-C goal is reached, consider adding medication to reach non-HDL-C goal:

- Intensify therapy with LDL-C-lowering medication, or
- Add nicotinic acid or a fibrate to further lower VLDL.

If triglycerides are ≥500 mg/dL, first lower triglycerides to prevent pancreatitis:

- Very low-fat diet (<15% of calories from fat)
- Weight management and physical activity
- A fibrate or nicotinic acid

When triglycerides are <500 mg/dL, turn to LDL-lowering therapy.

Abbreviations: LDL-C, low-density lipoprotein cholesterol; HDL-C, high-density lipoprotein cholesterol.

Based on National Institute of Health, 2001, *National Cholesterol Education Program*.

Treatment of Low HDL-C (<40 mg/dL)

First, reach LDL-C goal:

- Increase physical activity and intensify weight management.
- If triglycerides are 200 to 499 mg/dL, achieve non-HDL-C goal.
- If triglycerides are <200 mg/dL (isolated low HDL-C) in CHD or CHD equivalent, consider nicotinic acid or fibrate.

Abbreviations: LDL-C, low-density lipoprotein cholesterol; HDL-C, high-density lipoprotein cholesterol.

Based on National Institute of Health, 2001, *National Cholesterol Education Program*.

General Treatment Guidelines for the CHD Patient

The optimal LDL-C goal for patients with CHD or CHD risk equivalent is <100 mg/dL[1,14] or <70 mg/dL in people considered very high risk, such those with as with 3+ risk factors, poorly controlled risk factors, comorbidities, including vascular disease, diabetes, or metabolic syndrome.[1] Recommendations (figure 8.2) should be incorporated with pharmacologic therapy (figure 8.3). All patients with CVD should be on a statin if tolerated and followed closely to make sure the goal is attained. Additionally, the following treatments should be prescribed:

- Begin or intensify lifestyle and drug therapies to lower LDL-C.
- Initiate or intensify weight reduction and increased physical activity in persons with insulin resistance.

- Institute treatment of other lipid or nonlipid risk factors. If the patient has elevated triglycerides or low HDL-C, consider the use of nicotinic acid or fibric acid.
- Studies have shown that even if baseline LDL-C is <100 mg/dL, the patient with CHD will benefit from statin therapy as well as from controlling other lipid or nonlipid risk factors and treating insulin resistance if present.[1,2,4,14]

Pharmacologic Therapy

Details regarding pharmacologic therapy are beyond the scope of these guidelines and are covered comprehensively by the NCEP.[14] Pharmacologic therapy includes the use of one or more of the following drugs targeted to reduce LDL and triglycerides.

• HMG Co-A reductase inhibitors (statins). This class of drugs inhibits HMG Co-A reductase,

Figure 8.2   Model of Steps in Therapeutic Lifestyle Changes (TLC)

Visit 1	6 weeks	Visit 2	6 weeks	Visit 3	4 to 6 months	Follow-up visits
Begin TLC		Evaluate LDL-C. If it exceeds goal, intensify TLC.		Evaluate LDL-C. If it exceeds goal, consider adding lipid-lowering drug.		Monitor adherence to TLC.
Reduce intake of saturated fat and cholesterol; increase or begin physical activity; dietitian referral.		Reduce intake of saturated fat and cholesterol. Add dietary fiber and stanols and sterols; dietitian referral.		Initiate medication drug for metabolic syndrome, weight reduction, physical activity; dietitian referral.		

Abbreviation: LDL-C, low-density lipoprotein cholesterol.

Based on National Institute of Health, 2001, *National Cholesterol Education Program*.

Figure 8.3   Model of Progression of Drug Therapy in Primary Prevention

Visit 1	6 weeks	Visit 2	6 weeks	Visit 3	4 to 6 months	Follow-up visits
Evaluate LDL-C. Initiate LDL-C-lowering medication.		Evaluate LDL-C. If it exceeds goal, intensify LDL-C therapy.		Evaluate LDL-C. If it exceeds goal, intensify LDL-C therapy, refer to specialist.		Monitor response and adherence to TLC.
Start statin, bile acid sequestrants, nicotinic acid.		Consider change in medication dose or adding new agent.		If LDL-C goal is achieved, consider medication for other lipid abnormalities and risk factors.		

Abbreviations: LDL-C, low-density lipoprotein cholesterol; TLC, therapeutic lifestyle change.

Adapted, by permission, from National Cholesterol Education Program, 2003, "Executive Summary of the third report of the Expert Panel on Detection, Evaluation and Treatment of High Blood Cholesterol in Adults (Adult Treatment Panel III)," *JAMA* 289(19): 2560-2572.

the rate-limiting enzyme in cholesterol biosynthesis, causing upregulation of LDL-C receptors, decreasing LDL-C and VLDL-C, and increasing HDL-C. Aside from their effects on lipids, clinical investigations have revealed that statins can exert a number of cardioprotective and anti-inflammatory actions through upregulation of endothelial function and other physiological and biochemical effects.[31-37] These drugs are generally well tolerated but rarely can cause liver enzyme elevation

and creatine phosphokinase (CPK) elevation with myositis. They may also occasionally cause skin rash, stomach upset, and headaches. Additionally, statins should be used cautiously in persons with significant comorbidities who are on multiple medications. This class of drugs is considered first-line therapy in CAD patients.[1-6]

• Bile acid sequestrants. These drugs are ion exchange resins that bind bile acids; increase conversion of liver cholesterol to bile acids; and upregulate LDL receptors in the liver, thus decreasing plasma LDL by about 20%. Furthermore, because the resins are nonsystemic, this class of medications may be very useful in younger patients with CAD or at very high risk of developing CAD who face a lifetime of lipid-lowering therapies. Side effects include bloating and constipation; elevation of triglycerides; and interference with absorption of digoxin, tetracycline, D-thyroxine, phenylbutazone, coumadin, and potentially other medications.

• Niacin. Niacin decreases VLDL-C and LDL-C production and raises HDL-C. Additionally, while research continues to evaluate the efficacy of lowering lipoprotein(a) [Lp(a)] in persons with dyslipidemias, fibric acid derivatives, exercise, and alcohol-extracted soy protein have been shown to effectively lower Lp(a). Side effects include flushing; gastric irritation; and elevations in uric acid, glucose, and liver enzymes in patients. One aspirin per day minimizes flushing and can be used initially. Niacin should be avoided in patients with liver disease, a history of peptic ulcer, or diabetes. Although niacin is available over the counter, patients should take it under the direction of a physician.

• Fibrates. This class of medications is very effective in lowering triglycerides and VLDL-C by decreasing the production and enhancing the breakdown of triglycerides. They usually lower LDL-C, increase HDL-C by modest amounts, and are generally well tolerated; but muscle cramps and intermittent indigestion can occur, as well as cholesterol gallstone formation and myopathy. The drug may potentiate the action of coumadin. Fibrates should be used cautiously in patients with renal insufficiency; and, depending on the severity of the chronic renal disease, the dose of the fibrate may need to be lowered or may be contraindicated.[1] When used in combination with statin therapy, there is an increased risk for abnormal liver function tests and myopathies.

• Cholesterol absorption inhibitors. This class of drugs selectively inhibits dietary and biliary cholesterol absorption at the brush border of the intestine and does not affect absorption of triglycerides or fat-soluble vitamins. These drugs lower LDL-C and are most effective when used with a statin, allowing for an additional LDL-C decrease of 17% to 18%. They also lower triglycerides and increase HDL-C slightly. Side effects can include gastrointestinal distress, an increase in muscle soreness, and a small increase in hepatic enzymes (~1%) when used in combination with statin therapy.

• Omega 3-acid ethyl esters. n-3 fatty acids in higher doses lower triglycerides and can be an alternative to fibrates or niacin for treatment of hypertriglycerides. They are recommended for triglycerides >500 mg/dL.

Long-Term Follow-Up

Achieving long-term control of dyslipidemia requires application of the same interest and attention on the part of both the patient and the CR/SP staff to long-term management issues as to initial evaluation and treatment. The effective use of adherence-enhancing techniques combined with the effort and participation of a variety of skilled health care professionals, as found in the secondary prevention team, has the greatest potential for helping the patient achieve an optimal lipid profile. Specific strategies include the following:

• Teaching the patient how adhere to the treatment regimen

• Helping the patient identify ways to remember doses

• Teaching patients to identify, anticipate, and manage side effects

• Providing updates on the effectiveness of treatment

• Ensuring mechanisms for patients to contact the health care professionals who supervise the lipid management

According to the NCEP, follow-up of lipid measurements should include these elements:

• Reassessment at 4 to 6 weeks and again at 3 months if the patient has not reached the goal

• Follow-up at 8- to 12-week intervals through week 52 once the patient has reached the goal

• Follow-up with the patient at 4- to 6-month intervals after the goal has been maintained for 1 year (LDL-C should be measured once a year; at other times, total cholesterol measures will suffice)

Hypertension

One in three U.S. adults has hypertension, and two-thirds of persons 65 years of age or older are hypertensive.[1] Hypertension is more common in men than in women until age 55, when the prevalence in women becomes greater that that of men. Hypertension is more common among black Americans and, not surprisingly, is highly prevalent among people with initial MI (69%) or stroke (77%) and congestive heart failure (74%). Importantly, hypertension has been reported to be present in 48% of patients enrolled in CR/SP programs (guideline 8.3).[2] The CR/SP staff can effectively work with the primary physician or health provider to evaluate and manage this important modifiable risk factor. Table 8.4 lists the Joint National Committee VII (JNC-VII) classification of BP for adults.[3,4]

A pertinent medical history includes many items recommended for the initial evaluation of patients entering the secondary prevention program (see chapter 6), with a particular focus on dietary sodium intake, excessive alcohol and caloric consumption, and low levels of physical activity. The goals of this evaluation are to determine cardiovascular risk status and the presence (and extent) of target organ damage, as well as to determine if there are secondary causes that may be amenable to treatment. The initial physi-

Guideline 8.3   Diagnosis of Hypertension

- Hypertension should not be diagnosed on the basis of a single measurement.

- Initial elevated readings should be confirmed on at least two subsequent visits over a period of 1 to several weeks (unless systolic BP is >180 mmHg or diastolic BP is >110 mmHg); average levels of systolic BP ≥140 mmHg or diastolic BP ≥90 mmHg are required for diagnosis.

Table 8.4 Classification and Management of Blood Pressure for Adults Aged 18 Years or Older

	MANAGEMENT				INITIAL DRUG THERAPY	
BP classification	SBP, mm Hg*		DBP, mmHg*	Lifestyle modification	Without compelling indication	With compelling indications
Normal Prehypertension	<120 120-139	and or	<80 80-89	Encourage Yes	No antihypertensive drug indicated	Drug(s) for the compelling indications†
Stage 1 hypertension	140-159	or	90-99	Yes	Thaizide-type diuretics for most; may consider ACE inhibitor, ARB, BB, CCB, or combination	Drug(s) for the compelling indications Other antihypertensive drugs (diuretics, ACE inhibitor, ARB, BB, CCB) as needed
Stage 2 hypertension	≥160	or	≥100	Yes	Two-drug combination for most (usually thiazide-type diuretic and ACE or ARB or BB or CCB) ‡	Drug(s) for the compelling indications Other antihypertensive drugs (diuretics, ACE inhibitor, ARB, BB, CCB) as needed

SBP, systolic blood pressure; DBP, diastolic blood pressure; ACE, angiotensin-converting enzyme; ARB = angiotensin-receptor blocker; BB = beta-blocker; CCB = calcium channel blocker.

*Treatment determined by highest BP category.

†Treat patients with chronic kidney disease or diabetes to BP goal of <130/80 mmHg.

‡Initial combined therapy should be used cautiously in those at risk for orthostatic hypotension.

Reprinted, by permission, from National Cholesterol Education Program, 2003, "Executive Summary of the third report of the Expert Panel on Detection, Evaluation and Treatment of High Blood Cholesterol in Adults (Adult Treatment Panel III)," *JAMA* 289(19): 2560-2572.

cal examination should include two or more BP measurements taken 2 min apart after 5 min of rest with the patient seated and legs uncrossed, followed by verification in the contralateral arm (if values are different, the higher value should be used). The following are additional important aspects of the physical examination related to the evaluation of hypertension that an appropriately trained health care professional should perform and document:

- Examination of the eye, including fundoscopy, for presence of retinopathy or hemorrhage
- Examination of the neck for carotid bruits, distended jugular veins, or an enlarged thyroid gland
- Examination of the heart for increased rate or size, precordial heave, clicks, murmurs, arrhythmias, and third (S3) and fourth (S4) heart sounds
- Examination of the abdomen for bruits, enlarged kidneys, masses, and abnormal aortic pulsation
- Examination of the extremities for diminished or absent peripheral arterial pulsations or the presence of bruits or edema
- A complete neurologic assessment

Initial laboratory evaluation should be performed routinely before hypertension therapy is started. This includes urinalysis; a complete blood count; a fasting blood glucose (if possible); potassium, calcium, creatinine, and uric acid; and lipid profile. A 12-lead electrocardiogram should be used to identify the presence of left ventricular hypertrophy. Based on this evaluation, appropriate and tailored therapy can be started.

Expert opinion supports exercise and education as important components of a multifactorial intervention that should also include counseling, behavioral intervention, and pharmacologic approaches to the management of hypertension (guideline 8.4).[3]

Secondary prevention programs can greatly assist the primary care physician in the treatment and close monitoring of patients with hypertension. Lifestyle modifications are the foundation for treatment of hypertension (see table 8.5). Lifestyle modifications are effective in lowering BP for many people who follow them and can also reduce other risk factors for premature CVD, although their capacity to reduce morbidity or mortality has not been conclusively documented. Lifestyle modifications, if properly used, offer multiple benefits at little cost and with minimal risk. Even when not adequate in themselves to control hypertension, they may reduce the number and doses of antihypertensive medications needed to manage the condition.

The JNC-VII underscores the importance of lifestyle modifications, which include weight reduction (if the patient is overweight), increased physical activity, and moderation of diet, that can be used as definitive or adjunctive therapy for hypertension. Dietary modifications should include several components: (1) individualize diet to achieve and maintain a healthy body weight (see "Overweight and Obesity" section later in the chapter); (2) limit alcohol intake to less than 1 oz ethanol a day; (3) limit sodium intake; (4) emphasize intake of fruits, vegetables, and low-fat dairy products; and (5) reduce saturated fat and trans fat in general.[5] The AHA recommends that all American adults limit their sodium intake to 1500 mg/day.[6] However, the 2010 Dietary

---

Guideline 8.4 Hypertension Intervention

- CR/SP professionals should initiate intervention in all patients with BP ≥140 mmHg systolic or higher or ≥90 mmHg diastolic. This is done with a documented program of weight management, physical activity, alcohol moderation, and moderate sodium restriction.

- Antihypertensive medications that are individualized to other patient requirements and characteristics (i.e., age, risk factors, comorbidities, race, need for drugs with specific benefits) should be added if BP is ≥140 mmHg systolic or ≥90 mmHg diastolic in 3 months or if initial BP is ≥180 mmHg systolic or ≥110 mmHg diastolic.[1,2]

Table 8.5 Lifestyle Modifications to Manage Hypertension*

Modification	Recommendation	Approximate SBP reduction, range
Weight reduction	Maintain normal body weight (BMI = 18.5-24.9).	5 to 20 mmHg/10 kg weight loss
Adoption of DASH eating plan	Consume a diet rich in fruits, vegetables, and low-fat dairy products with a reduced content of saturated and total fat.	8 to 14 mmHg
Dietary sodium reduction	Reduce dietary sodium intake to no more than 100 mEq/L (2.4 g sodium or 8 g sodium chloride).	2 to 8 mmHg
Physical activity	Engage in regular aerobic physical activity such as brisk walking (at least 30 min/day, most days of the week).	4 to 9 mmHg
Moderation of alcohol consumption	Limit consumption to no more than two drinks per day (1 oz or 30 mL ethanol; e.g., 24 oz beer, 10 oz wine, or 3 oz 80-proof whiskey) in most men and no more than one drink per day in women and lightweight persons.	2 to 4 mmHg

*For overall cardiovascular risk reduction, stop smoking. The effects of implementing these modifications are dose and time dependent and could be higher for some individuals. SBP, systolic blood pressure; BMI, body mass index calculated as weight in kilograms divided by the square of height in meters; DASH = Dietary Approaches to Stop Hypertension.

Reprinted, by permission, from National Cholesterol Education Program, 2003, "Executive Summary of the third report of the Expert Panel on Detection, Evaluation and Treatment of High Blood Cholesterol in Adults (Adult Treatment Panel III)," *JAMA* 289(19): 2560-2572.

Guidelines for Americans recommend a sodium restriction of 1500 mg/day or 2300 mg/day, depending on age and individual characteristics.[7] The 1500 mg/day recommendation applies to groups known to be salt sensitive. These include African Americans; individuals with existing hypertension, diabetes mellitus, or chronic kidney disease; and adults over the age of 50. For all others, the dietary guidelines have established a sodium restriction of 2300 mg/day. The DASH diet (Dietary Approaches to Stop Hypertension) has been shown to reduce BP in both hypertensive and nonhypertensive people, and particularly in African Americans.[8-10] The DASH diet emphasizes five to nine servings of fruits and vegetables a day and two to four servings of low-fat dairy products a day. The plan includes whole grains, fish, poultry, and nuts and is low in fat, red meat, sweets, and sugar-containing beverages. This diet is also rich in potassium, magnesium, and calcium. Increased intake of these minerals, particularly potassium, has been associated with lower BP.[11] In addition to these recommendations, stress, which is associated with increased adrenaline and norepinephrine levels, must also be managed.

As mentioned previously, hypertension is very common in older patients. In addition, isolated systolic hypertension also frequently occurs in older persons (systolic BP consistently 140 mmHg or greater and diastolic pressure less than 90 mmHg). The goal of treatment in older patients should be the same as that in younger patients (<140/90 mmHg). The starting dose for older patients should be less than that used for younger patients, but frequently patients are prescribed one or more antihypertensive medications despite lifestyle modifications. Unfortunately, these medications may increase the occurrence of orthostatic hypotension, potentially leading to falls, which are already more common in older persons; thus blood pressure should always be measured in both the standing and seated positions.

Pharmacologic therapy should be started based on several factors, including these:

- The severity of BP elevation
- The presence of major risk factors (smoking, abnormal lipids, diabetes, age >60 years, male gender, postmenopausal women, a family history of premature CVD)
- Evidence of target end organ damage (heart, kidneys, cerebrovascular system, peripheral arterial disease, retinopathy) and clinical CVD
- The presence of comorbidities
- The side effects and costs of the medication and potential drug interactions

Table 8.5 also outlines lifestyle treatment strategies appropriate for individual risk factors. Initial monotherapy is usually successful in patients with Stage 1 hypertension. In the patient whose blood pressure readings are greater than 20/10 mmHg over goal (Stage 2 hypertension), a single drug will likely be ineffective, and combination therapy is recommended. Thiazide-type diuretics are indicated as initial therapy for most patients with hypertension, either alone or combined with one or more drugs in other classes, including ACE inhibitors, angiotensin-receptor blockers, beta-blockers, or calcium channel blockers. These medications are equally effective in reducing blood pressure.[3]

Hypertension is the most common major risk factor for CHD.[12] In a patient with documented coronary artery disease, there are well-established benefits for the use of beta-blockers to decrease recurrent ischemic events.[3] This class of medications may also be used for the treatment of hypertension in this population. ACE inhibitors are also commonly used in this patient population. In patients who have had a MI, this class of medications is used to help promote favorable left ventricular remodeling. With a combination of ACE inhibitors and beta-blockers, patients with CHD should be aggressively treated to goal.

Among patients with diabetes or chronic kidney disease, the BP goal should be below 130/80 mmHg. Combinations of the various classes of drugs are usually required to achieve this goal. ACE inhibitors are preferred for patients with diabetic nephropathy. In patients who cannot tolerate ACE inhibitors, angiotensin-receptor blockers (ARBs) are the preferred agents.

Poor adherence to long-term treatment, encompassing both lifestyle modifications and pharmacologic therapy, has been identified as the major reason for inadequate control of high BP. CR/SP programs can be particularly effective in providing education and support aimed at improving patient understanding of specific therapies and treatment goals, correcting misconceptions, adjusting the therapeutic interventions to patient lifestyles, and enhancing family or other social support. Thus, patients may achieve long-term adherence to treatment schedules and BP control.

Physical Inactivity

Recent reports consistently indicate that adult Americans do not engage in enough physical activity (PA) to favorably affect their health.[1,2] National statistics indicate that less than 50% of adults (47% of women and 49% of men) meet the minimal PA recommendations widely publicized by the federal government and other prominent health organizations.[2,3] This is particularly concerning since numerous observational studies and consensus statements[2-6] confirm that a sedentary lifestyle contributes to significantly increased risk for CVD. In addition, both low cardiorespiratory fitness (CRF)[7,8] and accumulated sitting time[9,10] have been associated with increased risk for CVD and all-cause mortality. Based on the accumulated body of evidence, it is clear that the relationships between CVD risk and levels of PA and CRF are inverse, graded, and most importantly, modifiable.[11] Furthermore, the evidence suggests that the risk associated with low PA or CRF is relevant to both primary and secondary prevention of CVD.[5,7,12] Therefore, allied health professionals should view increasing PA and CRF, as well as reducing overall sitting time, as important goals within CVD risk reduction programs. The following sections provide information related to

---

Guideline 8.5   Physical Activity Versus Exercise

Although the terms *physical activity* and *exercise* are often used interchangeably, they are not considered synonymous within the chronic disease risk factor literature or in public health statements. To delineate the risks and benefits associated with a sedentary lifestyle, operational definitions should be recognized.[13]

- *Physical activity* is any bodily movement produced by the contraction of skeletal muscle that increases energy expenditure above basal metabolic rate.

- *Exercise* is a subcategory of PA, that is, planned, structured, and repetitive bodily movement done to improve or maintain one or more components of physical fitness.

definitions, risks, assessment, and recommendations for PA and CRF.

Physical activity recommendations in recent public health statements[1-3,14] may be used to define a PA threshold below which one would be considered habitually *inactive*. There is general consensus that accumulating <150 min/week of moderate-intensity PA (or <60 to 75 min of vigorous-intensity PA) identifies an inactive lifestyle. However, at least two reports[9,10] have focused on physical inactivity from a different perspective, that is, time spent seated each day. Both of these studies reported that daily sitting time, independent of leisure-time PA, predicted CVD mortality. Therefore, operational definitions for physical *inactivity* will continue to evolve as better assessments of leisure-time PA become available and are deployed within population-based studies of CVD risk (see later section on physical activity assessment).

Unlike PA and exercise, which are *behaviors*, CRF is a *capacity*. Cardiorespiratory fitness is typically directly measured or predicted from the results of an exercise tolerance test. The most common definition of CRF is the capacity of the body to consume oxygen, often referred to as the peak oxygen uptake or $\dot{V}O_2$peak. Physical activity, exercise, and CRF are interrelated in that a chronic increase (or decrease) in PA and exercise often leads to a similar change in CRF.

Relative Risk of Physical Inactivity

Prospective observational studies have typically shown that the relative risk for CVD associated with inactivity is approximately two times greater when the least active individuals are compared to the most physically active within a study cohort.[6] This relative risk is similar to that reported for many of the other risk factors reviewed in this chapter. Furthermore, in studies that analyzed disease risk across multiple ordinal categories of reported PA (e.g., low, moderate, high), the risk was graded, indicating that CVD risk decreases across categories of PA from low through moderate to high. This is often referred to as a *dose–response* relationship and has been summarized in public health messages in the following way[6]:

- Important health benefits (CVD risk reduction) can be obtained by including a moderate amount of PA on most, if not all, days of the week.

- Additional health benefits (further CVD risk reduction) result from greater amounts of PA.

Given the combination of high prevalence of inactivity in the population (>50%) and the approximate twofold relative risk for CVD, interventions that target inactive lifestyles have significant potential to lower the overall CVD risk burden within society. Furthermore, PA is a unique risk trait in that it has both a direct and an indirect impact on CVD risk. While numerous studies have shown that the CVD risk associated with inactivity is independent of other CVD risk factors such as smoking, hypertension, and hypercholesterolemia, well-controlled clinical trials of exercise training have consistently shown that habitual PA favorably alters other CVD risk factors such as hypertension, hypercholesterolemia, obesity, and type 2 diabetes mellitus.[3] Therefore, the importance of targeting physical inactivity in risk reduction programs goes well beyond the independent influence that a more active lifestyle has on lowering CVD risk.

As already mentioned, observational reports have focused on inactivity from a different perspective, that is, the amount of time per day spent sitting. Katzmarzyk and colleagues[9] reported a progressively higher risk of CVD mortality across increasing hours of sitting time in 17,013 Canadians aged 18 to 90 years. Their findings were also independent of self-reported leisure-time PA. Stamatakis and coauthors[10] followed 4,512 Scottish men for about 5 years and quantified the amount of moderate- to vigorous-intensity PA at baseline as well as the television/screen viewing time per day. After adjustment for traditional CVD risk factors, including leisure-time PA, incident CVD was twice as likely among men who reported 4 or more h of screen time per day compared to those reporting less than 2 h/day. While these recent reports confirm the lower CVD risk associated with moderate to vigorous PA, they extend our understanding of the unique risks associated with significant amounts of time spent seated. In other words, even people who adopt a more active lifestyle can likely further reduce their risk by limiting the amount of time they spend watching television or engaging in other "screen-based" activities that typically coincide with sitting for prolonged periods.

Relative Risk of Low Cardiorespiratory Fitness

Numerous prospective studies have shown that lower CRF predicts all-cause and CVD morbidity and mortality independent of other CVD risk factors.[6,7] This finding is consistent for both primary and secondary prevention, as well as across studies that employed varying measures of CRF (i.e., measured vs. predicted $\dot{V}O_2$max, treadmill vs. cycle ergometer modalities, and maximal vs. submaximal test end point). Myers and colleagues[7] reported that each 1 metabolic equivalent (MET) increase in CRF was associated with a 12% reduction in mortality. Blair and coauthors[15] reported that modest improvements in CRF lowered mortality risk. Therefore, while an optimal CRF has not been defined, the focus within risk reduction programs has been to improve fitness through habitual PA, including regular endurance exercise training.

Assessment of Physical Activity

It is important to make an accurate assessment of the presence of all cardiovascular risk factors, including physical inactivity. As already stated, an individual is considered to be physically inactive without *sufficient PA,* defined as meeting the recommendations from the 2008 Physical Activity Guidelines for Americans.[2] As with smoking status, the length of time (e.g., months, years) a patient has been inactive should also be assessed. Although there is no established standard, a pattern of inactivity ≥3 months is often used to establish a sedentary lifestyle.

Physical activity is multidimensional and is a complex behavior to measure.[16] To determine whether an individual is obtaining sufficient PA, the components of PA (duration, frequency, and intensity) need to be assessed. One challenge in PA assessment involves measuring duration, since activity can be accumulated throughout a day in bouts of at least 10 min per session. Another challenge is determining the intensity of PA, which can be classified as either relative to the individual (i.e., % of maximal capacity) or absolute (moderate and vigorous intensity are operationally defined as 3-5.9 METs and ≥6 METs, respectively). Inappropriate or crude measures of PA are likely to yield misleading results.[16] Thus, it is important for CR/SP staff to carefully consider the methods they use to assess PA.

The two most common methods used to assess PA status are self-report questionnaires (subjective) and use of PA monitors (objective). The advantage of questionnaires is that they are inexpensive and require little time to administer. However, subjective methods are limited by the ability of the respondent to accurately remember PA behaviors and to accurately classify the intensity of PA. PA monitors can accurately assess (or measure) ambulatory movement, including intensity. The limitations to this objective approach are that nonambulatory PA is not captured and that purchasing monitors and replacing lost or damaged monitors entail an expense.

The International Physical Activity Questionnaire that follows (IPAQ, www.ipaq.ki.se) is suitable for standardizing the PA assessment in CR/SP. The instrument quantifies PA duration, frequency, and intensity. Moreover, the type of activities can be customized to those most common in the population being assessed. The IPAQ also provides information on sitting time, which as already discussed may be useful in determining an overall CVD risk profile.[9] It is easy to compare time and frequency reported for moderate and vigorous PA on the IPAQ to the recommended standards of >150 min/week (moderate) or >75 min/week (vigorous). The IPAQ can also provide a classification into one of three levels (see "IPAQ Classification Categories") and uses the MET · min^{-1} variable mentioned in the 2008 Physical Activity Guidelines for Americans to help quantify the total volume of PA.[2]

Although there are many different types of PA monitors, accelerometers have the most utility in CR/SP because they capture PA duration, frequency, and intensity and can also quantify duration of inactivity. Patients require standardized instructions for use of the PA monitor. The typical assessment period is 7 days. Criteria for acceptable data from a PA monitor include that it is worn a minimum of 12 h/day (note that time periods of >1 h with no activity are excluded) and that a minimum of 4 complete days are recorded. Accelerometer data can be stored on a computer and processed by device-specific software. A self-report log of patient activity can be very helpful in assessing data from the PA monitor. Examples of data reports from accelerometers which can be used to determine PA behavior are shown in figures 8.4 and 8.5 . The presentation of the daily PA and inactivity time profiles can be quite useful for helping patients understand their PA habits.

International Physical Activity Questionnaire

We are interested in finding out about the kinds of physical activities that people do as part of their everyday lives. The questions will ask you about the time you spent being physically active in the **last 7 days**. Please answer each question even if you do not consider yourself to be an active person. Please think about the activities you do at work, as part of your house and yard work, to get from place to place, and in your spare time for recreation, exercise, or sport.

Think about all the **vigorous** activities that you did in the **last 7 days**. **Vigorous** physical activities refer to activities that take hard physical effort and make you breathe much harder than normal. Think *only* about those physical activities that you did for at least 10 minutes at a time.

1. During the **last 7 days**, on how many days did you do **vigorous** physical activities like heavy lifting, digging, aerobics, or fast bicycling?

   _____ **days per week**

   ☐ No vigorous physical activities ⟶ *Skip to question 3*

2. How much time did you usually spend doing **vigorous** physical activities on one of those days?

   _____ **hours per day**
   _____ **minutes per day**

Think about all the **moderate** activities that you did in the **last 7 days**. **Moderate** activities refer to activities that take moderate physical effort and make you breathe somewhat harder than normal. Think only about those physical activities that you did for at least 10 minutes at a time.

3. During the **last 7 days**, on how many days did you do **moderate** physical activities like carrying light loads, bicycling at a regular pace, or doubles tennis? Do not include walking.

   _____ **days per week**

   ☐ No moderate physical activities ⟶ *Skip to question 5*

4. How much time did you usually spend doing **moderate** physical activities on one of those days?

   _____ **hours per day**
   _____ **minutes per day**

Think about the time you spent **walking** in the **last 7 days**. This includes at work and at home, walking to travel from place to place, and any other walking that you might do solely for recreation, sport, exercise, or leisure.

5. During the **last 7 days**, on how many days did you **walk** for at least 10 minutes at a time?

   _____ **days per week**

   ☐ No walking ⟶ *Skip to question 7*

6. How much time did you usually spend **walking** on one of those days?

   _____ **hours per day**
   _____ **minutes per day**

The last question is about the time you spent **sitting** on weekdays during the **last 7 days**. Include time spent at work, at home, while doing course work and during leisure time. This may include time spent sitting at a desk, visiting friends, reading, or sitting or lying down to watch television.

7. During the **last 7 days**, how much time did you spend **sitting** on a **week day**?

   _____ **hours per day**
   _____ **minutes per day**

More Information

More detailed information on the IPAQ process and the research methods used in the development of IPAQ instruments is available at www.ipaq.ki.se and in ML Booth, "Assessment of Physical Activity: An International Perspective," *Research Quarterly for Exercise and Sport,* 2000;71:s114-120. Other scientific publications and presentations on the use of IPAQ are summarized on the website.

IPAQ Classification Categories

Low (Category 1)

- Not active enough to meet criteria for Categories 2 or 3

Moderate (Category 2)

- ≥3 days of vigorous activity of ≥20 min/day **OR**
- ≥5 days of moderate activity or walking of ≥30 min/day **OR**
- ≥5 days of any combination of walking, moderate, or vigorous activity achieving a
- minimum of 600 MET·min/week

High (Category 3)

- Vigorous activity ≥3 days/week achieving at least 1,500 MET·min/week **OR**
- ≥7 days of any combination of walking, moderate, or vigorous activity achieving a minimum of 3,000 MET·min/week

Abbreviations: IPAQ, International Physical Activity Questionnaire; MET, metabolic equivalent.

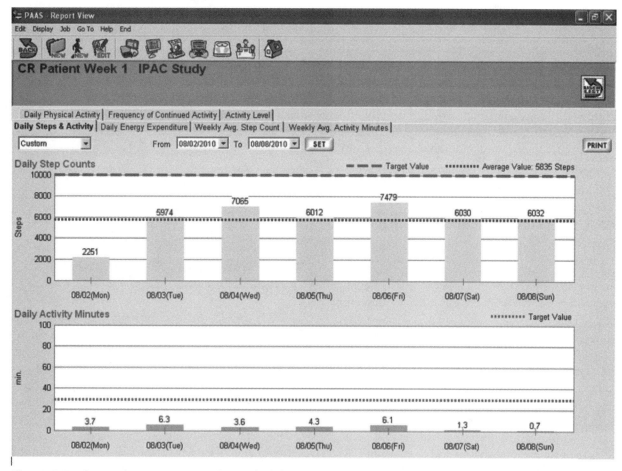

Figure 8.4 An accelerometer report from a baseline PA assessment at the beginning of a maintenance CR/SP. The results show the patient is insufficiently active (averaging only 5,835 steps a day and accumulating only 26 min/week of moderate to vigorous PA).

Courtesy of Ball State University Clinical Exercise Physiology Program.

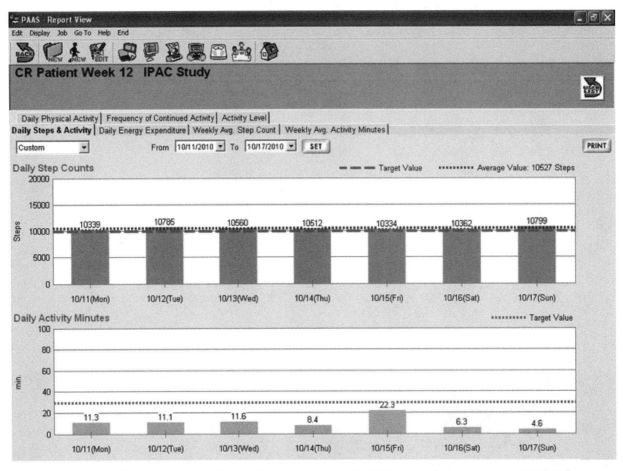

Figure 8.5 An accelerometer report from a PA assessment at the 12th week of a maintenance CR/SP. The results show the patient has significantly increased her PA level (now averaging 10,527 steps a day and now accumulating ≈75 min/week of moderate to vigorous PA).

Courtesy of Ball State University Clinical Exercise Physiology Program.

Assessment of Cardiorespiratory Fitness

As mentioned previously, CRF is typically assessed using an exercise tolerance test. Because exercise is a cornerstone of CR/SP, it is important to get a baseline assessment in order to most effectively "dose" the exercise prescription as well as to identify contraindications or potential limitations to exercise training[17] (see "Contraindications for Exercise" in chapter 6). Furthermore, assessment of CRF with sign- or symptom-limited exercise testing before and after an exercise intervention can yield important objective information related to appropriate exercise dose and changes in CRF. However, exercise testing data may not always be available, thus the need for assessing functional status of patients using tools described previously.

Recommendations for the use of exercise testing have been published.[17-20]

Recommendations for Physical Activity and Exercise

CR/SP should provide patients with knowledge and skills needed to enhance the adoption or resumption of an optimal level of PA. To this end, programs should give patients recommendations for both structured exercise training and leisure-time PA. It is generally accepted that the overall goal should be to increase habitual PA to a level that promotes health and reduces chronic disease risk. The goal of exercise training should be to increase CRF. Guideline 8.6 provides key variables that should be considered in preparation for the development of the exercise prescription.

Guideline 8.6 Considerations for the Prescription of Exercise and Physical Activity

To reduce the risk associated with exercise and to individualize the exercise prescription, CR/SP professionals must consider:

Safety Factors

- Clinical history
- Risk associated with CVD progression or instability and exercise participation
- Degree of left ventricular impairment
- Ischemic and angina thresholds
- Cognitive or psychological impairment

Associated Factors

- Vocational or avocational requirements
- Orthopedic limitations
- Previous and current activities
- Personal health and fitness goals

Other Noncardiac Diagnosis Considerations

This section presents recommendations for both structured exercise training and leisure-time PA.

An important initial consideration in exercise planning is safety. While most patients can engage in exercise without incurring undue risks, appropriate risk stratification should be performed. Safety and risk stratification are discussed in detail in chapter 6. Recommendations for supervision and ECG monitoring can be found in chapter 7. See tables 8.6 and 8.7 for basic exercise prescription information. A model for risk stratification of cardiovascular events is outlined in "Stratification of Risk for Cardiac Events During Exercise Participation" in chapter 7.[21] After risk stratification, recommendations for supervision, ECG monitoring and prescribed intensity and duration of exercise training can be made (see Recommendations for Intensity of Supervision and Monitoring Related to Risk of Exercise Participation).[21]

Comprehensive, evidence-based recommendations for structured exercise training in CR/SP are available from several prominent organizations[2,19,20,22] and are only summarized here. A comprehensive exercise program includes cardiorespiratory, musculoskeletal, and flexibility components. Specific elements for each component are summarized in tables 8.6 through 8.9 and include guidelines for intensity, duration (i.e., time), frequency, and type of exercise for training. Each of the elements should be pre-scribed relative to one another and in a way that effectively addresses predefined training goals (e.g., increased aerobic or musculoskeletal fitness, weight reduction, control of blood glucose, resumption of occupation).

Cardiorespiratory Endurance Training

Cardiorespiratory endurance (CRE) training should be the foundation of most exercise routines for adults with or at risk for CVD. This type of exercise training is the most effective way to increase CRF. Elements of an exercise prescription for CRE are presented in table 8.6. The relative training intensity may vary between 40% and 80% of maximal heart rate reserve or metabolic reserve ($\dot{V}O_2R$). Initial programs should focus on the lower part of the intensity range, with progression to higher intensities as patients adapt to the program. Ratings of perceived exertion are considered adjunctive to heart rate (HR) monitoring, but may become more important as a subjective intensity guide as patients gain experience with exercise training and learn how to use the scale. Exercise training duration varies as a function of the overall energy expenditure goals of the patient. Twenty continuous minutes of exercise per session is commonly recommended as a minimum within structured programs, although some patients follow an intermittent (i.e., interval) exercise regimen. Furthermore, some patients may need to accumulate shorter bouts (e.g., multiple 10 min bouts) throughout the day due to comorbidities or lifestyle factors. Ideally, patients should be active

Table 8.6 Components of the Exercise Prescription for Cardiorespiratory Endurance for Cardiac Patients Cleared for Participation

Component	Recommendation

Intensity	• 40% to 80% of Max HR or $\dot{V}O_2$ reserve or $\dot{V}O_2$ peak if maximal exercise data are available (see table 8.7 when exercise test data are not available)
	• RPE of 11 to 16 on 6 to 20 scale as adjunct to objective measure of HR
	• 10 bpm below HR associated with any of the following criteria:
	  • Onset of angina or other symptoms of cardiovascular insufficiency
	  • Plateau or ↓SBP; SBP >240 mmHg; DBP >110 mmHg
	  • >2 mm ST-depression, horizontal or downsloping
	  • Radionuclide evidence of reversible myocardial ischemia or echocardiographic evidence of moderate-to-severe wall motion abnormalities during exertion
	  • ↑frequent of ventricular dysrhythmias
	  • Other significant ECG disturbances (e.g., second- or third-degree AVB, atrial fibrillation, SVT, complex ventricular ectopy)
	  • Other signs or symptoms of exertional intolerance

Duration	• 20 to 60 min per session • Longer durations or multiple sessions accumulated throughout the day are recommended to enhance total energy expenditure for weight reduction
Frequency	• Ideally, most days of the week (4-7 days/week)
Type	• Rhythmic, larger muscle group activities (i.e., walking, cycling, stair climbing, elliptical trainers, and other arm or leg ergometers that allow controlled movement and consistent intensity

Abbreviations: HR, heart rate; $\dot{V}O_2R$, maximal oxygen uptake reserve; RPE, rating of perceived exertion; SBP, systolic blood pressure; DBP, diastolic blood pressure; ECG, electrocardiogram; AVB, atrioventricular block; SVT, supraventricular tachycardia.

Based on ACSM 2010.

Table 8.7 Components of Initial Exercise Prescription for Patients Without a Recent Symptom-Limited Exercise Tolerance Test

Component	Initial recommendation
Warm-up	• Stretching, low-level calisthenics • 5 to 10 min

Cardiorespiratory fitness	• Intensity (guides)
	  • 2 to 4 METs
	  • RPE 11 to 14
	• Duration
	  • 20 to 30 min
	• Frequency
	  • 3 to 5 days/week
	• Type
	  • Treadmill, leg or arm ergometer, stairs, ROM

Musculoskeletal fitness	• Resistance exercises: all major muscle groups • Appropriate for patients meeting criteria presented in Guideline 8.7 • See exercise components in table 8.10
Cool-down	• 5 to 10 min

Abbreviations: METs, metabolic equivalents; RPE, rating of perceived exertion; ROM, range of motion.

Based on ACSM 2010.

Table 8.8 Components of an Exercise Prescription for Muscular Strength and Endurance for Cardiac Patients Cleared for Participation

Component	Recommendation
Intensity	• Resistance that allows ~10 to 15 repetitions without significant fatigue • RPE of 11 to 13 on Borg 6 to 20 scale • Complete movement through as full a range of motion as possible, avoiding breath holding and straining (Valsalva maneuver) by exhaling during the exertion phase of the motion and inhaling during the recovery phase • Maintain a secure but not overly tight grip on the weight handles or bar to prevent an excessive BP response • RPP should not exceed that identified as threshold for CRE exercise
Volume	• Minimum of one set per exercise • May increase to two or three sets once accustomed to the regimen and, if greater gains are desired, ~8 to 10 different exercises using all major muscle groups of the upper and lower body: chest press, shoulder press, triceps extension, bicep curls, lat pull-down, lower back extension, abdominal crunch or curl-up, quadriceps extension, leg curls (hamstrings), and calf raise
Frequency	• 2 or 3 nonconsecutive days/week
Type	• Variable: free weights, weight machines, resistance bands, pulley weights, dumbbells, light wrist or ankle weights • Select equipment that is safe, effective, and accessible
Progression	• Training loads may be increased ~5% when the patient can comfortably achieve the upper limit of the prescribed repetition range

Abbreviations: RPE, rating of perceived exertion; BP, blood pressure; RPP, heart rate × systolic blood pressure product; CRE, cardiorespiratory endurance.

Adapted from ACSM 2010; Williams et al. 2007.

Table 8.9 Components of an Exercise Prescription for Musculoskeletal Flexibility

Component	Recommendation
Intensity	• Hold to a position of mild discomfort (not pain) • Exercises should be performed in a slow, controlled manner, with a gradual progression to greater ranges of motion
Duration	• Gradually increase to 30 s, then as tolerable to 90 s for each stretch, breathing normally • Three to five repetitions for each exercise
Frequency	• 2 or 3 nonconsecutive days/week
Type	• Static, with a major emphasis on the lower back and thigh regions

Adapted from ACSM 2010; Williams et al. 2007.

Guideline 8.7   Patient Selection Criteria for Participation in a Resistance Training Program[a]

• Minimum of 5 weeks after date of MI or cardiac surgery, including 4 weeks of consistent participation in a supervised CR/SP endurance training program

• Minimum of 3 weeks following transcatheter procedures (PCI, other), including 2 weeks of consistent participation in a supervised CR/SP endurance training program

• No evidence of the following conditions:

  ○ Acute congestive heart failure

  ○ Uncontrolled dysrhythmias

  ○ Severe valvular disease

  ○ Uncontrolled hypertension; patients with moderate hypertension (SBP >160 or DBP >100 mmHg) should be referred for appropriate management, although these values are not absolute contraindications for participation in a resistance training program

  ○ Unstable symptoms

[a]A resistance training program is defined here as one in which patients lift weights >50% one-repetition maximum (1RM). Elastic bands, 1 to 3 lb (.45 to 1.3 kg) hand weights, and light free weights may be used in a progressive fashion starting at outpatient program entry provided that no other contraindications exist.
Adapted from ACSM 2010; Williams et al. 2007.

most days of the week,[6] but structured programs are often designed with a frequency of three or four sessions per week. Note that longer exercise duration combined with increased training frequency is most effective for weight reduction programs,[23] since this serves to enhance the overall energy expenditure (see section titled The Energy Balance–Weight Loss Equation). Finally, common forms of CRE exercise are also listed in table 8.6.

Once the initial exercise prescription has been established, patients should progress gradually toward pre- or redefined program goals. There is no set format with respect to progression since many factors, including fitness level, motivation, and orthopedic limitations, influence the rate at

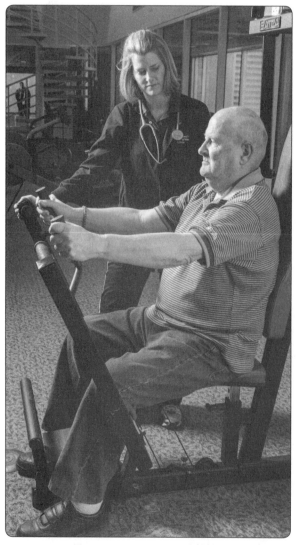

Cardiorespiratory endurance training should be the foundation of most exercise routines for adults with or at risk for CVD.

which a patient may progress. In general, it is prudent to change one variable and provide some time (a minimum of one exercise session) to assess the adaptation to the new level before progressing further. When time permits, increases in duration and frequency should precede increases in intensity. Modest increases in intensity, when appropriate, are likely to be tolerated and should be based on the observations of the staff and subjective responses of the patient, provided that the changes remain within the limits specified in the most recent evaluation.

A guiding principle should be progression of the total volume or dose of exercise such that the patient achieves desired energy expenditure thresholds within a 3- to 6-month period. The most appropriate volume of exercise depends on the individual CVD risk profile, training goals, and comorbidities (i.e., diabetes, hypertension, obesity, arthritis). An accumulating body of evidence affirms a dose–response relationship between the volume of PA and health outcomes.[2] It should be noted that thresholds of approximately 1,500 and 2,200 kcal/week have been associated with stable or regression of coronary artery lesions, respectively.[24] Unfortunately, multiple studies have documented that energy expenditure in structured CR/SP does not typically meet either of these thresholds.[25-29] Therefore, patients will likely need to engage in PA outside of the structured program to achieve the optimal levels of energy expenditure.

Few studies have supported the efficacy of structured exercise training as a singular strategy to normalize body weight and body composition in cardiac patients. This underscores the importance of multiple behavioral strategies in weight reduction programming for overweight patients. The volume or dose of exercise associated with the typical CR/SP training session may be the limiting factor. As mentioned previously, numerous studies have shown the weekly dose to be inadequate for weight or fat reduction. As an example, a typical exercise session for an outpatient with a peak functional capacity of 7 METs might be 30 min at a heart rate that would equate with about 4 METs (total metabolic equivalents). The following formula provides a method to estimate the caloric costs of the exercise session:

$$\text{Calories per minute} = [\text{METs} \times \text{Body weight in kilograms} \times 3.5]/200$$

It should be noted that the 4 MET value in this example includes the resting energy expenditure component (1 MET). Therefore, the *net* caloric cost of the exercise would be based on only 3 METs. If the hypothetical patient in this example weighed 100 kg (220 lb [91 kg]) and exercised 3 days per week for 30 min, the net caloric expenditure would be approximately 480 kcal/week (5.3 kcal/min × 30 min × 3 days/week). Though patients can clearly improve exercise tolerance with this regimen, the estimated caloric expenditure falls well short of contemporary recommendations for PA and in most cases would not be effective for weight or fat loss.[27] As an example, 40 min sessions, five times per week, would result in approximately 1,060 kcal/week. Thus, adjustments must be made with regard to frequency and duration of exercise to allow patients to achieve greater energy expenditures to enhance program outcomes. These adjustments must be made, however, with the caveat that although it is prudent to increase exercise volume progressively, staff must carefully consider the risk that a higher-volume program may lead to higher dropout rates. Therefore, overweight patients must be educated about the need to develop and maintain fitness as the core of their exercise regimen, with the additional volume of PA facilitating weight loss and other goals. Finally, it should be noted that as CRF improves, patients are able to exercise at a higher metabolic rate (i.e., kcal/min) at a given relative intensity (i.e., % maximal heart rate reserve). This allows patients to accumulate a greater caloric deficit over time.

Exercise Recommendations for Patients Without a Recent Exercise Test

For patients entering a secondary prevention program without an entry exercise test, staff should implement exercise programs conservatively with close patient surveillance. The medical director and referring clinician should advise on the upper safe training intensity. Initial exercise intensities can be determined according to the length of time from cardiac event, hospital discharge, and patient assessment (i.e., activities of daily living). At a minimum, monitoring should include electrocardiogram, signs and symptoms, BP, rating of perceived exertion (RPE), and signs of overexertion. A submaximal exercise evaluation with conservative end points can be helpful to determine exercise session parameters. Table 8.7 contains information regarding initial recommendations for patients entering a program without a recent exercise test.[20] A patient who responds normally to three to six exercise sessions as outlined in table 8.7 may gradually be progressed to an exercise prescription more consistent with that presented in the table. Progression should be individualized and based on a normal response to exercise along with the absence of abnormal signs or symptoms during and following exercise sessions.

A way to establish an initial exercise intensity is to begin with 2 to 4 METs and observe heart rate, blood pressure, and other physiological responses, including fatigue, at this workload. The RPE scale is helpful in determining how the patient tolerates the exercise load, with a suggested range of 11 to 13. However, such levels (i.e., METs, HR, or RPE) should be used with caution, as there is likely interindividual variation within each of the approaches.[20] Progression of the elements in table 8.7 should be based on the patient signs and symptoms, monitored response, and RPE. If the patient remains asymptomatic, exercise staff under the direction of the program medical or referring clinician may gradually increase exercise intensity to the upper safe limit as documented. Over time, stable patients typically progress to exercise plans similar to those presented in table 8.6. A study that compared training outcomes between patients with and without program entry exercise testing reported similar physiological improvements and no cardiovascular events.[30]

Physical Activity Outside of CR/SP

As noted earlier, many patients attending CR/SP do not achieve desired energy expenditure levels, especially when they attend only two or three sessions a week, typically expending <300 kcal per session.[31] Additionally, most cardiac patients perform even less PA on days they do not participate in CR/SP.[32-34] It is important to recognize that most patients who enroll in CR/SP have previously been insufficiently active. Thus, they face the challenge of changing another aspect of their lifestyle (along with possibly quitting smoking and changing their dietary habits to support weight loss, lipid or glucose control, blood pressure control, or anticoagulant control, for example) to become regularly physically active. Principles of behavior modification that apply to changing PA behavior are covered in chapter 3.

Although patients are routinely instructed to obtain more than 30 min of moderate-intensity PA on days they do not attend CR/SP, it is clear that many patients may need more support or alternative approaches to be more active. Having patients track and record their PA outside of CR/SP has been shown to be helpful in increasing PA.[35] Physical activity assessment instruments, similar to the one described earlier, can be used for this purpose. The ideal approach for tracking activity outside the CR/SP would be for patients to use a PA monitor to objectively record their PA habits. Pedometers are the lowest-cost option and have been shown to help individuals increase their PA.[36] Pedometer features range from only daily measures that need to be manually recorded to weekly or longer storage that can be downloaded to a computer. Although slightly more expensive, some pedometers also include an accelerometer mechanism, which allows patients to monitor both time spent in moderate- to vigorous-intensity PA and time spent inactive. Figures 8.4 and 8.5 show patient data from the first week of maintenance CR/SP and then again following 12 weeks of participation. This patient significantly increased PA measured as steps per day and moderate- to vigorous-activity minutes per day. Some of these PA monitors provide computer software to allow patients to store their data and produce various types of reports. CR/PP staff can review this information from patients to provide feedback and support to help them achieve their PA goals.

An alternative method that is simple and the least costly is for patients to complete a weekly log of their daily PA or use a weekly recall questionnaire like the IPAQ. These can be assessed by patients with support, as needed, by the CR/SP staff. Patients can be given clear goals (minimal: 150 min of moderate intensity per week; optimal: 300 min of moderate intensity per week) to be able to evaluate their PA status.

One additional approach is for patients to use the Internet to obtain resources and support for initially making the change to their lifestyle and then to maintain their regular PA behavior. Internet sites range from those that are free (e.g., www.supertracker.usda.gov), requiring patients to enter all their PA data, to those that are free with the purchase of a pedometer (e.g., www.thepedometercompany.com/everystepcounts.html) or accelerometer that allow for downloading of data directly from the PA monitor (e.g., www.theactigraph.com), to those that require a fee that supports either access to materials and or staff in assisting the user (e.g., www.activeliving.info).

Providing patients with an assessment of their PA habits can be invaluable. These assessments allow for clear feedback on whether patients are meeting the thresholds of >150 min/week (moderate) or >75 min/week (vigorous) for substantial health benefits. Similarly, these assessments can inform patients and their clinicians of inactivity (sitting time). Although there are no clear standards for sitting time, it is becoming increasingly clear that prolonged sitting is deleterious to health and should be avoided.[37]

Resistance Training

For appropriately screened patients with CVD, resistance training should be incorporated into the exercise program. The perception that resistance exercise is harmful to cardiac patients, or at the least is not beneficial, is not supported by the scientific literature.[22] Lower myocardial demand as compared to that with dynamic exercise, attenuation of ischemic responses, and increases in subendocardial perfusion have all been observed in studies of resistance exercise training in cardiac patients. Furthermore, although the caloric expenditure during resistance exercise is less than with CRE exercise, increased muscle mass correlates with an increased basal metabolic rate and may therefore be an important training adaptation contributing to attainment and maintenance of healthy body weight. Finally, attaining and maintaining strength and endurance may hasten return to vocational and recreational activities and may well prolong functional independence for older patients.

Although ample evidence supports the safety and efficacy of resistance exercise, careful selection of patients is prudent. Patient criteria for clearance for safe participation are identified in table 8.8. Patient clearance should be a staff decision with approval of the medical director and surgeon, as appropriate. Once a patient has been cleared for participation, a measure of baseline muscular strength is important to establish a safe initial routine and monitor adaptations over time. Patients should be monitored for HR, RPE, and electrocardiogram (ECG) response throughout the evaluation of baseline capacity. Blood pressure can be measured before and immediately after

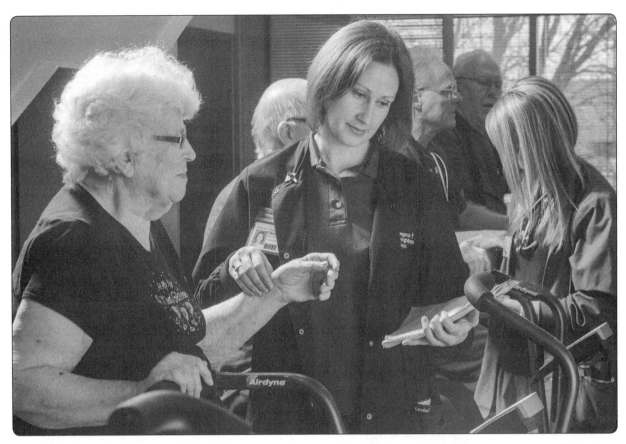

Once a patient has been cleared for participation in a resistance training program, a measure of baseline muscular strength is important to establish a safe initial routine and monitor adaptations over time.

completion of the final repetition. Methods for baseline assessment of muscular strength include the following:

- One-repetition maximum (1RM)—determines the maximal amount of weight that a patient can lift once, but not twice, while maintaining correct technique without straining

- Multiple RM (6RM to 15RM)—determines the maximal amount of weight that a patient can lift 6 to 15 times, maintaining correct technique and without straining

While the 1RM assessment is commonly used in healthy individuals, the multiple RM assessment is less stressful and can provide a reasonable baseline level of musculoskeletal fitness for most cardiac patients. The elements of a safe and effective resistance training routine are identified in table 8.8. As with CRE training, the prescriptive elements within the table must be individualized to the needs and goals of the patient.

Flexibility Training

Optimal musculoskeletal function requires that a patient maintain an adequate range of motion in all joints. It is particularly important to maintain flexibility in the lower back and posterior thigh regions. Lack of flexibility in these areas may be associated with an increased risk for the development of chronic lower back pain. Therefore, preventive and rehabilitative exercise programs should include activities that promote the maintenance of flexibility.[38] Lack of flexibility is prevalent in the elderly and contributes to a reduced ability to perform activities of daily living. Accordingly, exercise programs for the elderly should emphasize proper stretching, especially for the upper and lower trunk, neck, and hip regions. The elements of a musculoskeletal flexibility training routine are identified in table 8.9. As with CRE and musculoskeletal resistance training, the prescriptive elements within the table should be individualized to the needs and goals of the patient.

Diabetes

Diabetes mellitus is a complex metabolic disorder characterized by impaired glucose uptake caused by insufficient pancreatic insulin production (type 1) or loss of peripheral insulin sensitivity (type 2). Type 1 diabetes, usually diagnosed at a younger age than type 2, is generally not associated with obesity, and is less responsive to exercise as therapy. Type 1 diabetes is classified as an autoimmune disease. For the person with type 1 diabetes, exercise increases glucose disposal and decreases insulin requirements on exercise days. Type 2 diabetes typically, but not always, has its onset in adulthood and is often associated with obesity; hypertension; abnormal lipids; and a subclinical level of inflammation that effects coagulation, endothelial function, and other metabolic functions.

In 2010, the Centers for Disease Control and Prevention (CDC) reported that approximately 25.8 million Americans had diagnosed or undiagnosed diabetes.[1] It is estimated that almost 79 million Americans (35% of those 20 or older) have prediabetes, a condition in which blood glucose (BG) levels are elevated, which increases risk for type 2 diabetes. Approximately 90% to 95% of people with diabetes have type 2 diabetes. Weight loss and exercise have been shown to improve the insulin resistance associated with type 2 diabetes, although comprehensive treatment often involves oral hypoglycemic, antihypertensive, and lipid-lowering medications, especially in patients who are at risk for or who have CHD.

Type 2 diabetes is a significant contributor to premature mortality and morbidity related to CVD, blindness, kidney disease, nerve disease, and amputation.[1] Among patients with diabetes, CHD, stroke, hypertension, and peripheral arterial disease are the major causes of morbidity and mortality.[2] The biggest challenge faced by patients with diabetes is how to comply with complex treatment regimens. CR/SP professionals are in a key position to help monitor and motivate compliance with medications as well as with diet and exercise programs. CR/SP staff must work closely with the primary care physician or endocrinologist to help optimize the management of diabetes.

Type 2 Diabetes

The benefits of exercise for a patient with type 2 diabetes are substantial.[3] Regular exercise improves BG management, reduces the risk for CVD and its complications, and improves overall health and wellness in these patients. Exercise can prevent or delay the onset of type 2 diabetes in patients with prediabetes.[4] Most of the benefits of exercise and PA with respect to diabetes management are the result of enhancements in insulin sensitivity, accomplished through both cardiovascular endurance and resistance training.

A recent study demonstrated that for each metabolic equivalent (MET) increase in aerobic capacity, mortality is decreased by 19% and 14% for Caucasian and African American men diagnosed with type 2 diabetes.[5] It is well established that increased cardiovascular fitness is associated with increased insulin sensitivity after an exercise session.[6,7] The following list outlines the role of exercise for patients with diabetes.

The Role of Exercise in Improving Diabetes Management

- Improved sensitivity to insulin
- Improved BG control
- Decrease in required dose of insulin or oral hypoglycemic agents
- Decreased plasma insulin levels
- Improved glucose tolerance
- Lower hemoglobin A1c levels

Type 1 Diabetes

All levels of PA can be performed by people with type 1 diabetes who do not have complications and have good BG control. The ability to adjust the therapeutic regimen (insulin and medical nutrition therapy) to allow safe participation is an important management strategy in these individuals, including self-monitored BG data associated with PA response.[8] Hypoglycemia can occur during, immediately after, or be delayed for many hours after exercise or PA. Good knowledge of the activity-related metabolic responses, as well as sign and symptom awareness and self-management can minimize these episodes. Tailored insulin therapy provides patients with the flexibility to make appropriate insulin dose adjustments for various levels of exertion, rather than solely focusing on carbohydrate supplementation.

Risks of Exercise in Patients With Diabetes

Most patients with diabetes can exercise safely. However, exercise is not without risks for these patients; health care professionals should be aware of these risks,[3] which include the following:

Risks Associated With Exercise in Patients With Diabetes

Cardiovascular risks

- Cardiac dysfunction and dysrhythmias caused by subclinical or diagnosed ischemic heart disease (silent ischemia)
- Excessive increases or decreases in BP or HR caused by autonomic neuropathy
- Postexercise and orthostatic hypotension due to autonomic neuropathy

Metabolic risks

- Hypoglycemia in patients on insulin or most oral hypoglycemic agents
- Exacerbation of hyperglycemia

Musculoskeletal and traumatic risks

- Foot ulcers (especially in the presence of peripheral neuropathy)
- Orthopedic injuries related to peripheral neuropathy

Microvascular risks

- Retinopathy: Exercise that involves straining, jarring, or Valsalva-like maneuvers, as well as anaerobic exercise is contraindicated in patients with proliferative diabetic retinopathy.
- Nephropathy: Low- to moderate-intensity activities are safe, but high-intensity exercise should be discouraged.
- Peripheral neuropathy: Comprehensive foot care is required.

Preexercise Assessment and Testing of Patients With Diabetes for Exercise Programs

To maximize the benefits and minimize the risks of exercise in this patient population, it is necessary to provide appropriate screening of patients, emphasize adherence to program design guidelines, and offer education and tools to improve glucose monitoring and overall CVD risk factor modification. It is essential to determine individual patient knowledge and understanding of diabetes and its management, including the exercise regimen, as well as medication use and dietary considerations. This discussion should also specifically include

- insulin and oral hypoglycemic agents and all other medications including side effects and drug interactions,
- self-monitoring of BG levels, and
- current level of regular PA.

Due to an increased incidence of asymptomatic coronary artery disease in patients with diabetes, formal exercise testing is advisable if previously sedentary persons with diabetes are to undertake an exercise program. However, in patients with diabetes who are planning to participate in low-intensity forms of exercise such as walking, the physician or health care professional should use clinical judgment in deciding whether to recommend an exercise stress test. Persons intending to begin a more vigorous exercise program (e.g., activities more vigorous than everyday activities of daily living [≥5 metabolic equivalents, METs]) may benefit from being assessed before starting the exercise program. Complications from diabetes, including peripheral neuropathy, severe autonomic neuropathy, and retinopathy, may also contraindicate certain activities or predispose patients to injuries.[9] The preexercise evaluation should also include other important assessments, such as a review of current medications and any physical limitations and symptoms suggestive of the complications from diabetes (see chapter 2).

The following lists general indications for exercise stress testing in patients with diabetes.

General Indications for Stress Testing in Patients With Diabetes

- Age >40 years
- Age >30 years and any of the following:
  - Type 1 or 2 diabetes >10 years in duration
  - Hypertension
  - Cigarette smoking
  - Dyslipidemia
  - Proliferative or preproliferative retinopathy
  - Nephropathy including microalbuminuria
- Any of the following, regardless of age:
  - Known or suspected coronary artery disease (CAD), cerebrovascular disease, or peripheral artery disease (PAD)
  - Autonomic neuropathy
  - Advanced nephropathy with renal failure

Adapted from Colberg et al. 2010.

The exercise stress test should be performed with intention of evaluating the presence of ischemia, dysrhythmia, and abnormal blood pressure responses to exercise and recovery. Test results also provide more accurate information for the prescription of initial levels of exercise, along with corresponding training heart rates for specific activities, and identify any patient-specific precautions regarding exercise and physical activity.

Exercise Prescription for Patients With Diabetes

The exercise prescription for people with diabetes must be individualized according to a medication schedule, presence and severity of diabetic complications, and goals and expected benefits of the exercise program.[10] Food intake must be considered with respect to the timing of exercise. The primary goals for patients participating in a CR/SP program may include the following:

- Improved control of BG levels
- Minimizing complications of diabetes
- Increased self-management of other CVD risk factors
- Increased aerobic capacity, muscular strength and endurance, and flexibility
- Increased daily physical activity and decreased sitting time

The development and components of an exercise prescription for a patient with diabetes are similar to the standard methods for exercise prescription, with a few key exceptions (see "General Precautions for Patients With Diabetes" and "Instructions for Foot Care for Patients With Diabetes" sections).[3,11]

Education, Monitoring, and Management of Patients With Diabetes

There are a number of precautions and special instructions for exercise in persons with diabetes as listed in "General Precautions for Patients With Diabetes." Complications involving the feet are common in people with diabetes; therefore foot care is an important consideration. Problems most often develop in patients with peripheral neuropathy of legs and feet and when blood flow is compromised. Such problems can include extremely dry skin that may peel or crack; calluses that may ulcerate; and foot ulcers, particularly at the ball of the foot or at the base of the big toe. Patients should be routinely taught to inspect their feet and report any sores, infections, or inflammation to their health care provider. In addition to regular inquiry by the health care staff regarding foot health, initial assessment for peripheral neuropathies and pulses should be performed. CR/SP staff should instruct patients on routine foot care.[12] General precautions for patients with diabetes are covered in the following list.

General Precautions for Patients With Diabetes

- Avoid vigorous exercise before blood glucose has been adequately controlled.
- Have knowledge and awareness of the signs, symptoms, and management of hypoglycemia and hyperglycemia; exercise late in the evening may increase risk of nocturnal hypoglycemia.
- Some medications may mask or exacerbate exercise-related hypo- or hyperglycemia, including beta-blockers, diuretics, calcium channel blockers, and warfarin.
- Take appropriate precautions:
  - Always carry a carbohydrate (CHO) source.

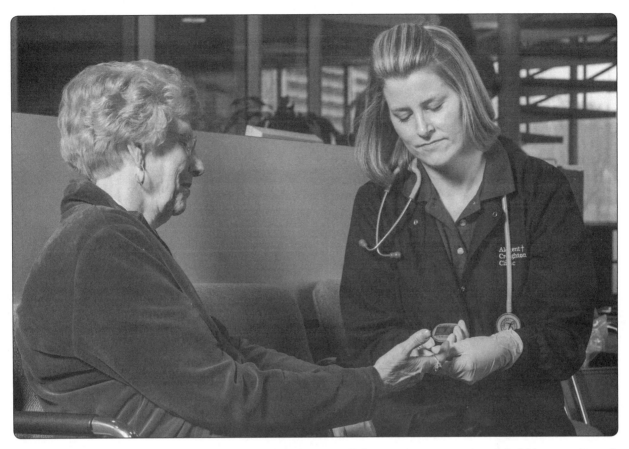

When patients with diabetes begin an exercise program, BG response to exercise should be monitored closely.

○ Avoid exercise at time of peak insulin effect; alternatively, consume a CHO snack 30 min before exercise or decrease insulin or oral hypoglycemic dose before exercise; schedule exercise 1 to 2 h after meals.

○ Test blood glucose frequently; responses may vary with each individual and day to day.

○ Hydrate adequately before, during, and after exercise.

○ Use caution when exercising in the heat. Temperature regulation may be impaired in some patients with diabetes.

○ Carry a personal ID at all times specifying diabetes along with emergency contacts.

○ Public or cell phone access is important.

○ Inject insulin abdominally before exercise commencing within 30 min; do not use active muscles as injection sites for insulin preexercise.

• Patients with neuropathy

○ may require alternatives to palpating pulse for controlling intensity (e.g., commercial heart rate monitor or use of rating of perceived exertion),

○ may have abnormal heart rate and blood pressure responses to exercise,

○ are at increased risk of orthostatic hypotension, and

○ should routinely care for their feet and hands.

Instructions for Foot Care to Patients With Diabetes

Foot hygiene

• Inspect your feet daily for blisters, cuts, and scratches; report any issues to your health care provider immediately. If appropriate, a family member may assist with foot inspection.

- Inspect the interior and the soles of your shoes on a daily basis for roughness or inconsistent wear.
- It is helpful to have and alternate two pairs of shoes on a daily basis for exercise.
- Wash and dry feet carefully every day, giving special attention to areas between the toes.
- Dry skin may be relieved with application of baby oil after bathing and drying feet or hands.
- Do not soak your feet.
- Avoid bathing in extreme temperatures.
- Cut toenails straight across.
- Do not cut or trim corns; do not treat corns and calluses with chemical agents.
- Do not use adhesive tape on feet.

Note: The health provider or physician should examine feet at each visit.

Footwear

- Wear properly fitted, synthetic or wool socks, pantyhose, and so on. Avoid mended stockings or stockings with seams that may irritate the feet. Change socks and stockings daily.
- Wear wool socks with protective footwear in the winter.
- Wear socks if your feet are cold at night.

- Buy comfortable shoes made of materials that provide protection for your feet and keep your feet dry.
- Do not wear sandals with thongs between the toes.
- Do not walk barefoot, especially on hot surfaces.

Monitoring BG levels is vital for the long-term maintenance of glycemic control and is especially important during exercise given that beta-blocker therapy can mask the onset of an impending insulin reaction. Monitoring BG levels during exercise may also provide positive feedback regarding the regulation or progression of the exercise prescription, which may result in subsequent long-term adherence to exercise. This is particularly important since exercise is a cornerstone of treatment for diabetes.

Summary

The exercise prescription for persons with diabetes should be tailored according to the timing of their medications, presence of diabetes complications, and individual exercise goals. The benefits of regular exercise go beyond increasing insulin sensitivity and lowering BG levels. A comprehensive exercise program performed consistently and progressively will help persons with diabetes manage the disease and improve their quality of life.

 Guideline 8.8   Monitoring Blood Glucose in CR/SP

When patients with diabetes begin an exercise program, BG response to exercise should be monitored closely.[13] Monitoring and recording BG levels before and after exercise is important because it may

- help identify risk for hypo- or hyperglycemia,
- help identify appropriate preexercise BG levels for decreasing risk of hypoglycemia (It is not necessary to postpone exercise based simply on hyperglycemia, provided the patient feels well or blood ketones are negative.),[14]

- help identify patients who should monitor BG during exercise,
- provide information for adjusting the exercise prescription on a daily basis, and
- provide feedback regarding the effects of exercise.

Tables 8.10 through 8.16 describe the procedures for monitoring BG in a CR/SP setting.

Table 8.10 Preexercise Hypoglycemia Care

Preexercise	Plan of care	Intervention
Patients using insulin or oral agents that increase the risk of hypoglycemia should maintain BG levels during exercise at 100 mg/dL or higher[2]	Assess patient for individual risks for low BG: • Medication use • Time and content of last meal or snack	Increase or maintain appropriate BG levels during exercise by eating a meal or a snack of 15 g carbohydrate (with some fat and protein; e.g., 1 tbsp peanut butter and six crackers) before exercising
BG should be taken immediately before exercise	Establish strategies for BG values of 100 mg/dL or less; encourage patients to look for patterns in their BG response	Individual BG targets should be set
Patients with a history of hypoglycemia unawareness or frequent symptomatic hypoglycemia	Assess patient level of understanding and discuss signs and symptoms of low BG and treatment if needed[32]	Patient may require a higher pre-exercise BG target, increased testing, or both during the exercise session; treat appropriately
Patients using insulin pumps	Consult with endocrinologist or CDE for instructions on insulin dose adjustment related to exercise	Every effort should be made to set appropriate BG targets to prevent hypoglycemia from interfering with the exercise session and performance[32]

Abbreviations: BG, blood glucose; CDE, certified diabetes educator.

Reprinted, by permission, from F. Lopez-Jimenez et al., 2012, "Recommendations for managing patients with diabetes mellitus in cardiopulmonary rehabilitation. An American Association of Cardiovascular and Pulmonary Rehabilitation Statement," *Journal of Cardiopulmonary Rehabilitation and Prevention* 32: 101-112.

Table 8.11 Postexercise Hypoglycemia Care[13]

Postexercise	Plan of care	Intervention
Glycemic goal postexercise should be individualized.	BG should be taken within 15 min after exercise.	Encourage patients to test BG frequently after exercise to be aware of the potential for a hypoglycemic response that can last 24 to 48 h after exercise session.
A postexercise BG goal of 100 mg/dL or higher can be used to discharge an asymptomatic patient until a BG pattern and response have been established.	Use clinical discretion regarding the discharge of patients on oral hypoglycemic medication if BG is lower than 100 mg/dL and the individual is asymptomatic; caution should be used in discharging patients on insulin if BG is lower than 100 mg/dL.	Carbohydrate snacks to prevent hypoglycemia may contain some protein, fat, or both; carbohydrate snacks to treat hypoglycemia are more rapidly digested and absorbed if they are pure carbohydrate; to prevent hypoglycemia during extended activity, a snack of 15 to 30 g carbohydrate should be eaten for every 30 to 60 min of physical activity.
Patients using insulin pumps	Patients using pumps should consult with their endocrinologist or CDE for instructions on insulin dose adjustment related to exercise and BG targets.	Discuss with patient's physician whether insulin or other medication needs to be reduced before the exercise session; obtain specific goals for exercise BG.

Abbreviations: BG, blood glucose; CDE, certified diabetes educator.

Reprinted, by permission, from F. Lopez-Jimenez et al., 2012, "Recommendations for managing patients with diabetes mellitus in cardiopulmonary rehabilitation. An American Association of Cardiovascular and Pulmonary Rehabilitation Statement," *Journal of Cardiopulmonary Rehabilitation and Prevention* 32: 101-112.

Table 8.12 Hypoglycemia Recommendations[13]

Points for consideration	• Treatment of hypoglycemia (blood glucose [BG] <70 mg/dL) requires ingestion of glucose- or carbohydrate-containing foods; rapid glycemic response correlates better with the glucose content than with the carbohydrate content of the food; ongoing activity of insulin or insulin secretagogues may lead to recurrence of hypoglycemia unless further food is ingested after recovery[2]; people on an alpha glucosidase inhibitor (Precose [acarbose] or Glyset [miglitol]) must use dextrose only (such as glucose tablets) for treatment of hypoglycemia. • The "15 grams of a rapidly digested (such as apple juice) carbohydrate, wait 15 minutes" rule, that is, giving 15 to 20 g of a rapidly digested carbohydrate, is the preferred treatment for the conscious individual with hypoglycemia, although any form of carbohydrate that contains glucose may be used; if BG 15 min after treatment shows continued hypoglycemia, the treatment should be repeated; once BG returns to normal, the individual should consume a meal or snack to prevent recurrence of hypoglycemia.[2]
Examples of 15 g glucose	• 1/2 cup, or 4 oz (120 mL), of fruit juice • 1/2 cup, or 4 oz (120 mL), of a regular, not diet, soft drink • 1 cup, or 8 oz (240 mL), of milk • Five or six pieces of hard candy • Three or four glucose tablets (check label for how many tablets equal 15 g)
Intervention	• Help patient determine amount of food or drink or number of glucose tablets that equals 15 g carbohydrate; differentiate carbohydrate used to treat a hypoglycemic episode from appropriate carbohydrate intake to prevent hypoglycemia; added fat may retard and then prolong acute hypoglycemic episode; explain to patient that overtreating low BG can lead to hyperglycemia and weight gain. • Validate patient glucose meter by comparing with institution-calibrated glucose meter. • In unresponsive people with diabetes experiencing a hypoglycemic event, follow institution policy regarding glucagon injection or intravenous administration of dextrose.

Reprinted, by permission, from F. Lopez-Jimenez et al., 2012, "Recommendations for managing patients with diabetes mellitus in cardiopulmonary rehabilitation. An American Association of Cardiovascular and Pulmonary Rehabilitation Statement," *Journal of Cardiopulmonary Rehabilitation and Prevention* 32: 101-112.

Table 8.13 Preexercise Hyperglycemia Care for Patients With Type 1 Diabetes[13]

Preexercise	Plan of care	Intervention

• Avoid exercise if fasting BG is 300 mg/dL or higher or ketosis is present.
• A person with type 1 diabetes who is deprived of insulin for 12 to 48 h can become ketotic[2]; exercise can aggravate the hyperglycemia and ketosis.
• Vigorous activity is not recommended in the presence of ketosis; it is not necessary to postpone exercise based simply on hyperglycemia if urine, blood ketones, or both are normal.[12]
	1. With repeated BG levels of 300 mg/dL or higher, with or without ketones, obtain BG goals and medication adjustments from the physician for planning treatment, interventions needed for an exercise session, or both.
	2. Help patient determine possible causes of increased BG:
	  • Medication compliance
	  • Insulin pump malfunction
	  • Signs or symptoms of an infection or dehydration
		• Obtain individualized BG range for patient if warranted; it would be useful to have physician order for instructions regarding ketone testing.
		• If fasting BG or postprandial BG continues to be elevated, consider an adjustment in insulin dosing; refer patient to physician, CDE, or both for further intervention.
		• Assess patient knowledge and proficiency in following prescribed dosing.
		• Check medication and test strip expiration dates.
		• Follow instructions given for checking pump operation.
		• Patient should postpone exercise and follow up with physician.

Abbreviations: BG, blood glucose; CDE, certified diabetes educator.

Reprinted, by permission, from F. Lopez-Jimenez et al., 2012, "Recommendations for managing patients with diabetes mellitus in cardiopulmonary rehabilitation. An American Association of Cardiovascular and Pulmonary Rehabilitation Statement," *Journal of Cardiopulmonary Rehabilitation and Prevention* 32: 101-112.

Table 8.14 Preexercise Hyperglycemia Care for Patients With Type 2 Diabetes[13]

Preexercise	Plan of care	Intervention
• Patients with type 2 diabetes should exercise with caution if BG is 300 mg/dL or higher. • Routinely testing ketones is not indicated in patients with type 2 diabetes unless they are instructed to do so by their physician.	1. With repeated BG levels of 300 mg/dL or higher, obtain BG goals from the physician for planning treatment, interventions, or both for an exercise session. 2. Help patient determine possible causes of increased BC: • Medication compliance • Signs or symptoms of an infection • Dehydration	• Obtain individualized BG range for patient if warranted. • If fasting BG or postprandial BG continues to be elevated, consider an adjustment in medications; refer patient to physician, CDE, or both for further intervention. • Assess patient knowledge and proficiency in following prescribed dosing. • Check medication and test strip expiration dates. • Patient should postpone exercise and follow up with physician. • If elevated BG is caused by timing of meal and patient is asymptomatic, advise exercise with caution; in the absence of very severe insulin deficiency, exercise may decrease the BG level. • BG can be evaluated during exercise to make sure it is not increasing; if BG increases, exercise may need to be stopped until patient is within goal range. • If hyperglycemic hyperosmolar state is suspected, contact physician immediately.

Abbreviations: BG, blood glucose; CDE, certified diabetes educator.

Reprinted, by permission, from F. Lopez-Jimenez et al., 2012, "Recommendations for managing patients with diabetes mellitus in cardiopulmonary rehabilitation. An American Association of Cardiovascular and Pulmonary Statement," *Journal of Cardiopulmonary Rehabilitation and Prevention* 32: 101-112.

Table 8.15 Postexercise Hyperglycemia Care[13]

Postexercise	Plan of care	Intervention
• Patients with diabetes may have an increase in BG values after exercise if undertreated or if physical activity is performed at intense aerobic levels; this results from an increased catecholamine response to this level of exertion, leading to an exaggerated release of glucose for fuel. Hyperglycemia may last for several hours before BG returns to desired levels.[28] • In some patients, the BG supply can exceed demand; this can be seen after intense physical activity such as weightlifting. This response does not erase other fitness benefits, but the individual may feel discouraged or have concerns about doing harm.	Assess patient and extenuating circumstances (e.g. consuming a meal just before exercise.)	Instruct the patient to continue monitoring and follow usual treatment guidelines for high BG. If significant hyperglycemia remains or if the patient is symptomatic, the physician should be contacted.

Abbreviation: BG, blood glucose.

Reprinted, by permission, from F. Lopez-Jimenez et al., 2012, "Recommendations for managing patients with diabetes mellitus in cardiopulmonary rehabilitation. An American Association of Cardiovascular and Pulmonary Statement," *Journal of Cardiopulmonary Rehabilitation and Prevention* 32: 101-112.

Table 8.16 Signs and Symptoms of Hypo- and Hyperglycemia

Hypoglycemia	Hyperglycemia
Rapid heart rate	Frequent urination
Sweating	Extreme thirst
Anxiety	Extremely dry skin
Shakiness	Drowsiness
Dizziness	Nausea
Weakness and fatigue	Infections that do not heal
Headache	Hunger
Irritability	Blurred or impaired vision
Hunger	
Blurred or impaired vision	

Psychosocial Considerations

Recovering from cardiac disease and adjusting to subsequent life changes is a challenge for most cardiac patients and their families.[1] Several psychosocial factors, including depression, anxiety, and social isolation, can impede recovery.[2,3] In contrast, successful psychological adjustment enhances the recovery process as evidenced by increased adherence to recommendations and decreased morbidity and mortality (guideline 8.9).[4]

Clinicians in secondary prevention settings should address the psychosocial needs of patients in a manner that conveys empathy and builds on their existing strengths.[5] These needs can be addressed using assessment, feedback, brief interventions, and specialized interventions and referrals as appropriate. The structure and focus of psychosocial services may differ in inpatient and outpatient settings; however, assessments in both settings should answer the following questions:

- Has a crisis been caused by the illness or by entry into secondary prevention?
- Has the ability to adapt to daily demands of living been disrupted by the illness?
- Does the patient show affective or cognitive impairment in the ability to cope with the adaptive demands of illness or those of secondary prevention?
- Is the patient receiving adequate psychosocial support to aid in coping with the stressors of medical intervention or secondary prevention?

 Guideline 8.9   Assessment and Outcomes Related to Psychosocial Concerns

Assessment

- Staff should identify clinically significant levels of psychosocial distress using a combination of clinical interview and psychosocial screening instruments at program entry, exit, and periodic follow-up.

Outcomes

- Clinical: Patient should experience emotional well-being as evidenced by the absence of
  - psychosocial distress indicated by clinically significant levels of depression, social isolation, anxiety, anger, and hostility;
  - drug dependency; and
  - chronic or excessive psychophysiological arousal.
- Behavioral: Program services should enhance the ability to

- describe the recovery and CR/SP process;
- develop realistic health-related expectations;
- assume responsibility for behavior change;
- demonstrate problem-solving capabilities;
- engage in regular physical exercise and incorporate relaxation techniques, such as meditation, into the daily schedule;
- demonstrate effective use of other cognitive–behavioral stress management skills;
- obtain effective social support;
- adhere to psychotropic medication regimen if prescribed;
- reduce or eliminate alcohol, tobacco, caffeine, or other nonprescription psychoactive drugs; and
- return to meaningful social, vocational, and avocational roles.

- Does the patient show any behavioral patterns that warrant aggressive, immediate psychosocial intervention? Behaviors such as smoking, overeating, or substance abuse may be considered here.

- What are the major concerns of the patient and family regarding anticipated psychosocial adjustment challenges in the immediate future?

With these questions as a backdrop, the following specific guidelines can help clinicians provide psychosocial services in inpatient and outpatient settings. Additionally, affiliation with a mental health care provider improves access to resources that can assist patients with addressing identified needs. Thus, programs are encouraged to identify local behavioral health resources and cultivate relationships with them.[3]

Evaluation

The most current statement of core competencies for CR/SP professionals advises that staff should be able to provide a comprehensive evaluation including assessment of psychosocial correlates of heart disease such as depression, anxiety, social isolation, and anger or hostility.[5] Since many patients are grieving the loss of health, youth, employment, and role functioning, some level of distress is quite common. However, long-term prognosis is generally better in those adapting well to the CR/SP process. It is therefore helpful to identify individuals with maladaptive coping styles early in the evaluation. Assessing certain issues can help determine the level of intervention warranted (guideline 8.10).

Adjustment

Adjusting to any major life change can be challenging, and the onset or exacerbation of a major medical problem often affects multiple aspects of life. Feelings of sadness, anger, and grief are common, but may signify normal adjustment rather than clinical concern. However, these same emotions may also signify a clinical level of distress, as discussed in the next subsection. Denial may buffer a patient from the initial distress of an event, but it can be harmful when it impedes care or when it becomes a long-term coping strategy.[6] Note, however, that even short-term denial can be detrimental.[7] Understanding the greater context of the adjustment made by a patient helps clinicians to determine if denial is of concern.

Signs and Symptoms

Evaluating patients for the following signs and symptoms assists staff in understanding whether a patient is adjusting normally or if further intervention is necessary. In addition to the presence or absence of specific symptoms, the clinician should focus on the number and severity of symptoms, as well as their impact on daily functioning.

Guideline 8.10 Evaluation

CR/SP staff should

- determine the manner in which and the success with which the patient is coping with the medical crisis;

- determine the perception of health status on the part of the patient and family;

- assess for the presence of significant negative affect, particularly depression;

- determine if there is evidence of posttraumatic stress disorder;

- assess the ability to relax and manage stress;

- assess for excessive anger and hostility and a tendency to experience excessive distress;

- determine the level of social support;

- assess spiritual needs; and

- determine whether referral for specialized consultation is needed due to the presence of depression, smoking, alcohol abuse, significant anxiety, excessive frustration or anger, or spiritual crisis; and

- identify the goals with regard to sexual adjustment and problem behaviors (e.g., type A behavior, smoking, overeating, hostility).

Clinical Depression Does the patient exhibit signs or symptoms of clinical depression? These may include

- dysphoria;
- ongoing struggle to control mood or sustain sufficient energy to cope with daily stressors;
- preoccupation with fears, regrets, insecurities, and thoughts of death;
- loss of the ability to enjoy previously pleasurable activities;
- changes in sleep and eating patterns;
- decreased sexual drive;
- recurring sense of being overwhelmed by current stressors;
- agitation, irritability, and frustration;
- self-blame, pessimism, and hopelessness;
- psychomotor retardation;
- disrupted concentration and memory; and
- failure of supportive interaction with others to alleviate symptoms of depression.

Assessment for depression is essential since there is evidence that depression is a risk factor both for the development of heart disease and for subsequent poor prognosis.[8]

Anxiety Does the patient exhibit signs or symptoms of anxiety disorders? General signs and symptoms may include

- nervousness, agitation, irritability;
- worry;
- weakness, numbness, and fatigue;
- headache, muscle tension or ache;
- stomach churning;
- shortness of breath;
- blurred vision;
- feeling unable to cope;
- dizziness;
- heart palpitations;
- trembling and shaking;
- feelings of paralysis;
- sweating;
- pressure in head or chest; and
- feeling that things are not real.

Anxious patients with CVD may report any combination of these; however, fears of dying, fainting, going crazy, having a heart attack, losing control, causing a scene, or not being able to get back to a safe environment (i.e., home) may be most notable. In addition, some patients with heart disease become hyperattuned to visceral or body feedback perceived to be consistent with these fears.

Posttraumatic Stress Disorder Signs and symptoms of posttraumatic stress disorder (PTSD) often develop after a dramatic event involving significant actual or threatened physical harm. Individuals who have persistent frightening memories or thoughts, are emotionally numb, are easily startled, or present with a sleeping disorder should be further assessed for the presence of PTSD.

Anger and Hostility Longstanding excessive anger (an emotional state) and hostility (a persistent negative attitude) are associated with poor prognosis for persons with heart disease.[9] Similar to anxiety and depression, anger and hostility may precede the development of heart disease as well as accentuate its course. However, unlike anxiety and depression, in which physical symptoms of these problems may overlap with symptoms of heart disease, anger and hostility do not include signs and symptoms characteristic of heart disease. While the relationship between anxiety or depression and heart disease is bidirectional, anger or hostility in this context is a longstanding personality pattern that may precede the onset of heart disease. Patients with high levels of anger and hostility may present as delightful until they are displeased or provoked; thus the presence of these characteristics may be hidden unless the behavior patterns are formally assessed.

Type D Personality Similar to anger and hostility, a general pattern of distress characterized by negative affect and social inhibition (type D personality pattern), resulting in a tendency to become distressed while inhibiting expression of the distress, puts patients at risk for cardiovascular morbidity and mortality.[10] This pattern can also diminish quality of life.[11] The fact that patients who withhold expressing suffering may appear to be well adjusted makes it even more critical to formally assess for this distressed pattern.

Sexual Dysfunction Sexual dysfunction is relatively common in patients with heart disease. It is therefore essential to incorporate questions regarding past and present sexual function when obtaining the general medical and health history. Interviews with both the patient and the partner can be helpful, both in eliciting a complete history and facilitating communication and understanding regarding this sensitive topic.

Factors contributing to erectile dysfunction (ED) or low libido (or both) include anxiety regarding the safety of sexual activity, depression, medication side effects (e.g., antidepressants, antihistamines, antihypertensives), hormonal changes associated with menopause, vascular insufficiency, poor physical fitness, and altered body image associated with chronic illness. Of particular note is the use of medications prescribed for the relief of ED, for example sildenafil (Viagra), vardenafil (Levitra), and tadalafil (Cialis). The potential interaction between ED medications and nitrates leading to a hypotensive emergency is often not fully appreciated by patients, and appropriate caution is indicated. In addition, it is not uncommon for patients taking these medications to believe that erections will automatically occur even in the absence of intimacy and sexual stimulation. Hence, brief education and counseling may be helpful in facilitating the successful resumption of sexual activity.

Managing Psychosocial Concerns

The management of psychosocial issues can range from those which CR/SP staff may have the skills to be helpful and to guide patients, to those difficulties which require professional referral. The managing physician should always be advised of these situations and provide guidance for staff. Likewise, CR/SP staff should be cognizant of their own limitations and of the appropriate referral process.

Stress Management and Relaxation

The ability to manage stress and the ability to relax are important skills for recovery. These skills can facilitate coping with fear, anxiety, and pain. The CR/SP professional should assess for signs and symptoms of stress and investigate how the patient attempts to relax. In the inpatient setting, patients are often coping with the acute aspects of illness, while in the outpatient setting the mid-

and long-term effects of cardiac disease begin to emerge. Thus, assessment in both settings is important for understanding the current needs.

Social Support

Each person experiences heart disease within a greater social context. Although professional CR/SP staff provide a level of support, as do other patients at times, assessment of the overall social support system and functioning is vital. Poor functional support is associated with increased mortality.[2] Several of the psychosocial concerns listed here, such as depression, hostility, and type D personality pattern, may have an impact on the level of social support and ability to access those resources as needed. Thus, when one is evaluating the social support system, low social support may suggest that other psychosocial factors are also in play.

Spiritual Needs and Counseling

Many patients experience spiritual crises during the course of secondary prevention. The crisis may be manifested as questioning or anger directed toward God, urgent appeal to a higher power for help in coping, or anxiety over being separated from the spiritual support system. Some patients believe that anxiety equates with a lack of spiritual strength or trust. This can result in even greater anxiety and stress. Other patients may cope relatively well but could benefit from the extra support of pastoral counseling. Here, as in all aspects of psychosocial intervention, the CR/SP professional should provide responses appropriate to the needs but remain within a personal comfort zone. Minimally, patients should be asked whether they wish consultation from a pastoral counselor or religious leader.

Need for Specialized Consultation

Specialized consultation from a mental health professional is suggested for any patient who has protracted adjustment struggles, who does not respond to brief interventions geared toward crisis management, or whose recovery may be impeded by psychosocial problems. When signs and symptoms of distress are clinically significant, the patient should be referred back to the primary care provider or to a mental health specialist. The findings of a formal psychological evaluation can greatly aid the efforts of CR/SP staff who are not mental health professionals. Such assessments typically incorporate data from extended clinical interviews with patients and spouses and the results of a battery of standardized personality, neuropsychological, and family systems inventories.[12] Furthermore, the CR/SP professional can provide significant input into this evaluation through direct observation and documentation of patient behaviors that may contribute to psychosocial distress.

Need for Medication

Is the patient in need of evaluation for psychotropic medication and psychotherapy? Between 30% and 50% of cardiac patients suffer clinically significant levels of anxiety or depression. These symptoms dissipate spontaneously within 6 to 9 months in many patients. However, depressed patients remain at a higher level of cardiovascular risk until remission or dissipation of the symptoms. Hence, CR/SP professionals should very carefully consider medical evaluation of the need for antidepressant or anxiolytic therapy for a patient who has a history of anxiety or depression, who exhibits an elevated score on a questionnaire assessing negative affect (e.g., Beck Depression Inventory,[13] Symptom Checklist-90-Revised [SCL-90R],[1] Profile of Mood States,[15] Center for Epidemiologic Studies Depression Inventory [CES-D],[16] Spielberger State-Trait Anxiety Inventory[17]), or whose current functioning is significantly compromised by any combination of the signs and symptoms. While it remains unclear whether pharmacologic treatment of psychological distress decreases overall mortality, there is evidence that it can lower psychological distress as exemplified by the use of selective serotonin reuptake inhibitors (SSRIs) for the treatment of depression.[18]

Tobacco and Alcohol

Patients who continue to smoke following a coronary event experience twice the risk of death as their counterparts who quit. Efforts to promote smoking cessation begun during the inpatient stay appear to be particularly effective.[19] Appendix K presents a questionnaire that may be useful in eliciting a comprehensive smoking history.

It is estimated that 25% of patients in the hospital abuse alcohol or are alcohol dependent.[20] The increased risk associated with excessive alcohol intake and other substance abuse makes this an important area for assessment. Persons abusing substances routinely downplay the severity and effect of their use, making it all the more difficult to uncover. The CAGE Questionnaire (appendix L) has a particularly helpful set of standardized questions that can be used during a clinical interview in both the inpatient and outpatient settings.

Adherence: Attendance, Risk Factor Modification, and Medication

Adherence to recommendations including CR/SP program attendance, risk factor modification, and medication is essential for addressing CVD. However, several of the factors discussed earlier, such as depression, can impair adherence. Hence, early identification and treatment of significant psychosocial distress is essential in optimizing patient outcomes.

Interventions

Inpatient CR/SP services present an early opportunity to assist transition into the home environment while providing support, education, and counseling related to those areas identified in guideline 8.11.

Support, Education, and Guidance

While supportive counseling for the patient and family begins at the first professional contact, a structured program of education and psychosocial support tailored to the needs identified in the initial evaluation should be developed. Early interactions should emphasize active listening to patient and family concerns and the development of rapport. Patients should be assured that their questions and fears are normal and should receive practical suggestions for the management of novel stressors that accompany hospitalization. The CR/SP professional should provide multiple, brief interventions consisting of education and anticipatory guidance.[21] Conceptualization of the illness as an opportunity for physical, mental, and spiritual growth can lead to more optimistic thoughts and increases the likelihood of successful outcomes. Adaptive coping should be encouraged, and patients may be empowered through recall of previous success they may have had in dealing with other life challenges.

Family members or friends identified by the patient as a significant part of their social support system should be invited to participate in

Guideline 8.11 Interventions

CVR staff should

- provide individual counseling or small-group education (or both) regarding
  - adjustment to illness;
  - stress management;
  - coping with depression, anger, and anxiety or PTSD;
  - overeating;
  - medication adherence;
  - exercise;
  - sexual health;
  - and smoking cessation;
- provide a supportive environment to enhance the level of social support; and
- refer patients experiencing clinically significant posttraumatic stress, depression, substance abuse, anxiety, or hostility for further mental health evaluation and treatment.

the education and counseling sessions. Such involvement facilitates a common understanding regarding secondary prevention recommendations and an appreciation of the importance of social support. The difference between effective social support (i.e., active listening, mutual participation in behavior change, positive reinforcement of healthy lifestyle changes) and ineffective or even harmful actions (i.e., excessive policing, monitoring, blaming, shaming, or criticizing) should be emphasized.[22,23] Long-term behavior change is facilitated when the entire family system is viewed as an integral component of the rehabilitation process.

Relaxation Training

A variety of brief interventions geared toward teaching the patient to relax can be incorporated into routine care. For example, instruction in abdominal breathing and moderate-intensity progressive muscle relaxation may be helpful. Where applicable, patients can be encouraged to recall and use previously learned relaxation strategies, such as the breathing techniques used in Lamaze training. Patients can also be instructed to focus attention on soothing stimuli or visual imagery. Preparatory education regarding prognosis and scheduled interventions seems to have a positive effect on tension levels for many patients. Some, however, may actually respond with higher levels of anxiety when presented with more details related to their conditions. Thus, clinicians should assess the effect of such education on anxiety levels and adjust the level of detail accordingly.

Specialized Consultation and Referral

Signs and symptoms of clinical depression, anxiety, hostility, or substance abuse noted during the clinical interview, or elevated scores on psychometric measures of these conditions, suggest the need for specialized consultation.[24] Individuals with these characteristics may need psychotropic medications, psychotherapy, or spiritual counseling. In the event that referral for specialized counseling is necessary, the CR/SP professional should initiate and maintain communication with the counselor whenever possible. For example, where alcohol abuse counseling is indicated, the CR/SP professional should, within the limits of confidentiality, inform the counselor of any observed changes in tolerance, symptoms of withdrawal, or odor of alcohol on the breath.

Tobacco Cessation

Patients with a recent history of smoking or other forms of tobacco use should receive clear guidance regarding the need for cessation. Education about the effects of nicotine on the cardiopulmonary system should be provided along with information about the impact that smoking continuation or resumption is likely to have on prognosis. Previous attempts at smoking cessation should be discussed, and the patient should be made aware of contemporary pharmacologic and behavioral interventions. The physician or other health care provider should be consulted regarding the appropriateness of prescribing a nicotine receptor partial agonist (e.g., varenicline), nicotine

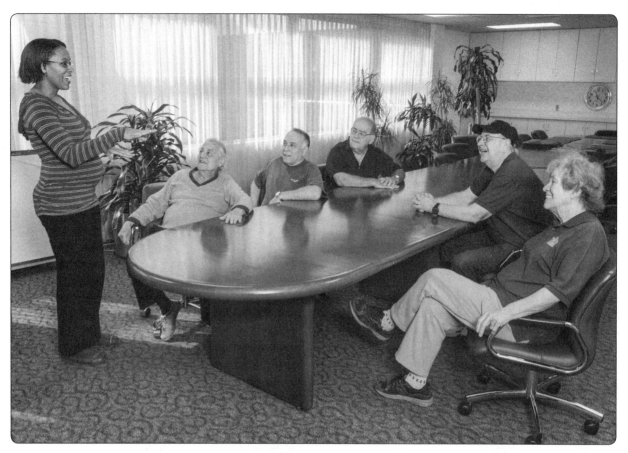

Early counseling interactions with patients who may be experiencing depression should emphasize active listening to concerns and the development of rapport. Patients should be assured that their questions and fears are normal and should receive practical suggestions for the management of novel stressors that accompany hospitalization.

replacement therapy (NRT), or buproprion. Recent evidence suggests that varenicline is particularly effective, though adverse effects, primarily nausea, may limit full adherence.[25] Behavior change counseling is an important adjunct to pharmacologic intervention, regardless of the specific agent used.

Discharge Planning

The discharge planning session sets the stage for further CR/SP efforts that may or may not include outpatient CR/SP. Discharge planning is best delivered simultaneously to patients and significant others.[26] They should be warned of the possibility of homecoming depression, anxiety, and increased family tensions as they attempt to adjust to the illness, the demands of secondary prevention interventions, and the consequences of relapse.[22,23,27] In addition, the CR/SP professional should proactively address concerns regarding the sexual consequences of illness and medications, offering reassurance and practical advice.[27-29]

Specific plans should be made for secondary prevention interventions involving changes in exercise, diet, and smoking. Methods to ensure adherence to medication regimens (e.g., a written schedule of medications, instruction on the use of pill boxes or medication dispensers) should also be reviewed in detail. After a review of these recommendations, the opportunity to ask questions should be provided, and comprehension and willingness to comply should be assessed.

Where possible, a brief follow-up phone call regarding psychosocial concerns should be made within the first month after discharge, particularly for those with elevated levels of psychological distress or depression and also for those not entering CR/SP.[19] If a follow-up call is not possible, a written reminder of key points covered in the discharge plan should be sent.

Outpatient Services

Secondary prevention programs greatly benefit from a relationship with a mental health provider who is knowledgeable about secondary prevention of CVD and who is willing to become an active member of the team. Such professionals can serve as outpatient therapists or group leaders. Their contributions can enhance the intensity and comprehensiveness of psychosocial interventions. All patients and their families should be encouraged to participate in these services as appropriate to their needs. These activities should be a major therapeutic thrust for patients with clinically significant levels of emotional or interpersonal distress.

A broad range of interventions supporting recovery and secondary prevention can be provided in individual and group formats. The type of format used is based on learning objectives, topic sensitivity, and logistics. Formats include 15 to 60 min classes delving deeply into specific topics; 3 to 5 min group mini-sessions immediately before or after exercise; counselor-led group support sessions; and one-on-one or family counseling for sensitive or patient-specific issues such as depression, sexual dysfunction, and anger management. Although interventions are often prepackaged, efforts should be made to tailor the message as much as possible to the needs of individual patients and families. Typical topics include the following:

- Linking behavior change objectives (e.g., increasing exercise to enhance fitness) to desired life goals (e.g., being able to return to work, participate in favorite hobbies, play with grandchildren)
- Strategies for modifying problem behaviors such as smoking or overeating
- The dangers of unchecked anger and depression and ways to modify these experiences
- Sexual adjustment throughout the life cycle and the effects of CVD, medications, and poor physical fitness on mood and sexual response
- General stress management strategies including time management, relaxation techniques, positive "self-talk," and exercise
- Giving and receiving effective social support
- Managing medications
- Recognizing when to ask for help

An increasing number of resources are available to guide CR/SP professionals in the development and implementation of psychosocial services.[28,30-32]

Finally, a crucial and often overlooked aspect of the psychosocial component of secondary prevention is follow-up. CR/SP staff should include questions regarding psychosocial adjustment in all follow-up interviews, mailed questionnaires, or phone contacts. Persistent psychosocial distress or poor adherence to lifestyle and medical regimens should be communicated to the primary care physician.

Overweight and Obesity

Obesity is an independent risk factor for CHD.[1] Excess adiposity predisposes individuals to other risk factors for CHD such as hypertension, dyslipidemia, and diabetes mellitus.[2] Therefore, it is not surprising that more than 80% of patients enrolled in CR/SP programs are overweight.[3-5] Unfortunately, the prevalence of overweight individuals enrolling in CR/SP programs increased by a remarkable 33% between 1996 and 2006,[6] requiring CR/SP programs to include weight management as one of their primary program objectives .

Despite the prevalence and strong link to other risk factors, overweight and obesity have not been a primary focus of intervention for many CR/SP programs. Instead, physicians caring for individuals with CHD have primarily treated the metabolic consequences of overweight pharmacologically without an emphasis on lifestyle changes. Less than half of CR/SP programs self-report providing a weight management program.[7] This paucity of scientific data on treatment programs in the CR/SP literature is further evidence of the lack of focus on obesity. A consequence is that the amount of weight loss among CR/SP patients is minimal, only about 1 to 2 kg.[3-5]

While the weight loss is far less than what is needed to optimize CHD risk reduction, participation in CR/SP is associated with significant reductions in the prevalence of metabolic syndrome characteristics,[8,9] has been shown to reduce the incidence of new cases of CHD in otherwise healthy individuals with coronary risk factors,[10] and is associated with a reduced rate of cardiac events.[11] Specifically, weight loss in individuals with CHD, accomplished with a comprehensive behavioral weight loss intervention, is associated with marked improvements in abdominal obesity, insulin resistance, lipid profiles, blood pressure,[12] endothelial function,[13] platelet aggregation,[14] and self-reported quality of life.[15] Since an overall goal of CR/SP is to favorably alter lifestyle-related markers of CHD, programs should concentrate efforts on the careful evaluation and treatment of overweight patients and integrate programs to yield meaningful and long-lasting weight reduction.

Identifying Overweight Patients

The first step in a treatment strategy is to identify overweight patients (guideline 8.12).

At a minimum, all patients entering CR/SP should have height and weight measured and recorded and BMI calculated (weight in kilograms/ height^2 in meters) (see table 8.17). Weight can then be measured on a weekly basis and serve as one index to evaluate program effectiveness.[16] Similar to BMI, waist circumference measurement is an effective means of identifying individuals who would benefit from a weight loss intervention.[16] Gender-specific, high-risk criteria for waist circumference have been identified (table 8.17).[17]

BMI is frequently used as a surrogate measure of body composition (see table 8.17). For adults, overweight is defined as a BMI 25.0 to 29.9 kg/m^2; obesity is defined as a BMI ≥30.0 kg/m^2. Both are risk factors for developing metabolic syndrome. Metabolic syndrome is in turn an overweight-related medical disorder that increases individual risk of developing CVD.[17] Metabolic syndrome is defined by the presence of three of the following five risk factors: large waist circumference, high blood pressure, elevated fasting glucose and triglyceride levels, and reduced HDL-C (see table 8.18).[17] Metabolic syndrome

Guideline 8.12   Weight Management

- Weight management interventions should be targeted to those patients whose weight and body composition place them at increased risk for, or exacerbation of, cardiometabolic disease, including CHD, diabetes mellitus, hypertension, and dyslipidemia.

- Patients generally at risk include those with a body mass index (BMI) ≥25 kg/m² and a waist circumference >40 in. (102 cm) in males and >35 in. (88 cm) in females.

Table 8.17   Classification of Overweight and Obesity

Weight class	BMI (kg/m^2)
Normal	18.5-24.9
Overweight	25.0-29.9
Class 1 obesity	30.0-34.9
Class 2 obesity	35.0-39.9
Class 3 obesity	≥40

Table 8.18   Clinical Identification of Metabolic Syndrome[7]

Risk factor	Defining level
Abdominal obesity (waist circumference)	
• Men	>102 cm (>40 in.)
• Women	>88 cm (>35 in.)
Triglycerides	>150 mg/dL
High-density lipoprotein cholesterol	
• Men	<40 mg/dL
• Women	<50 mg/dL
Blood pressure	≥130 / ≥85 mmHg
Fasting glucose	≥110 mg/dL

Reprinted, by permission, from National Cholesterol Education Program (NCEP), 2003, "Executive Summary of the third report of the Expert Panel on Detection, Evaluation and Treatment of High Blood Cholesterol in Adults (Adult Treatment Panel III)," *JAMA* 289(19): 2560-2572.

and associated insulin resistance are particularly prevalent among CR/SP patients.[17] The incidence of metabolic syndrome among patients in CR/SP is more than 50%,[18] twice that of the general population.[19] Excess adiposity associated with metabolic syndrome predicts an increased risk of death and recurrent events following a MI.[20-25] Thus, overweight should be viewed as a highly prevalent and serious medical condition.

The Energy Balance–Weight Loss Equation

Overweight is a heterogeneous problem stemming from genetic, biologic, and behavioral factors that affect the balance between energy intake (calorie content of food consumed) and total energy expenditure. Total energy expenditure is partitioned into three components: (1) resting metabolic rate (~60-75% of total); (2) thermic effect of food (~10% of total); and (3) physical activity, the most variable of the three components and the one that can be voluntarily modified (~15-30% of total) through lifestyle changes.[26] To accomplish weight loss, a net caloric deficit, achieved through increased energy expenditure or dietary restriction or both, needs to occur. A caloric deficit of 3,500 kcal equates with a weight loss of 0.45 kg (1 lb) of fat.[27]

Program Components of Weight Loss

Effective behavior change is integral to the success of any weight loss program and must address reductions in energy intake and increases in energy expenditure through physical activity. Initially practitioners should assess motivation and patient readiness for change to ensure that the patient is at least contemplating making a change.[28] The three standard components of behavioral weight control programs are behavioral modification, dietary patterns, and exercise and physical activity.[29-31]

Behavioral Modification

Behavioral modification principles focus on changing factors that control behavior. Attention is directed toward identifying environmental antecedents or cues that set the stage for behavior or reinforcers that lead to its reoccurrence. Common program components for weight reduction are shown in table 8.19.

Typically, treatment sessions in a group setting for approximately 60 min are provided by a trained facilitator (registered dietitian, behavioral psychologist, nurse, exercise professional, or related health care professional). Evidence suggests that group therapy is more effective than individual treatment.[27] Treatment visits use a structured curriculum and sessions focused on reviewing patient progress and problem solving related to barriers to changes in behavior.

The ultimate goal of a behavioral weight loss program is to produce lifelong changes in dietary and exercise behaviors resulting in permanent weight loss. Patients treated via a comprehensive behavioral approach over a 4- to 6-month period lose approximately 10 kg, or 11%, of initial weight.[32] A significant challenge for CR/SP is that behavioral weight loss programs are typically 16 to 24 weeks, while the duration of most early CR/SP is 12 weeks or less. Individual programs should develop creative approaches that fit within the constraints of limited resources and that best serve their patient population with a strong emphasis on a long-term continued program. Possible alternatives include developing and referring patients to medical-based weight loss programs that serve the general population, adapting the curriculum so that requisite information is provided in fewer sessions, allowing individuals to attend classes even if they are not formally enrolled in CR/SP, using web-based weight loss programs, and referring patients to existing community-based programs.

Table 8.19 Behavior Modification Techniques[27]

Self-monitoring	Systematic observation and recording of eating behaviors
Stimulus control	Altering the environment associated with eating and exercise
Problem solving	Proposing strategies to control factors that may precipitate excessive caloric intake
Assertiveness training	Teaching assertiveness regarding social situations involving eating and exercise
Goal setting	Establishing realistic short- and long-term weight loss and exercise training goals
Relapse prevention	Developing strategies to prevent or recover from relapse into behaviors associated with weight gain
Positive reinforcement	Emphasizing positive behaviors while avoiding negative thoughts

Adapted, by permission, from K.D. Brownell, 2000, *LEARN program for weight control* (Dallas, TX: American Health Publishing Co.).

Dietary Pattern

Long-term weight loss should be managed by a dietitian. In general, patients should have a caloric reduction goal approximately equivalent to 500 to 1,000 kcal less than their estimated daily maintenance energy requirements. Maintenance energy requirement is estimated by multiplying baseline body weight by 12.[29] Thus, for a 200 lb person, the daily maintenance caloric requirement would be 2,400 kcal and a targeted daily caloric intake between 1,400 and 1,900 kcal. An initial goal of reducing body weight by approximately 10% from baseline should be considered, but the time frame to accomplish this must be individualized.

Individualized recommendations for dietary modification should be made with consideration of reasonable goals and likelihood of compliance. Patients should be encouraged to consume a lower-fat diet (in particular, low in saturated and trans fats) that emphasizes whole grains, vegetables, and fruits[33] with the overall goal of a reduction of caloric intake. Patients must be educated regarding appropriate caloric reduction. Food journaling, if done correctly, is effective for recognition of current eating habits and documentation of caloric intake. Diets with different macronutrient compositions have proven to be compatible with weight loss and CHD risk reduction.[34-37] For weight loss to be maintained, foods consumed must be compatible with long-term adherence focusing on different food choices that ensure adequate nutrients and essential vitamins. Group sessions and individualized counseling should be conducted by a dietitian.

Exercise and Physical Activity

The primary objective of an exercise and physical activity program designed for optimal weight loss is to increase daily caloric expenditure. It is important to recognize that standard CR/SP exercise alone is of limited benefit in inducing significant weight loss over a 3- to 4-month time frame.[3-5] It has been demonstrated that increased calorie expenditure using exercise, alone[38,39] or combined with a comprehensive behavioral weight loss strategy,[12] results in significantly more weight loss than standard CR/SP. Moreover, high calorie expenditure exercise training is well tolerated, is perceived to be as enjoyable as standard CR/SP exercise,[15] and is similar in volume to training that supports long-term weight loss maintenance.[40]

Formal exercise sessions should focus on exercises that use large muscle groups—thus maximizing caloric expenditure—performed in a continuous fashion. Patients must be counseled on ways to increase their overall daily activity in addition to the formal exercise training.

Intensity Initially, exercise intensity should be approximately 60% to 70% of peak heart rate, which for most individuals equates to a fairly light to moderate intensity (11 to 12 on a rating of perceived exertion). This exercise intensity is safe, is well tolerated, provides an adequate stimulus to improve cardiovascular fitness,[41,42] and can usually be performed in a continuous fashion for a prolonged duration. With regard to progression, the focus should be on increasing duration first, followed by increases in exercise intensity.

Frequency Initially, an every-other-day exercise schedule is recommended. After a few weeks, frequency of training should be increased to 5 to 7 days/week. Exercise therapy should be viewed as a medicine that is "dosed" nearly every day. Exercise performed nearly every day maximizes caloric expenditure and reinforces exercise as a consistent part of the daily routine. In addition, the importance of increasing overall daily physical activity must be reinforced.

Modality Barring musculoskeletal limitations, weight-bearing activities provide the greatest caloric expenditure and should be recommended whenever possible.[43] Activities such as walking, as well as machines such as treadmills or elliptical exercisers, are generally associated with greater calorie expenditure than arm or leg ergometers. If weight-bearing exercises are difficult, modalities that employ large muscle groups should be selected, such as upright or recumbent cycles that use both upper and lower extremities. Caution is warranted with the use of modalities that may be biomechanically difficult for overweight individuals, such as elliptical trainers or other modalities that may increase the risk of loss of balance or falling.

Duration Gradual increases in duration from 30 to over 45 to 60 min are recommended for overweight patients. Intermittent exercise may be necessary for those who are limited in duration or intensity. Patients should be closely monitored and questioned regarding signs of overuse.

Lifestyle Activity People can achieve additional significant caloric expenditure by increasing physical activity levels separate from formal, prescribed exercise.[44] The amount of physical activity required for weight loss or for sustaining weight loss may be greater than the recommendations for general public health. Therefore, overweight and obese adults may need to be gradually progressed from initial recommendations of 150 min/week (1,000 kcal/week) to 250 to 300 min/week (>2,000 kcal/week).[45,46] Other effective recommendations include simply decreasing the amount of time spent being sedentary.[47] Guidance and encouragement are in order regarding the avoidance of energy-saving devices, taking stairs instead of elevators, parking at the outer perimeter of parking lots, and walking or biking as alternative modes of transportation. Patients should be taught that many home activities, such as lawn mowing, yard work, and housework, all increase overall caloric expenditure. For weight loss and eventual weight maintenance, patients should be advised and instructed regarding how to increase their levels of lifestyle physical activity on all days of the week and to decrease their sedentary time.

Summary

CR/SP programs cannot ignore the challenge of treating overweight and obese patients. These programs need to be innovative; staff needs to work cooperatively with other health care professionals, and the programs should be designed to provide effective behaviorally based interventions for weight loss and long-term weight maintenance.

Emerging Risk Factors

Although numerous studies have confirmed that traditional risk factors explain 90% or more of atherosclerotic events, several additional factors have emerged.[1-6] In general, these risk factors relate directly or indirectly to thrombus formation and dissolution, as well as to inflammation or endothelial dysfunction—processes that promote initiation and progression of atherosclerosis. The three factors discussed here have received considerable attention and may be helpful for quantifying risk among persons with or at risk for CVD.

Homocysteine

Altered homocysteine metabolism can lead to elevations in the plasma concentrations of homocysteine beyond the normal level of 10 mmol/L. A large series of cross-sectional and retrospective case–control studies indicated that levels >15 mmol/L are associated with increased risks of CHD, peripheral artery disease, stroke, and venous thromboembolism. Elevated homocysteine levels may be linked to atherosclerosis and thrombosis by several pathophysiologic mechanisms, including endothelial cell injury and impairment of endothelial function, increased proliferation of vascular smooth muscle cells, adverse modification of LDL particles, increased propensity for coagulation, and increased oxidative stress. Although treatment of hyperhomocysteinemia with vitamin supplementation (folic acid, vitamin B_6, and vitamin B_{12}) is effective in lowering the plasma levels of homocysteine, several randomized trials have reported no reduction in clinical cardiovascular events within 5 years.[6-9] As a result, population-wide screening for elevated homocysteine levels is not recommended. In selected patients with personal or family history of premature CVD, especially those without other known risk factors, evaluation of homocysteine levels may be prudent. In patients with levels >10 mmol/L, it may be advisable to increase their intake of vitamin-fortified foods (vegetables, fruits, legumes, fortified grains and cereals) and to suggest the use of supplemental vitamins (folate, vitamin B_6, and vitamin B_{12}). In summary, although studies have shown a relationship between blood levels of homocysteine and CVD events, the evidence does not support supplementation with folic acid, vitamin B_6, or vitamin B_{12} for treatment of hyperhomocysteinemia.

Lipoprotein(a) and Other Factors Related to Thrombosis

Although Lp(a) is technically a lipid, this molecule plays a regulatory role in atherothrombosis. Unlike other lipid molecules that participate in the process of atherosclerosis, Lp(a) has a structural homology with plasminogen and is thought to compete with plasminogen in binding to fibrin. This results in a potential direct inhibition of endogenous fibrinolysis. Clinical case–control and cohort studies have suggested a role of Lp(a) in development and progression of atherosclerosis. However, the association has been shown to be moderate at best.[10-12] Although niacin, fibric acid derivatives, exercise, alcohol-extracted soy protein, and a few other treatments have been associated with lower levels of Lp(a), the question whether these treatments are effective in reducing coronary risk remains unresolved.[10,11,13] Elevated fibrinogen levels, as well as elevated levels of tissue-type plasminogen activator (tPA), have also been shown to be associated with increased cardiovascular risk. Tziomalos and colleagues[14] concluded that no clinical evidence supports the implementation of specific therapies to lower Lp(a) to reduce the risk for clinical cardiovascular events. These authors suggested that the risk associated with Lp(a) may be reduced by aggressively managing other traditional vascular risk factors such as LDL-C. Finally, the European Atherosclerosis Society consensus panel concluded that Lp(a) should be measured in those whose risk level is intermediate to high and that a level of 50 mg/dL should be targeted with niacin as the recommended treatment.[15] As methods for detection of thrombogenic factors improve, future studies may provide additional evidence that supports or argues against the need for their continued consideration as important targets for evaluation and possible treatment.

C-Reactive Protein and Other Markers of Inflammation

Because it is now recognized that atherosclerosis is an inflammatory process, several plasma markers of inflammation have been evaluated as potential tools to predict the risk of coronary events. Many of those are now being studied, including high-sensitivity C-reactive protein (hs-CRP), heat shock protein, interleukin-6, and soluble intercellular adhesion molecule type 1 (sICAM-1). Of these, hs-CRP has been the most widely studied and is the only marker of vascular inflammation that has an established World Health Organization standard. In addition, the National Academy of Clinical Biochemistry Laboratory Medicine practice guidelines concluded that only hs-CRP met all of the stated criteria required for acceptance as a biomarker for risk assessment in primary prevention.[16] Moreover, high-sensitivity assays for this parameter appear to provide valid and reliable results. Recent meta-analyses have shown that increased hs-CRP levels are associated with higher risk for in-stent stenosis and increased absolute risk for CVD-related events.[17,18] A follow-up report from JUPITER demonstrated that apparently healthy men and women with elevated hs-CRP but normal LDL-C (<3.4 mmol/L) have a 44% reduction in CVD events with 20 mg/day of rosuvastatin.[19] Therefore, hs-CRP has potential for future clinical use as a readily obtainable marker that may guide preventive treatment strategies.

Summary

In conclusion, since several studies have reported that traditional risk factors for atherosclerosis explain the vast majority of cases of CVD, the clinician and practitioner in CR/SP should focus on these in primary and secondary prevention of CVD events. It appears that at this time, only hs-CRP among the emerging risk factors has any relative significance among the risk factors for CVD events.

Summary

The interaction of the various risk factors discussed in this chapter contribute to the overall potential for the development of and events resulting from CHD. CR/SP staff assessment of these risk factors, and ultimately, providing patients with tools for modifying their risk for future events, are of paramount importance. To accomplish risk reduction, patients must be educated as to the significance of these factors, and in conjunction with patient input, an individualized, case-management strategy developed for implementing the various interventions. Clearly, the elimination of habitual tobacco use; the control of hypertension, dyslipidemia, diabetes, and obesity; increasing physical activity, and treating anxiety and depression are keys to reducing subsequent MI and death resulting from heart disease.

Special Populations

Contemporary cardiac rehabilitation and secondary prevention (CR/SP) delivers individualized programs of prescribed exercise and risk factor modification that focus on the attainment of well-defined, measurable goals. The attainment of these specific goals predicts improved clinical and quality-of-life outcomes. This model emphasizes the roles of education and behavior modification aspects of CR/SP as equal to that of exercise and individualizes available rehabilitation services. The resulting services for both exercise and behavioral change individualize CR/SP to the particular collection of problems and needs that each cardiac patient brings to the rehabilitation setting. This personalized approach works well in a case management environment in which an increasing number of subgroups of cardiac patients are in CR/SP (see guideline 9.1).

The purpose of this chapter is to provide an overview of patient evaluation considerations and strategies to successfully implement secondary prevention services for selected subgroups of cardiac patients, with emphasis on strategies that

- maximize patient safety,
- individualize rehabilitation services, and
- optimize patient outcomes.

OBJECTIVES

This chapter describes the basis for assessment and intervention strategies related to specific groups of patients within the overall CR/SP model, providing individualized program considerations for

- older and younger patients;
- women;
- patients of racial and cultural diversity;
- patients who have undergone revascularization or valve surgery;
- patients with a history of complex arrhythmias or placement of a pacemaker or implantable cardioverter-defibrillator (ICD);
- patients with heart failure;
- patients who have undergone cardiac transplantation; and
- patients with diabetes, pulmonary disease, or peripheral arterial disease.

> ### Guideline 9.1   Implementation of CR/SP in Special Populations
>
> CR/SP specialists should
>
> - prepare a list of special population groups likely to attend their facility, for example older and younger adults; women; patients of ethnic diversity; patients who have undergone revascularization or valve replacement; and patients with a history of dysrhythmias, heart failure, heart transplant, diabetes, chronic obstructive pulmonary disease and heart disease, and peripheral arterial disease;
> - identify major safety concerns and outline strategies to minimize safety problems and respond to safety incidents should they occur for each group;
> - prepare a plan of care outlining how secondary prevention services, encompassing both exercise and education, will be adjusted to the unique problems and issues of a given group;
> - develop a competency plan to ensure that staff members have the requisite knowledge and skills to work with the special groups;
> - include an assessment for special physical and psychosocial needs in the initial evaluation; and
> - identify and maintain a list of other professionals and support services that staff may need to call on to assist with implementation of secondary prevention services in special populations or with patients with special needs.

Older and Younger Adults

Recognizing the potential impact of widely varying patient age as it may affect program development, delivery, and effectiveness of CR/SP services is a critical component to the overall success of the program. With the progressive aging of the American population and advances in both the acute treatment and secondary prevention of coronary heart disease (CHD), the number of older adults eligible for CR/SP programs is increasing steadily.[1] By 2006, close to 50% of individuals participating in CR/SP were age 65 or older ("older"), and one in six was over the age of 75 years ("older old").[1] Older patients with CHD have very high rates of disability, recurrent CHD events, comorbid medical conditions, and health resource use.[2-4]

Conversely, younger patients (<40 years of age) have issues that can be characterized in general but are often specific to gender, including vocation and family as the highest priorities. Obesity is common;[5,6] but muscle mass, strength, and physical functioning are more often in the normal range compared to values in older people. Time pressure and anxiety are common with the addition of unexpected illness, potential lifestyle adjustments, and the time required for CR/SP program participation. Younger patients with CHD often present with complex risk factor profiles and an urgency with regard to decreasing risk-associated behavior.

Characterizing patients simply on the basis of age is clearly an oversimplification of potential individual patient presentation. Nonetheless, there are considerations that can reasonably be made in considering potential special needs of patients in general, particularly on both ends of the age continuum.

CR/SP in Older Patients

Substantial evidence documents beneficial effects of CR/SP in older patients, including improved physical function[7] and improved survival,[8] with a very favorable cost-effectiveness profile.[9,10] Yet use of CR/SP in older patients is very low, with U.S. participation rates in the Medicare population at 14% after myocardial infarction and 31% after coronary bypass surgery.[9] Within the older population, women, the older old, and minorities are particularly unlikely to participate (table 9.1).[11] Reasons for nonparticipation in CR/SP include a low rate of physician referral,[12] geographic maldistribution of programs,[11,13] and systems-based barriers such as a poor degree of automation in hospital systems in securing CR/SP referrals.[14] Active identification and recruitment of patients who are less likely to participate in CR/SP are indicated, as these subsets of patients obtain substantial benefits from CR.

High disability rates in older coronary patients are due to a number of factors beyond

Table 9.1 Cardiac Rehabilitation Participation in Older Patients

	Number of patients	Participation rate (%)
Age ≥65 years	267,427	18.7
Age 65 to 74 years	84,089	26.6
Age 75 to 84 years	54,012	18.6
Age ≥85 years	11,282	4.6
Male	149,383	22.1
Female	118,044	14.3
White	245,504	19.6
Nonwhite	21,923	7.8
Coronary artery bypass surgery	74,501	31.0
Myocardial infarction	192,926	13.9
Myocardial infarction and percutaneous intervention	27,431	20.9

Data from Suaya et al. 2007.

the deconditioning effect of the acute coronary event itself (particularly coronary bypass surgery). These include the presence of comorbidities such as peripheral vascular disease, chronic obstructive lung disease, arthritis, mental depression, and type 2 diabetes mellitus (T2DM).[15,16] In addition, advancing age within the older population is associated with lower levels of physical function.[2,16]

The baseline evaluation for CR/SP participation in older CHD patients should go beyond the standard clinical review, stress test, and risk factor review performed in younger patients. Elements of the baseline evaluation specific to older patients should include a cognitive status assessment; an evaluation of gait, balance, mobility, hearing, and sight; and a psychosocial assessment specific to older patients.

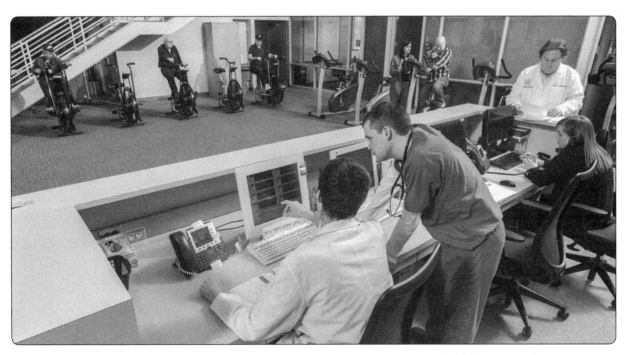

The baseline evaluation for CR/SP participation in older CHD patients should go beyond the standard clinical review, stress test, and risk factor review performed in younger patients.

Baseline Evaluation Components Specific to Older Cardiac Patients

- Mental status
- Gait and balance
- Vision and hearing
- Physical function and home activity requirements
- Transportation requirements
- Psychosocial assessment:
  - Social isolation
  - Depression and anxiety
- Ability to physically navigate the rehabilitation facility
- Nutritional assessment

Severely deconditioned older persons are often incapable of performing a standard exercise tolerance test and need to be individually assessed, often by a physical therapist or clinical exercise physiologist. Submaximal evaluations of the performance of specific activities such as the 6-minute walk, timed stair climbing, or simulated activities of daily living can also be used to evaluate the functional status of the older individual.[17,18]

Exercise training programs for older CHD patients should optimally include both resistance training and walking: resistance training because it leads to improvements in physical functioning, balance, coordination, and walking endurance;[19-21] walking because it leads to improved aerobic fitness and prognosis and is the most basic home physical activity requirement.[22] Resistance training intensity should optimally be based on carefully performed measures of single-repetition maximal (1RM) lifts in the CR/SP environment, though it can also be guided by perceived exertion using the Borg scale.[23,24] Maximal lift assessments using 1RM should be carefully supervised and determined by CR/SP staff with close attention to proper technique and safety. Specific exercises should include strengthening exercises of the major muscle groups of the lower and upper body (table 9.2). Resistance training stations are safer to use than loose dumbbells, whereas dumbbells may provide more flexibility and individualization at lower weight levels.

At program entry, severely deconditioned older patients may be unable to sustain exercise through a full session and need to be closely monitored and guided through CR/SP sessions. Several programmatic safety issues are specific to older patients.

Optimizing the Cardiac Rehabilitation Experience in Older Patients

General

- Consider increased musculoskeletal dysfunction, decreased mobility, slower reflexes, impaired senses, diminished short-term memory, limitations of balance and range of motion, and comorbidities.
- Floor surfaces require slip prevention.

Exercise

- Stabilize equipment; add safety accessories for mounting and dismounting (step stool for bike, grab bar for rower); allow room to

Table 9.2 Resistance Training Prescription in Older Coronary Patients

Intensity	50% to 80% of 1RM
Repetitions	10 to 15, with appropriate body mechanics, avoiding breath holding or straining, and not to failure
Sets	One or two
Frequency	Two or three times per week

Modality	Minimum of two from each of these groups:
	Lower body: leg extension (quadriceps)
	    • Leg press (gluteals, quadriceps)
	    • Leg curls (hamstrings)
	  • Upper body: bench press (pectoralis)
	    • Shoulder press (deltoids, triceps)
	    • Arm curls (biceps)
	    • Triceps extension (triceps)
	    • Lateral pull-down (latissimus)

Based on Williams et al. 2007.

mount and dismount; allow more time for progression of activities to prevent overuse.

- Repeat instructions; post reminders; use cue cards.
- Focus on activities of daily living, preferred recreational activities, and functional independence.

Education

- Educational materials should take into account impaired senses; for example, use printed instructions for hearing-impaired people, large-type print for visually impaired people.
- Offer daylight classes, as older patients may be reluctant to drive after dark.
- Offer small amounts of information, repeated often, and individualized to maximize learning.
- Consider social isolation by involving personal caregivers.
- Identify barriers to learning.

Exercise areas must be cleared of clutter, such as seated walkers or canes, to minimize falls. Exercise equipment like rowing and cycle ergometers should be stabilized to avoid tipping, loss of balance, and injuries. The presence of a cognitive impairment in any patient usually requires greater one-on-one supervision, particularly in people less able to independently manage exercise duration or intensity on a given piece of equipment.

The role of spouses or other family members in assisting the patient can be a help or a hindrance, and the latter should be considered.

Intermittent walking bouts on the treadmill with rest periods and weight-supported exercises, such as those on a seated stepper cycle or rowing ergometer, are usually sufficient to gradually advance the duration and intensity of exercise based on a target heart rate or ratings of perceived exertion. Social benefits of early outpatient and longer-term maintenance CR/SP should not be minimized. The socialization may counter some of the deleterious effects of social isolation and mental depression. Indeed, improvements in depression score while people are in CR/SP closely correlates with improvements in home-based physical functioning.[25] Exercise duration and frequency should be advanced before exercise intensity, but seniors rarely advance exercise intensity on their own. Exercise intensity should be progressed as fitness improves. Older patients do particularly well in longer-term CR/SP maintenance programs with respect to both the physical and the psychosocial benefits and should be strongly encouraged to participate.

Secondary Prevention in Older Cardiac Patients

While lifestyle treatments for lifestyle-related risk factors should predominate (table 9.3),[21] it is important for CR/SP programs to support

Table 9.3 Lifestyle Treatment for Secondary Prevention in Older Patient

Cardiac risk factor	Lifestyle treatment
Dyslipidemia	• Dietary counseling (eliminate trans fats, decrease saturated fats, increase soluble fiber and monounsaturated oils) • Weight reduction • Cardiovascular endurance exercise
Hypertension	• Weight reduction • Limit sodium intake • Dietary Approaches to Stop Hypertension (DASH) diet • Aerobic exercise
Type 2 diabetes, insulin resistance, obesity	• Weight reduction • Aerobic and resistance exercise
Physical inactivity	• Physical activity
Psychosocial dysfunction	• Group exercise programming • Psychological counseling
Tobacco use	• Nicotine replacement pharmacologic therapy • Group smoking cessation program

Based on Fleg et al. 2002.

appropriate use of pharmacologic therapy when indicated.

Dyslipidemia

Substantial data support the effectiveness of lipid-lowering therapy for improving morbidity and mortality in older patients with CHD.[26,27] The beneficial results of lipid lowering in older patients are similar to those in younger patients, but the absolute risk reduction for both all-cause and CHD risk is approximately twice as high for older patients. The National Cholesterol Education Program (NCEP) III guidelines should be followed with almost all patients aiming for low-density lipoprotein cholesterol <100 mg/dL; <70 mg/dL is considered an "option."[28] Efforts at optimizing the dietary pattern for older patients should include nutrition education for all CR/SP patients and nutritional consults for selected older patients with T2DM or a clinical indication for weight reduction. The CR/SP role should include obtaining a lipid profile at entry and actively assisting in the management of pharmacologic lipid-lowering therapy through frequent contact with the primary care physician.[29] Note that in certain older patients (such as those with a prolonged and complicated postoperative course, weight loss, and sarcopenia [diminished muscle mass]), the provision of taste-intensive calories to improve calorie intake to maximize weight and muscle regain should supersede the dietary treatment of dyslipidemia in the near term, given the poor prognosis associated with sarcopenia and frailty.

Hypertension

More than 65% of individuals age 65 or older have HTN; and in a recent survey, 71% of individuals entering CR/SP carried a diagnosis of HTN.[1] The role of CR/SP in HTN control includes a baseline assessment of blood pressure control, assistance with the diagnosis of newly discovered HTN with referral back to the primary physician for appropriate therapy, and frequent surveillance of blood pressure during participation. Perhaps most important is intervening with lifestyle-related treatments to assist with blood pressure control. Interventions include weight loss when appropriate; aerobic exercise; and the Dietary Approaches to Stop Hypertension (DASH) diet, which effectively overlaps with heart-healthy diets.[30-32] Frequent reporting of blood pressure

measures in CR/SP is always helpful in assisting physicians with long-term control.

Diabetes, Insulin Resistance, and Obesity

T2DM, insulin resistance syndrome, and abdominal obesity are common in older patients with CHD and together occur in more than 50% of patients.[33] These three factors are part of a continuum and from a lifestyle point of view are addressed with similar lifestyle interventions. T2DM and insulin resistance cluster with other obesity-related risk factors including dyslipidemia, HTN, inflammation, and clotting abnormalities.[34] The metabolic syndrome has been shown to be common in patients with coronary artery disease (CAD) and is strongly and inversely related to age.[35] Furthermore, therapeutic lifestyle change delivered through CR/SP and exercise training improved multiple parameters association with metabolic syndrome. The CR/SP program is an optimal site for lifestyle treatment of inactivity and obesity, since patients have essentially agreed to participate in the requisite aerobic exercise component. A more recent study demonstrated a decrease in the rate of metabolic syndrome from 59% to 31% when exercise was combined with a behavioral weight loss program in overweight patients with CHD.[36] The optimal exercise approach is a low-intensity, longer-duration, high-frequency (almost daily) walking program.[36] A structured weight loss program, however, is necessary and can be organized in the CR/SP setting based on previously described models.[37,38] For patients with established T2DM, frequent assessment of blood glucose is advised. Exercise and weight loss often requires adjustment of medication to avoid hypoglycemia.

Physical Inactivity

Physical inactivity is a risk factor for the development and progression of CHD. Older patients who begin physical activity in the CR/SP setting or elsewhere have an improved overall health status and prognosis.[8,21] Note that older CHD patients entering CR/SP programs are remarkably inactive, with less than 15% falling into an "active" range as reflected in daily step counts.[39] Additionally, older CHD patients are significantly less fit, as measured by peak aerobic capacity, than middle-aged patients at entry into CR/SP.[15] Recommendations for increasing exercise participation should not be limited to structured CR/

SP sessions but should employ a broader interpretation of exercise programming and include leisure activities, as well as an active approach to daily activities such as taking stairs and doing housework. The harmful effects of prolonged sitting should be emphasized and patients should be encouraged to interrupt periods of sitting at 20-30 minute intervals with brief (even 2-3 minutes) episodes of activity.

Psychosocial Dysfunction

Rates of mental depression, social isolation, and anxiety are high in older CHD patients.[40] These factors not only affect quality of life but are significant predictors of long-term medical outcomes and may be influenced by psychosocial interventions and exercise.[41-43] CR/SP programs need to screen for these factors at baseline using instruments such as the Geriatric Depression Questionnaire or the Patient Health Questionnaire-9 (PHQ-9), although the presence of true depression is usually diagnosed at a formal psychiatric interview.[44,45] Furthermore, psychosocial dysfunction needs to be monitored as patients progress in CR/SP, with active referral of high-risk and nonresponding individuals for counseling or medical therapy. CR/SP providers should also address end-of-life issues including resuscitation (code/no-code) status and advance directives (end of life).[46]

Tobacco Use

Smoking cessation reduces cardiac morbidity and mortality even when accomplished over the age of 70 years.[47,48] Interventions that have proven effective in younger patients, such as nicotine replacement therapy and group and individualized counseling, have also been shown to be safe in patients with CHD, including those who are older.[48,49]

Cardiac Rehabilitation in Younger Patients

Younger patients (<40 years of age) have issues that can be characterized in general but are often specific to gender, including vocation and family as the highest priorities. Obesity is common; but muscle mass, strength, and physical functioning are more often in the normal range compared to values in older people. Time, pressure, and anxiety are common with the addition of unexpected illness, potential lifestyle adjustments, and the time required for CR/SP program participation. Younger patients with CHD often present with complex risk factor profiles and an urgency with regard to decreasing risk-associated behavior.

Younger Women

Whereas women overall compose roughly 25% of CR/SP participants in contemporary programs, participation of younger women (age <40 years) is exceedingly rare (only about 1-2% of all participants).[1] The younger women are a heterogeneous group, with approximately 50% carrying a diagnosis other than obstructive CHD. These include congenital heart disease, chronic heart failure, primary pulmonary HTN, and coronary artery spasm in the setting of normal coronary arteries. Younger women with standard obstructive CHD are characterized by high rates of obesity, T2DM, and cigarette smoking.[6] Depression and anxiety are common, and a proactive program of exercise and risk reduction is preferable to denial and lack of preventive action (see the section on tobacco use in chapter 8 for more detail).

Younger Men

Younger men constitute about 4% to 5% of all patients attending CR/SP.[1] Compared with older men, younger men with CHD have higher rates of obesity with its associated metabolic risk factors of insulin resistance (or T2DM), dyslipidemia, and HTN.[50] Younger men also have higher measures of anxiety, anger, and hostility.[50] If weight loss can be accomplished, insulin resistance, hyperlipidemia, and HTN all improve; thus this should be a high priority in the CR/SP process.[35] The importance of risk reduction and long-term exercise adherence in these individuals needs to be recurrently emphasized. For younger men who perform physical work, such as construction work, reproducing work requirements in the CR/SP setting with close cardiovascular monitoring decreases patient anxiety regarding return to the workforce. Creative solutions to CR/SP scheduling can be important for younger patients given that work and family issues often preclude thrice-weekly sessions at the CR/SP center. Once-weekly visits to the center, with prescription of home exercise, as well as arrangements for preventive teaching and risk factor treatment, are important considerations versus the provision of no services at all.

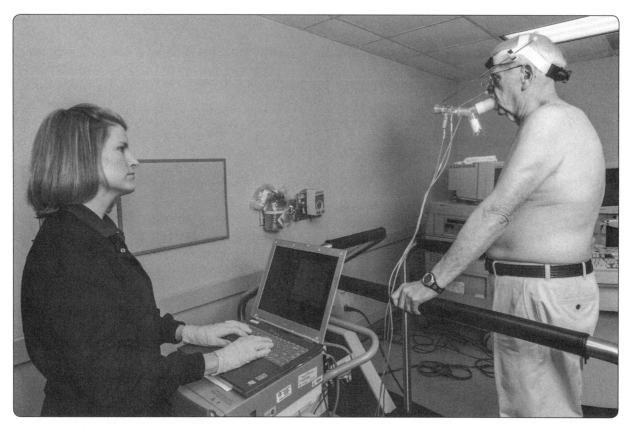

In the CR/SP setting, close cardiovascular monitoring decreases patient anxiety regarding return to normal activities and the workforce.

Women

Coronary heart disease is the leading cause of death in women[1]; its manifestations carry enormous personal and societal burdens in an increasingly diverse CHD population.[2] Nearly half a million American women are hospitalized annually with an acute coronary syndrome (ACS); women are twice as likely as men to have poor outcomes after coronary artery bypass graft (CABG) surgery and 1.5 times more likely to die within a year of a myocardial infarction (MI).[1] The reasons particular subgroups of women have more angina, higher mortality, higher rehospitalization rates, or increased prevalence of MI compared to men are unclear.[3-5] Women typically experience their first MI about 9 years later in life than men.[6] Various risk factors are more prevalent and associated with greater mortality risk in women with CHD than in men with CHD (see table 9.4). These factors include HTN, obesity, smoking, T2DM, glucose intolerance, hypercholesterolemia, and elevated triglycerides.[1,7]

Compared to men, women younger than 50 years have a higher incidence of risk factors and comorbidities such as diabetes.[8] Young women with sudden cardiac death are more likely to have coronary plaque erosion, whereas plaque rupture is more common in men and in older women.[9] Coronary angiography is used less often in women because their risk of death from CHD has been historically underestimated; yet women have significantly higher mortality rates than do men, regardless of age.[10] Compared to men, women ≤45 years with MI are significantly more likely to present without chest pain and have higher in-hospital mortality.[4] The reason for this excess risk is unclear, but the absence of chest pain may be more predictive of mortality in younger women with MI than in other similarly aged groups. Glaring escalations in CHD mortality of young women are emerging, with rates having increased an average of 1.3% between 1997 and 2002 among women aged 35 to 44 years.[11] Among over 10,000 hospitalized MI patients, the short-term death rates were much higher in younger women than

Table 9.4 Physiological Presentations of Younger and Older Women With Coronary Heart Disease Compared to Men[1,4,13,22-25]

	Younger women	Older women
PHYSIOLOGICAL		
Less obstructive coronary heart disease	✓	✓
Less Q-wave infarction	✓	✓
Prevalent congestive heart failure		✓ ✓
RISK FACTORS		
Diabetes	✓ ✓	✓
Obesity	✓ ✓	✓
Hypertension	✓	✓ ✓
Tobacco consumption	✓ ✓	✓
Musculoskeletal limitations	✓	✓ ✓
Inactivity	✓ ✓	✓
Dyslipidemia	✓	✓ ✓
Family history	✓ ✓	✓
Elevated C-reactive protein	✓ ✓	✓
ISCHEMIC SYMPTOMS		
Unusual fatigue	✓ ✓	✓ ✓
Dyspnea	✓ ✓	✓
Nausea or vomiting	✓ ✓	✓
Chest pressure	✓ ✓	✓
Sleep disturbance	✓ ✓	✓ ✓
Anxiety	✓ ✓	✓
Weak or heavy arms	✓ ✓	✓
Hand or arm tingling	✓ ✓	✓
Dizziness or fainting	✓ ✓	✓

Note: There is no standard definition of "younger women," but the term typically refers to premenopausal women. Checkmarks indicate that the presentation or symptom is more common in women than men; two checkmarks a greater incidence.

in younger men.[12] Young women plausibly possess biological and genetic factors predisposing them to more aggressive CHD.[13-16] Consequences of the obesity epidemic, the dramatic increase in the metabolic syndrome and T2DM, and inadequate use of efficacious therapies suggest a serious future public health burden of CHD in young women predisposed to early-onset MI.[17-19]

Intensive public education efforts by the American Heart Association, the American College of Cardiology, and the National Heart, Lung and Blood Institute have led to an increased awareness of CHD as the leading cause of death among women, from 30% in 1997 to 54% in 2009.[20] African American and Hispanic women, compared to white women, have less awareness, which poses continued challenges for education campaigns.[21]

Women are more likely than men to have a higher cardiovascular disease risk presentation and less likely than their male peers to have typical central chest pain.[22-24] Clusters of ischemic symptoms in women, particularly in young African American women, can include unusual fatigue, shortness of breath, any chest pain or discomfort, weak or heavy arms, frequent indigestion, palpitations, or tingling in the hands or arms.[23] In contrast, older women, more often white, tend to have fewer symptoms, smoke less, and manifest less obesity. Despite having unique symptoms and more physical limitations, women have less obstructive CHD than men along the spectrum of acute coronary syndromes[25] and when referred for revascularization.[26]

An important aspect of CR/SP programs is the assessment of functional capabilities and perceptions of health status, frequently measured with the SF-36 Health Survey[27] at program entry to individualize patient treatment plans and after program completion to evaluate improvements gained from participation.[28] Women with CHD report poorer perceptions of health than men, both at entry and after completing CR/SP.[29] Improving patients' perceptions of their health, in addition to their objective clinical health status, may foster long-term lifestyle behavior change and enhance their overall quality of life.[30]

Psychosocial Considerations

Women with CHD not only manifest particularly adverse psychosocial profiles and suboptimal social support but also report distinctive gender-specific CR/SP preferences and needs (see table 9.5).[31-33] Socioeconomically disadvantaged women are particularly plagued with psychosocial stressors that interfere with the self-management of CHD.[34] These stressors can manifest in fear, anger, social isolation, and a perceived burden to family and friends. Depressive symptoms are pervasive in women with CHD,[34-37] particularly at younger ages.[33,38-42] Depression reportedly confers up to a fourfold increased risk of CHD mortality[43,44] and more adverse cardiovascular outcomes in women than in men.[45-46] Women with depressive symptoms have a twofold increased risk of noncompletion of CR/SP.[47] Evidence supports the association between depression and poor behavioral compliance in CR/SP patients, conceivably because depression thwarts motivation for behavior change.[48-50] Nonadherence to CR/SP, including medication use and CR/SP completion,[51-52] exacerbates unfavorable outcomes associated with depressive symptoms. Of 30,000 elderly Americans with CHD, patients attending all 36 prescribed CR/SP sessions compared to those attending one session had a 47% lower risk of death and a 31% lower risk of MI.[53] Published guidelines[54] recommend routine screening of all CHD patients using the two-item Patient Health Questionnaire (PHQ-2);[55] patients with a positive PHQ-2 can then be evaluated with the nine-item PHQ-9,[56] with treatment referral for patients with elevated scores. Women should also be assessed for psychological or psychosocial considerations such as anxiety, anger or hostility, social isolation, marital or family distress, sexual dysfunction, and substance abuse; and appropriate referrals for psychiatric or psychological care should be made when needed.[57]

Gender-Specific Barriers to CR/SP Participation

Referral to CR/SP is a class I recommendation (useful and effective) for women with CHD.[58] Despite international endorsement of CR/SP[28,59-60] and strong evidence of improved morbidity and mortality with CR/SP participation,[47,61-62] only 15% to 20% of eligible women use these programs.[63-66] Patient-oriented, system-level, and environmental factors partially account for poor CR attendance among eligible women (see table 9.6).[60,65,67] Lack of physician endorsement of CR/SP continues to be a predictor of poor attendance,[68-70] while female gender is a significant patient-level predictor.[64,71] Women particularly underrepresented in CR/SP include those who are elderly, who are obese and sedentary, who smoke, who are socioeconomically disadvantaged, who are unmarried, or who are nonwhite, as well as women with greater comorbidity, lower exercise capacity, less social support, less education,

Table 9.5 Psychosocial Considerations for Women With Coronary Heart Disease Compared to Men[22-25,33-41]

Psychosocial considerations	Younger women	Older women
Depressive symptoms	✓✓	✓
Anxiety disorder	✓✓	✓
Anger or hostility	✓	✓
Marital or family dysfunction	✓✓	✓
Social isolation	✓	✓✓
Substance abuse	✓✓	✓
Suboptimal quality of life	✓✓	✓
Sexual dysfunction	✓	✓
Low self-efficacy	✓	✓
Sleep disruption	✓	✓
Fear	✓	✓

Note: Checkmarks indicate that the presentation or symptom is more common in women than men; two checkmarks indicate a greater incidence.

Table 9.6 Barriers to CR/SP for Women With Coronary Heart Disease

Barrier	Potential solution
PATIENT FACTORS[60,64,67,78,102,103]	
1. Uninterested or uninformed of CR/SP benefits, believe that CR is unnecessary or that home exercise is sufficient	Determine knowledge deficits, dispel myths, respect values and preferences, clearly inform and educate patient and family
2. Short hospital stay, poor recall of discharge information	Provide clear discharge instructions, promote CR/SP, coordinate continuous care, shared decision making
3. Low educational attainment, low health literacy	Determine understanding of CHD, preferences, and goals and provide health literacy–appropriate materials
4. Inadequate self-efficacy and confidence	Determine stage of readiness to change behavior, explore ambivalence using motivational interviewing counseling style
5. Racial or ethnic minority	Deliver culturally sensitive care
6. Extremes of age	Personalize program for young and elderly women
7. Psychosocial stressors, anxiety, social isolation, divorced or widowed, caregiving obligations	Screen and assess for psychological distress, particularly depression, anxiety, anger, and marital distress, and deliver counseling interventions for stress management and coping skills
8. Work-related obligations	Have flexible facility hours and meeting times
9. Dislike mixed-gender CR/SP groups, perceive exercise as painful and tiring	Consider gender-specific sessions with creative aerobic and resistance exercise options or home-based community programs
MEDICAL FACTORS[54,60,104]	
1. Depression	Screen and consult with clinical psychologist
2. Limiting comorbidities or musculoskeletal limitations	Individualize aerobic and resistance exercise program
HEALTH CARE SYSTEM FACTORS[60,69,104]	
1. Lack of referral, weak endorsement	Use automatic referral systems in hospital
2. Competing priorities among health care professionals	Identify a CR/SP champion and coordinator, implement performance measures
3. Time-consuming enrollment process	Streamline referral and enrollment process
4. Lack of CR/SP program within 60 min from home, limited parking and transportation access	Use home-based programs, telemedicine, Internet, mobile phone, community program delivery options
5. Hours of operation	Increase coverage and resources for center-based programs

competing family obligations, transportation barriers, and incomplete medical insurance coverage.[64-65,67,72-78] Depressive symptoms are linked to suboptimal CR attendance as well.[48,50,72,79-81] It has also been posited that women find CR/SP exercise tiring and painful,[69] dislike public or mixed-gender exercise,[82] and perceive unmet emotional needs, all of which deter women from enrolling, attending, and completing CR/SP.[83] Raising awareness among physicians regarding the benefits of CR/SP for women could provide more women the opportunity to achieve optimum health following a cardiovascular event.

Implications for CR/SP Program Delivery for Women

Creative strategies to address issues relevant to women, an underserved segment of CR/SP populations, are needed (see table 9.7).[84] Recognition of unique gender-based psychosocial issues potentially affecting quality of life has motivated recommendations for efficacious CR/SP programs designed for women.[70,85-86] Though some lament that gender-tailored risk reduction approaches for women are largely absent,[87] others have championed the concept of gender-specific tailoring in

CR/SP programs.[86,88] Where feasible, gender-specific programs, tailored to individual needs and readiness to change, may be more effective than traditional CR/SP programs in meeting the unique needs of women.[65,83,86,88,89] A gender-tailored, stage-of-change–matched CR program exclusively for women was found to be an effective attendance-enhancing strategy for women referred to CR/SP.[78] This program also led to significant improvements on four dimensions of health, specifically vitality, social functioning, mental health, and general health.[90] This theoretically driven CR/SP intervention tailored for women, compared to a mixed-gender CR/SP program, also led to a greater improvement in depressive symptoms[81] and quality of life.[91] It has been postulated that mechanisms other than, or in addition to, exercise and education likely account for the observed improvements. The gender-exclusive social support exchanged between women receiving exercise training and psychoeducational sessions as a cohesive cohort may foster motivation for change through shared support for behavior change and psychosocial need fulfillment.

The progressive nature of CHD requires persistent management of behavioral risk factors. However, the impact of CR/SP can begin to fade within six months of completion. Women need information and skills in disease self-management that empower them with confidence and self-efficacy after CR/SP completion. Theoretically based behavior change strategies (see chapter 3, on behavior modification) and counseling styles, including motivational interviewing and readiness-to-change–staged strategies,[92-94] may be effective for women who are ambivalent about adherence to therapeutic regimens. Encouraging women to voice their reasons for making positive behavior changes can assist them in taking greater responsibility for moving in the direction of lifelong change. Women are more likely to be engaged in activating their own motivations when CR/SP professionals listen to their preferences and address obstacles to changing health behavior that they express. The loss of professional contact after completion of CR/SP may be less detrimental to behavioral and psychological gains achieved during active intervention.

When transportation or home obligations limit center-based CR/SP participation, consideration of a home program is necessary. Home-based models may be an effective and realistic alternative for women with significant barriers related to structured outpatient programs.[95-96] There are also health care delivery models that use mobile phones, Internet, and communication technologies to deliver CR/SP services to outpatients in their homes.[97-98] Individually tailored, Internet-based interventions could provide women with tools and applications for setting goals and improving risk factors for CHD through behavioral self-management. Interaction between women at a distance and the CR/SP case manager remains critical to program efficacy. Additional interventions to assist with promoting behavior change include self-monitoring of food intake and exercise behavior as well as computer-assisted reminders and other electronic communications to support behavior change.[99-101]

Racial and Cultural Diversity

Over the past decade, health and health care disparities, along with the mandate for cultural competency in health care, have become central themes in health care education, research prac-

Table 9.7 CR/SP Considerations for Women With Coronary Heart Disease[23,99,105]

Exercise	Education and counseling
Exercise choices to accommodate musculoskeletal limitations	Recognition of symptom cluster unique to women
Creative exercise alternatives according to personal preference	Promotion of early health care seeking
Strength training for functional independence and bone health	Management of psychosocial issues
Encourage daily aerobic physical activity	Training for disease self-management
Foster self-confidence and self-efficacy for safe exercise	Peer support groups
Emphasize lifelong need for exercise	Chronicity of coronary heart disease

tices, clinical care, and policy. *Health disparities* refers to the differences in health and health care between groups of people. A health disparity can be defined as a particular type of health inequality, arising from race, culture, environment, gender, age, or socioeconomic status, that places the individual at a disadvantage regarding health.[1] Health disparities have been identified in a wide range of health measures, including access to health insurance; life expectancy; and prevalence of specific diseases, such as HTN, diabetes, and cardiovascular disease.[2] Health and health care disparities within racial and ethnic minority groups have plagued health care access and use of services, and have captured the attention of the federal government, regulatory organizations, providers, academic institutions, and community-based organizations. National concerns regarding

social determinants, social injustices, and their impact on health care disparities have raised an awareness of the understanding of culture in health care delivery from a patient, provider, and system perspective.[3]

One of the most challenging issues for the health care system is the fact that over 30% of the total population is composed of ethnicities other than non-Hispanic whites. By the year 2050, this proportion is expected to reach more than 50%.[4] In this regard, the U.S. Census Bureau in 2010 revealed that the vast majority of the growth in the total population had come from increases in persons who reported their race as other than white and their race or ethnicity as Hispanic or Latino in various counties across the United States (figure 9.1).[5-6] In 2010, there were 50.5 million Hispanics in the United States, representing 16%

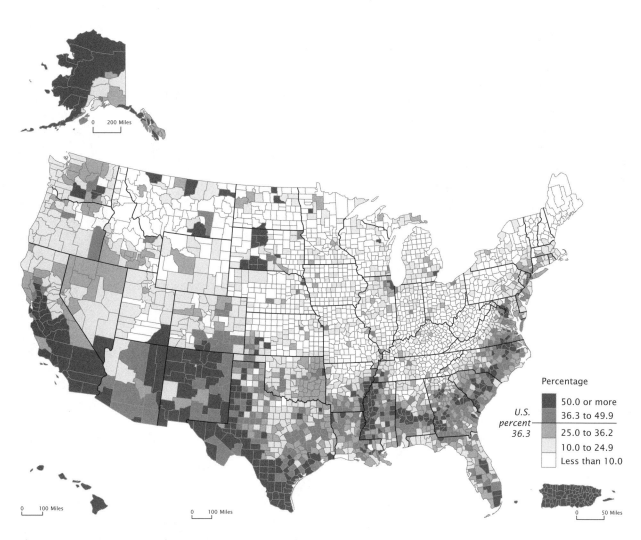

Figure 9.1 Minority population as a percentage of county population, 2010.

of the total population.[5-6] According to the U.S. Census, the Hispanic population was projected to nearly triple, from 46.7 million to 132.8 million, between 2008 and 2050, making one in three U.S. residents Hispanic or Latino. The African American population is also expected to increase and to represent 22% of the total population, while Asian Americans are predicted to constitute 10% of the total U.S. residents.[5-6] Therefore, a national health care action plan for a culturally competent health care delivery system needs to be endorsed and implemented.

Historical Perspective

In 1999, the U.S. Congress requested that the Institute of Medicine (IOM) examine the realities of racial and ethnic disparities in the health care system. The findings were published in 2002 in a document titled *Unequal Treatment: Confronting Racial and Ethnic Disparities in Health Care.*[7] The report highlighted the body of research that documents significant variation in access to care and quality of care provided to racial and ethnic minority patients in the United States.[7] The conclusions indicated that biases and prejudices of health care providers could contribute to the racial and ethnic disparities among minorities.[7] Therefore, the IOM strongly advocated that cross-cultural education and cultural competency be included in all health care provider programs to address provider biases and prejudices.[8] The IOM recommended initiatives to increase awareness among the general public, health care providers, academic institutions, insurance companies, and policy makers about disparities in order to align equity across all boundaries of industries and organizations involved in the delivery of health care services.[8]

Healthy People is a science-based public health initiative that provides national goals and objectives with 10-year targets designed to guide national health promotion and disease prevention efforts to improve the health of all people in the United States. During the past two decades, one of the overarching goals of Healthy People has focused on disparities. In Healthy People 2000, the aim was to reduce health disparities among Americans. In Healthy People 2010, it was to eliminate, not just reduce, health disparities. In Healthy People 2020, that goal was expanded even further: to achieve health equity, eliminate disparities, and improve the health of all groups.[9]

A review of Healthy People 2010 reported that despite significant improvements in health in the United States, health disparities persisted and had seen only minimal improvements.[10] In a 2004 report, *Missing Persons: Minorities in the Health Professions,* the Sullivan Commission prioritized the importance of including minorities in the health care workforce and the significance of setting standards in cultural competence.[11] The commission emphasized the importance of minority health care workers to provide care in underserved communities and to eliminate language barriers that may affect patient safety and quality of care. The American Association of Cardiovascular and Pulmonary Rehabilitation (AACVPR) conducted a survey of all of its members in 2010, which revealed that race of both staff and patients was predominantly white (~96%).[12] Diversity of patient populations who are referred and enrolled and who attend CR/SP, as well as of CR/SP professionals who care for this population, is a focus of study for AACVPR.

Cardiovascular Disease, Risk Factors, and Access to Health Care

According to the Office of Minority Health of the Department of Health and Human Services, heart disease is the leading killer among racial and ethnic minorities in the United States, accounting for 26% of all deaths in 2006.[13] Individuals in specific subgroups defined by race, ethnicity, socioeconomic status, and geography (zip codes) have disproportionate cardiovascular risk factor burden and risk of MI, heart failure, stroke, and other cardiovascular events (table 9.8). These individuals also have a worse outcome after these events, due to unrecognized and untreated risk factors that increase their cardiovascular risk burden and mortality.[13] One risk factor, obesity, has a high prevalence in minorities (table 9.8); hence, effective policies and environmental strategies that promote healthy eating and physical activity are needed for all populations and geographic areas, but particularly for populations and areas disproportionally affected by obesity.[14] Unfortunately, as of 2007, no state had met the Healthy People 2010 objective to reduce to 15% the prevalence of obesity among U.S. adults.[14]

The literature consistently demonstrates underuse of medical therapy, diagnostics, and revascularization procedures in women and multiple racial and ethnic groups. For example, African

Table 9.8 Cardiovascular Risk Burden (Percentages Are Prevalence of the Disease or Risk Factor)

	Asian and Pacific Islander (A/PI)	American Indian and American Native (AI/AN)	Hispanic	Non-Hispanic white (NHW)	Non-Hispanic black (NHB), African American (AA), and Black Caribbean
CAD	3.9%[13]	AI/AN have 1.2 times greater CAD prevalence than NHW; AN have highest PHD (36%) of all minorities[13]	5.8%	6.5%[27]	6.7%[13]
HTN	24%[13]	AI/AN have 1.3 times greater HTN prevalence than NHW[13]	Mexican Americans have 21.5% prevalence; Prevalence in women > men[13]	23%[27]	• 32.5% of NHB have HTN • NHB have 1.5 times greater HTN prevalence than NHW • NHB have >32% increase in stroke over any other minority group • NHB have 1.7 times greater chance of stroke than NHW • 60% of NHB with hypertension progress to ESRD[13]
Diabetes	8%[13]	9%[13]; prevalence is two times greater than in NHW[13]	10.6% prevalence; only 36% of Hispanic adults with diabetes receive all three recommended routine diabetes services (routine monitoring of blood glucose levels with hemoglobin A1c, dilated eye exam, foot exam), which is significantly lower than the 42% of non-Hispanic whites who would have received these services[13]	6.2%[13]	10.8% of NHB NHB have greater prevalence of DM, are 2.4 times more likely to die from DM than NHW, and have 1.7 times more hospitalizations related to DM complications than NHW[13]
Obesity	9%[13]	AI/AN have a 1.6 times greater prevalence than NHW[13]	Mexican Americans 28.7%[27]	25.6%[27]	51%[13]
Smoking	11.6%[27]	AI/AN have a prevalence of 33.5%[13]	Mexican American men 18.7% Mexican American women 9.7%[27]	22.8%[27]	Men 25.5% Women 17.1%[27]
Heart failure					• NHB are diagnosed at average age of 39 with HTN, obesity, CRD • At age 50 years HF is more prevalent in NHB than NHW[31]
Lipids	28.%[13]		Mexican American men 17.6% Mexican American women 14.4%[27]	Men 15.5% Women 18%[13]	Men 10.9% Women 13.3%[27]

Abbreviations: CAD, coronary artery disease; PHD, premature heart disease; CHD, coronary heart disease; ESRD, end-stage renal disease; HTN, hypertension; DM, diabetes mellitus; HF, heart failure; CRD, chronic renal disease.

Americans and women are less likely to receive cardiac angiograms or revascularization following a heart attack. Minorities and women are also less likely to have follow-up revascularization procedures after cardiac catheterization compared with Caucasians and men.[13] Hernandez and colleagues[15] reported that women and black patients were significantly less likely than white patients to receive implantable cardioverter–defibrillator therapy, independent of other characteristics such as patient preferences, age, hospital characteristics, and comorbidity.

Social economic status (SES) has also been shown to be an important and independent factor in the etiology and progression of cardiovascular disease (CVD). When SES is characterized in terms of education, employment, and income, a consistent inverse relationship exists between these indicators and risk factors for CVD. Even after controlling for SES, health insurance, and clinical factors, racial and ethnic inequalities in health status and care exist.[16]

The disparities in access to health care and quality of care are accompanied by disparities in awareness and access to knowledge about a healthy cardiovascular lifestyle. An American Heart Association (AHA) survey revealed that African American and Hispanic women have the lowest risk factor awareness of any racial or ethnic group but have the highest risk burden.[17] Cardiovascular and CR/SP outcomes were analyzed in 72,817 patients (2000-2007) from 156 hospitals participating in the AHA "Get With the Guidelines program."[18] Overall, 56% were referred to outpatient CR/SP at discharge. Older age and non–ST-segment elevation MI were associated with decreased odds of CR/SP referral, despite the fact that the benefits of participation are proportionally greater in many of these patients. Only 7% and 5% of African Americans and Hispanics, respectively, were referred to CR/SP. Variables associated with reduced referrals for nonwhites included language barrier; transportation problems; lack of culturally appropriate information on nutrition, lifestyle modification, and other educational topics; learning styles and values and beliefs relating to adherence; need to return to work; and funding for people in financial need. Dropout rates in CR/SP among both African American and Hispanic women were higher than for whites. Reasons cited included work conflicts, child care, and domestic issues.[18]

In summary, differences in health status across racial and ethnic groups have been widely documented. However, disparities should be now be analyzed from different perspectives, including epidemiologic, genetic, clinical, geographic issues; lifestyle choices; psychological profile; socioeconomic inequalities; and sociopolitical issues. Care providers can close the CVD gap by improving their knowledge and understanding of the interactions between culture, environment, socioeconomic status, and health and by implementing education programs in underserved communities.

Cultural Diversity and Competent Care

Cultural diversity refers to the differences between people based on a shared ideology and valued set of beliefs, norms, customs, and meanings evidenced by a particular way of life.[19] *Cultural competency* was defined by Cross and colleagues[20] as "a set of congruent behaviors, attitudes and policies that come together in a system, agency or professional and enable that system, agency or professional to work effectively in cross-cultural situations." Cultural competency is a continuous, evolutionary process of embracing cultural awareness and knowledge to effectively communicate in a cross-cultural manner. Communication models directed at cultural competency include the LEARN Model,[21] which provides the following cultural competency framework:

L: Listen with sympathy and understanding to your patient's perception of the problem.

E: Explain your perceptions of the problem.

A: Acknowledge and discuss the differences and similarities.

R: Recommend treatment.

N: Negotiate agreement.

Another communicative model is the mnemonically named ETHNIC Model,[22] a framework for practicing culturally competent care:

E: Explanation (How do you explain your illness?)

T: Treatment (What treatment have you tried?)

H: Healers (Have you sought any advice from folk healers?)

N: Negotiate (mutually acceptable options)

I: (Agree on) Intervention

C: Collaboration (with patient, family, and healers)

Health care providers who have been exposed to this educational framework and have incorporated these models into the normal structure of the therapeutic encounter have been able to improve communication, heighten awareness of cultural issues in health care, and obtain better patient acceptance of treatment plans. The IOM[8] also suggests that the following five elements are essential to providing culturally competent health care:

- Valuing diversity
- Developing the capacity for self-assessment
- Raising awareness of dynamics inherent when cultures interact
- Using organizational processes to institutionalize cultural knowledge
- Striving to develop individual and organizational adaptations to diversity

In 1998, Tervalon and Murray-Garcia advocated that medical training embrace "cultural humility" rather than "cultural competence" in educational initiatives for physicians training in the 21st century.[23] Cultural humility is a process that requires an individual to continually engage in self-reflection, self-awareness, and self-critique as a lifelong reflective learner when assessing, treating, and evaluating patients who are not culturally congruent with the provider in race and ethnicity. Ongoing self-reflection and examination of provider biases and personal prejudices are important in order to skillfully engage patients in self-care activities to increase their cardiac and pulmonary wellness. This is a process that helps health care providers develop respectful, dynamic partnerships with their patients.

In the continuum of coronary care, CR/SP has been modeled to provide effective secondary prevention. Evidence-based research has demonstrated that CR/SP programs reduce mortality, improve functional capacity and quality of life, and decrease rates of rehospitalization for cardiac complications as well as overall medical costs in both women and men.[24] Davidson and colleagues[25] illuminate key strategies for increasing access of multiculturally diverse groups to CR/SP services. These include (1) increasing and recruiting participation of health professionals and health workers from target populations; (2) implementing strategies to promote engagement and participation of local communities through the training of community health care workers who share a race and ethnic concordance with the local population; (3) providing culturally appropriate resources and support to local services; and (4) acknowledging the impact of historical, social, and economic circumstances on adverse health outcomes in minority populations. A mandate for ongoing cultural competency training from governmental regulatory bodies and multispecialty health care professional organizations is critical to the success of these targeted strategies to decrease the cardiovascular burden of care in minority groups through referral, access, and enrollment of minorities to CR/SP programs.

Eliminating Health Care Disparities

According to the 2000 U.S. Census, an estimated 47 million people in the country spoke a language other than English.[26] In 2001, the U.S. Department of Health and Human Services, Office of Minority Health, published its National Standards for Culturally and Linguistically Appropriate Services (CLAS) to ensure cultural competence in health care. The 14 quality care standards incorporated three themes: culturally competent care (standards 1-3); language access services and proficiency in interpreter services (mandated) (standards 4-7); and organizational supports for cultural competence (standards 8-14) (see "Office of Minority Health's Recommended National Standards for Culturally and Linguistically Appropriate Services in Health Care").[27]

The National Institutes of Health (NIH) is developing and supporting research activities relevant to health and health care disparities, including training of underrepresented individuals, in order to promote a culturally diverse biomedical research enterprise.[28] Several approaches have been implemented. These include (1) the National Center for Minority Health Disparities Centers of Excellence, which conducts research on health disparities within several disease areas and conditions, such as cancer, cardiovascular diseases, stroke, diabetes, nutrition, obesity, and maternal and infant health; (2) Community-Based Participatory Research awards to engage scientists and communities in health disparities research; (3) Loan Repayment awards to promote

The fundamentals of culturally competent care

1. Health care organizations should ensure that patients/consumers[†] receive from all staff members effective, understandable, and respectful care that is provided in a manner compatible with their cultural health beliefs and practices and preferred language.

2. Health care organizations should implement strategies to recruit, retain, and promote at all levels of the organization a diverse staff and leadership that are representative of the demographic characteristics of the service area.

3. Health care organizations should ensure that staff at all levels and across all disciplines receive ongoing education and training in CLAS delivery.

Speaking of culturally competent care

1. Health care organizations must offer and provide language assistance services, including bilingual staff and interpreter services, at no cost to each patient/consumer with limited English proficiency at all points of contact and in a timely manner during all hours of operation.

2. Health care organizations must provide to patients/consumers in their preferred language both verbal offers and written notices informing them of their right to receive language assistance services.

3. Health care organizations must ensure the competence of language assistance provided to limited English proficient patients/consumers by interpreters and bilingual staff. Family and friends should not be used to provide interpretation services (except on request by the patient/consumer).

4. Health care organizations must make available easily understood patient-related materials and post signage in the languages of the commonly encountered groups and/or groups represented in the service area.

Structuring culturally competent care

1. Health care organizations should develop, implement, and promote a written strategic plan that outlines clear goals, policies, operational plans, and management accountability/oversight mechanisms to provide CLAS.

2. Health care organizations should conduct initial and ongoing organizational self-assessments of CLAS-related activities and are encouraged to integrate cultural and linguistic competence-related measures into their internal audits, performance improvement programs, patient satisfaction assessments, and outcomes-based evaluations.

3. Health care organizations should ensure that data on the individual patient's/consumer's race, ethnicity, and spoken and written language are collected in health records, integrated into the organization's management information systems, and periodically updated.

4. Health care organizations should maintain a current demographic, cultural, and epidemiological profile of the community as well as a needs assessment to accurately plan for and implement services that respond to the cultural and linguistic characteristics of the service area.

5. Health care organizations should develop participatory, collaborative partnerships with communities and use a variety of formal and informal mechanisms to facilitate community and patient/consumer involvement in designing and implementing CLAS-related activities.

6. Health care organizations should ensure that conflict and grievance resolution processes are culturally and linguistically sensitive and capable of identifying, preventing, and resolving cross-cultural conflicts or complaints by patients/consumers.

7. Health care organizations are encouraged to make available regularly to the public information about their progress and successful innovations in implementing the CLAS standards and to provide public notice in their communities about the availability of this information.

CLAS standards are nonregulatory and therefore do not have the force and effect of law. The standards are not mandatory, but they greatly assist health care providers and organizations in responding effectively to their patients' cultural and linguistic needs. Compliance with Title VI of the Civil Rights Act of 1964 is mandatory and requires health care providers and organizations that receive federal financial assistance to take reasonable steps to ensure that persons with limited English proficiency have meaningful access to services.

†CLAS standards use the term "patients/consumers" to refer to "individuals, including accompanying family members, guardians, or companions, seeking physical or mental health care services, or other health-related services" (comprehensive final report, p. 5; see http://minorityhealth.hhs.gov/templates/browse.aspx?lvl=2&lvlID=15).

Reprinted from Department of Health and Human Services Office of Minority Health, 2000, *National standards for culturally and linguistically appropriate services in health care*. Available: http://minorityhlates/browse.aspx?lvl=2&lvlID=15.

research careers in basic, clinical, and behavioral research for young scientists from underserved communities; (4) the Minority Health and Health Disparities International Research Training awards to support young scientists conducting scientific research abroad; and (5) The Bridges to the Future Program, which helps students transition from an associate degree to a baccalaureate degree and from a master's degree to a doctoral degree.

Several studies addressing CVD in racial and ethnic minorities and individuals with low socioeconomic status have been published. The Multi-Ethnic Study of Atherosclerosis (MESA) was conducted from July 2000 to 2008 to investigate the prevalence, correlates, and progression of subclinical CVD in a population-based sample of 6,500 African Americans, Hispanic Americans, and Asian Americans aged 45 to 84 years.[29] The Jackson Heart Study assessed the physiological, environmental, social, and genetic factors related to CVD and the high rates of complications from HTN in African Americans, including stroke, kidney disease, and congestive heart disease.[30]

Other studies evaluating CVD in racial and ethnic minorities include the Strong Heart Study[31] of American Indians and the Genetics of Coronary Artery Disease in Alaska Natives study.[32]

Conclusion

CR/SP has been shown to reduce mortality, improve functional capacity and quality of life, decrease rates of rehospitalization for cardiac complications, and decrease medical costs in all patients regardless of gender, race, and ethnicity. However, in the CVD spectrum of care, health care disparities have been consistently reported in primary and secondary prevention, for example in referral and enrollment to CR/SP programs.[25] Health care disparities represent a significant problem in the health care system in the United States. Raising awareness of the problem and establishing comprehensive multilevel policies and strategies to improve the cultural competence of the health care delivery system are imperative. The sidebar "Useful Resources in Raising Racial and Cultural Awareness" provides examples of resources which can be helpful in raising

Useful Resources in Raising Racial and Cultural Awareness

Culturally and Linguistically Appropriate Services in Health Care Resources

www.thinkculturalhealth.hhs.gov

Cross Cultural Health Care Program

1200 12th Ave. S.

Seattle, WA 98144

206-621-4161

www.xculture.org

Diversity Rx

www.diversityrx.org

Initiative to Eliminate Racial and Ethnic Disparities in Health

U.S. Department of Health and Human Services

www.raceandhealth.hhs.gov

National Center for Cultural Competence

3307 M St. NW, Ste. 401

Washington, DC 20007-3935

1-800-788-2066

e-mail: cultural@gunet.georgetown.edu

Office of Minority Health

Health Resources and Services Administration

5600 Fishers Lane, 10-49

Rockville, MD 20857

301-443-2964

www.hrsa.dhhs.gov/dmh

Office of Minority and Women's Health Cultural Competence Program

Bureau of Primary Health Care

Health Resources and Services Administration

4350 East West Hwy., 3rd Floor

Bethesda, MD 20814

301-594-4490

www.bphc.hrsa.gov/omwh/omwh_20.htm

awareness. The whole of the health care system must be prepared to meet the cultural, linguistic, and educational needs of the diverse and changing population.

Revascularization and Valve Surgery

Contemporary CR/SP delivers individualized programs of prescribed exercise, education, and risk factor modification that focus on specific outcomes and performance measures.[1] The specific components of a comprehensive program have been previously published.[2] These programmatic core components should be applied and individualized to accommodate patients following revascularization and valve replacement or repair. In addition, program staff should have the aggregate knowledge and skills to safely and effectively implement programs in these kinds of patients.[3] For each patient subgroup in this chapter, this section addresses the following topics:

- Status of referral to CR/SP programs
- Special considerations for exercise prescription and training
- Exercise testing
- Secondary prevention

The number of patients undergoing procedures to improve coronary blood flow or to correct damaged valves continues to increase. The most recent statistical report from the AHA[4] stated that the number of patients undergoing CABG, percutaneous coronary intervention (PCI), and valve surgeries annually was 242,000, 596,000, and 139,000, respectively. Males accounted for 58% to 72% of the procedures, and the majority of the procedures (53-64%) were performed on persons 65 years of age or older.

CR is a service covered by the Centers for Medicare and Medicaid Services for PCI (percutaneous transluminal coronary angioplasty, with or without stenting, and atherectomy), CABG, and heart valve repair and replacement.[5] These regulatory and legislative changes should significantly increase the number of patients being referred to CR following revascularization or valve surgery. Procedures include traditional open-chest coronary artery bypass graft surgery (CABGS) and valve replacement or repair, as well as newer minimally invasive procedures without cardiopul-

monary bypass. Percutaneous coronary interventions include balloon angioplasty, coronary artery stenting, atherectomy, or more than one of these. Summaries of special considerations for patients who have undergone these procedures are presented in "Special Considerations for Revascularization or Valve Repair Patients During Cardiac Rehabilitation" and "Intervention Strategies for Revascularization or Valve Patients."

Revascularization

Several revascularization procedures are used to treat patients with significant atherosclerotic lesions in the coronary artery circulation. These include CABG and minimally invasive coronary bypass (MID-CAB), as well as PCI.

Practice Considerations for Patients Who Have Undergone CABG

Traditional CABG requires a sternotomy and can be performed with or without the use of a cardiopulmonary bypass machine that delivers oxygenated blood through the circulatory system during surgery. CABG typically uses a section of saphenous vein (SVG) or an internal mammary artery (IMA) as a conduit to deliver blood distal to the lesion being bypassed. Radial or gastroepiploic arteries may also be used for this purpose. Saphenous vein grafts (SVGs) can develop intimal fibroplasia and vein graft atherosclerosis. SVGs have 1-year and 10-year patency rates of 75% to 90% and 50% to 60%, respectively. In contrast, IMA grafts have a 10-year patency rate greater than 90%.[6]

MID-CAB involves access to the heart via small incisions between ribs on the side of the chest and is performed without a cardiopulmonary bypass machine ("off-pump"). During off-pump procedures, the heart continues to beat, but the surgical area of the heart is immobilized using stabilizers. Compared to CABG, MID-CAB procedures have the clinical advantages of less blood loss, reduced trauma and pain, faster recovery, and decreased risk of infection. MID-CAB can also be performed using a robot; while a surgeon controls the surgical instruments using robotic arms.

The use of CR/SP services is a Class I recommendation in the 2011 American College of Cardiology Foundation (ACCF)/AHA practice guideline for CABG,[6] and referral to an outpatient CR/SP program is an AACVPR/ACC/AHA

Special Considerations for Patients Following Various Interventions

CABG

- Whether the procedure resulted in complete versus incomplete revascularization
- Whether the procedure included bypass of previous CABGS graft occlusion
- Precautions for upper extremity exercise and sternal healing
- Patient minimization of seriousness of CHD and idea that the patient has been "cured"
- Importance of comprehensive services for secondary prevention of CHD

PCI

- Potential for restenosis or coronary thrombosis at PCI sites and ongoing disease progression
- Patient minimization of seriousness of CHD and idea that patient has been "cured"
- Importance of comprehensive services for secondary prevention of CHD

Valvular Heart Disease (VHD)

- Importance of anticoagulation therapy and precautions for exercise-related injuries and bleeding
- Precautions for upper extremity exercise and sternal healing
- Avoidance of resistance-type exercise with severe aortic stenosis or insufficiency

Abbreviations: CABGS, coronary artery bypass graft surgery; CHD, coronary heart disease; PCI, percutaneous coronary intervention; VHD, valvular heart disease.

Intervention Strategies for Revascularization or Valve Patients

- The goal for each patient is the prevention of reocclusion and advancing atherosclerosis, as well as optimal exercise tolerance.
- The common problem for rehabilitation staff is to help patients understand that the disease has not been cured by the procedure and that secondary prevention is important for preventing subsequent clinical issues.

CABG WITH MIDLINE STERNOTOMY		
Safety	**Exercise**	**Education**
• Incision care, infection prevention	• Avoid heavy arm exercises until healed; upper body stretches and flexes and light resistance exercises are appropriate to promote mobility	• "Normal" postoperative signs and symptoms • Cerebral anoxia—temporary memory loss*
MINIMALLY INVASIVE DIRECT CORONARY ARTERY BYPASS (MID-CAB) AND PCI		
Safety	**Exercise**	**Education**
• Risk of reocclusion or coronary thrombosis	• Less deconditioning at outset may allow greater activity level	• Antiplatelet, anticoagulation • Early recognition of signs and symptoms of reocclusion
VALVE SURGERY		
Safety	**Exercise**	**Education**
• Incision care, infection prevention • Long-term anticoagulant therapy for mechanical valves	• Increased deconditioning and older—gradual start at outset; may result in conservative exercise prescription	• Medications, motivation, and encouragement to become more active • Anticoagulation and antibiotic prophylaxis issues

*If cardiopulmonary bypass machine was used.

performance measure.[7] However, use of CR/SP by patients following CABG tends to be low. A study of Medicare beneficiaries found that 31% of CABG patients used CR/SP, with significant variation by state and region.[8]

Physical activity including early ambulation and range of motion, as well as walking and cycling, is indicated during hospitalization for CABG to help avoid the deleterious effects of bed rest, including decreased functional capacity and thromboembolic complications. Specific exercise prescription information for CABG inpatients can be found in the *ACSM's Guidelines for Exercise Testing and Prescription*.[9(pp:236-240)] Providing structured inpatient CR/SP services is a challenge because of the 3- or 4-day hospital stay for uncomplicated patients, but multiple daily ambulation sessions for these patients are critical to recovery. Elderly patients and those with complicated postoperative courses are often transferred to a transitional program, such as one in an acute inpatient rehabilitation or subacute facility. In these programs they receive continued medical care; they also receive occupational and physical therapy to improve endurance strength, balance, and cognitive status for independence in self-care, household ambulation (including stairs), and home and food management activities (see chapter 4).

The rate of recovery for CABG patients is dependent on age, gender, and surgical techniques. Exercise testing is a Class II recommendation when performed after discharge for the purpose of activity counseling or exercise training as a component of CR/SP.[10]

Exercise prescription methodology is generally the same as that for CVD patients.[9(pp:241-244)] Initially, some patients may need lower-intensity or modified exercise prescriptions because of musculoskeletal discomfort or healing issues at the site of the sternal or vein harvesting incision. Patients should not engage in upper extremity resistance training before 5 weeks following a sternotomy. In addition, a resistance training program should be preceded by 4 weeks of regular participation in supervised cardiovascular endurance exercise training. In the absence of sternal instability (evidenced by sternal movement, cracking, or popping), caution is advised with upper body exercise for up to 8 weeks following surgery.[9(p:250)] Cardiothoracic surgeons typically issue very specific instructions for patients related to upper extremity exercise and resistance training. It is important for CR/SP program staff to be knowledgeable about these instructions and to incorporate them into the exercise prescription for those patients.

Staff should assess sternal and vein harvest site wound healing in all new patients referred after CABG or other heart surgery. Signs of wound infection include redness, swelling, and drainage; patients with an infected wound require a sterile dressing to avoid cross-contamination of other patients in the program. Because of the possibility of early saphenous vein graft closure, program staff should also be alert for new patient complaints of angina pectoris or angina-equivalent symptoms, signs and symptoms of exercise intolerance, and new electrocardiogram (ECG) signs of myocardial ischemia. Patients should be informed about and alert for these as well.

Dysrhythmias, including atrial fibrillation, are not uncommon within the first several days after open heart surgery, and can also occur during outpatient CR/SP. Complex dysrhythmias and new onset of atrial fibrillation should be reported promptly to the program medical director and referring physician (see the dysrhythmia section of this chapter).

Pleural and pericardial effusions, generally related to postoperative inflammation, may also occur postsurgery, generally within the first several weeks, and can be detected during early outpatient CR by evidence of decreasing exercise capacity, chest discomfort, and increasing dyspnea. These symptoms should be promptly reported to the program medical director, surgeon, and referring physician.

It is important to know whether the revascularization procedure was complete or incomplete in order to ensure a full assessment of signs and symptoms. This information is generally available in a surgical report or discharge summary. Complete revascularization (patent bypass grafting of all significant atherosclerotic lesions) should alleviate all associated signs and symptoms of myocardial ischemia. Vessels that are small or diffusely diseased are more likely to result in incomplete revascularization. This increases the likelihood of postsurgical signs and symptoms of residual myocardial ischemia during exercise.

It is important that all CABG patients practice all appropriate secondary prevention measures to help minimize the progression of the atherosclerotic process. Atherosclerotic lesions will almost certainly advance in native coronary arteries or vein grafts, necessitating further revascularization procedures, without implementation of aggressive lifestyle and other secondary prevention measures. Of note, lipid values may be falsely low for several weeks following surgery; thus lipid lowering should be based on preoperative lipid profiles.

Practice Considerations for Patients Who Have Undergone PCI

The other major revascularization procedure is PCI. Of the estimated 596,000 patients annually undergoing PCI procedures in 2008, 66% were males and 53% were 65 years of age or older.[4] When stents were implanted during PCI procedures, the vast majority (76%) were drug-eluting stents (DES).

As with CABG patients, referral of patients following PCI to CR/SP is a Class I recommendation,[11] is an endorsed performance measure,[7] and is a covered service for Medicare patients.[5] In one study, referral rates to CR/SP after PTCA were reported to be 60%,[12] and another study reported participation of 40% of eligible patients.[13] Because PCI patients are frequently discharged within 24 h of the procedure, opportunities for inpatient CR/SP services are very limited. Thus, the use of an automatic referral strategy to outpatient CR/SP at the time of discharge is particularly helpful, especially if it is facilitated by adequate communication between the referring providers, CR/SP program staff, and postdischarge contact with patient.

Exercise testing after discharge post-PCI is a Class II recommendation when used to guide activity counseling or exercise training (or both) in a CR/SP program. Additionally, results of exercise testing performed 1 to 3 days following PCI may be beneficial for the prediction of subsequent restenosis and may facilitate earlier return to work and daily living activities.[10]

Post-PCI patients can begin exercise training as outpatients almost immediately after hospital discharge. If the groin was used for catheter access, care should be taken to ensure that the access site is healing appropriately before the patient begins lower extremity exercise. Incomplete revascularization is also possible with PCI, which increases the possibility of exercise-induced signs and symptoms of residual myocardial isch-

emia. CR/SP staff should stress to patients who have undergone PCI the importance of adherence to preventive medications, particularly antiplatelet agents. Exercise prescription methodology is similar in MI and CABG patients. Resistance training exercises may be started 2 to 3 weeks following the PCI and completion of 2 weeks of supervised endurance training in CR/SP.[9(p:252-255)] Compared to patients who have undergone CABG or primary PCI for an acute ST-segment-elevation MI, patients who undergo elective PCI may be able to progress at a faster rate because they have not recently sustained myocardial damage or had a sternotomy.

Stressing the importance of secondary prevention is especially important for PCI patients, particularly in those without a previous MI or angina pectoris. Without a history of myocardial ischemia symptoms or an event, these patients may feel as though their coronary atherosclerosis has been "cured" by the PCI and therefore believe that secondary prevention and behavior modification measures are unnecessary.

Valve Replacement and Repair Surgery

According to the most recent AHA statistics, an estimated 139,000 patients underwent valve surgeries in 2008. Of this total, 58% of the surgeries were performed on males, and 64% were performed on persons 65 years of age or older. The number of annual hospital discharges for patients with a diagnosis of valvular heart disease (VHD) was nearly equal for aortic and mitral valve disease, an estimated 48,000 and 42,000, respectively.[4]

VHD may involve either stenosis or regurgitation and can affect any of the four cardiac valves, although valve dysfunction (mitral, aortic) on the higher-pressure left side of the heart requires intervention much more frequently than the tricuspid or pulmonic valves in the lower-pressure right side. Valvular stenosis is a narrowing or obstruction of the valve orifice, resulting in a valve that does not open adequately. The causes of stenosis include degenerative calcification, rheumatic disease, and congenitally malformed valves (e.g., bicuspid aortic valve). Regurgitation is the result of an incompetent valve that allows retrograde flow. It may be caused by rheumatic heart disease, infections, or congenital diseases (e.g., Marfan syndrome). Aortic insufficiency can also be caused by an ascending aortic aneurysm from atherosclerotic disease. In the case of the mitral valve, regurgitation can also be the result of mitral valve prolapse or MI leading to ruptured chordae or papillary muscles. Surgical interventions for valvular dysfunction include annuloplasty or valve replacement using a prosthetic valve. Annuloplasty tightens the annulus in an effort to restore the competence of the valve. Prosthetic heart valves are divided into two main categories: bioprostheses and mechanical prostheses. Bioprosthetic valves are further classified as heterografts, homografts, and stentless heterografts. Types of mechanical prosthetic heart valves include the caged-ball, tilting-disk, and bileaflet valves.[14] Before surgery, the surgeon typically discusses the choice of valve with the patient, reviewing the fact that mechanical valves are more durable but require lifelong anticoagulation due to much higher risk for clotting and therefore embolism.

Catheter-based procedures have emerged as alternatives to surgery for selected high-risk patients. Transcatheter aortic valve replacement (TAVR) compared to surgical replacement was studied extensively in the PARTNER study, and outcomes up to 2 years indicated that these two procedures resulted in similar mortality, reduction of symptoms, and valve hemodynamics[15-16] Another type of catheter-based procedure involves repairing mitral regurgitation by percutaneously implanting a clip that realigns the mitral valve leaflets.[17] Patients who undergo either of these procedures would not have a sternotomy and may be able to progress more rapidly during CR/SP.

VHD can sometimes involve multiple valves that require combined surgical or interventional management. Common combinations of VHD include mitral stenosis and tricuspid regurgitation, mitral stenosis and aortic stenosis, and aortic stenosis and mitral regurgitation. VHD can also coexist with CAD, especially in elderly patients.

Practice Considerations

Referral of patients to CR/SP following valve replacement or repair is an AACVPR/AHA/ACC-endorsed performance measure[7] and is a covered indication for Medicare patients.[5]

The exercise prescription and training of VHD patients following valve replacement are similar to those for CABG patients. However, the physical activity of some VHD patients may have been restricted for an extended period because of symptoms before valve repair or replacement. The resulting low functional capacity requires these patients to start and to progress slowly during the early stages of an exercise training program. CR/SP professionals should use standard exercise prescription methodology with these patients but should take care to avoid upper extremity exercise (including resistance training involving the upper extremities) until the sternum is stable and there are no sternal wound healing issues.

Patients who have undergone valve replacement surgery are not cured of VHD but instead have exchanged native valve disease for prosthetic valve disease. Prevention of infections at prosthetic valve sites and management of anticoagulation medications are important issues for the postsurgical patient. Patients who have undergone combined valve replacement and CABG have the same secondary prevention issues regarding reducing CAD risk profiles as discussed earlier for the CABG-only patients.

Patients with VHD, but without valve repair or replacement, may also be referred for CR/SP for other coexisting conditions, such as MI, PCI, angina, or CABG. In these patients, critical aortic stenosis is a contraindication for both inpatient and outpatient CR/SP. Patients with less severe aortic stenosis can exercise but may develop symptoms (e.g., dyspnea, angina, or syncope) during exercise. Exercise training intensity should be kept under the threshold that precipitates the onset of symptoms because these symptoms indicate that the cardiac output is not meeting the demands of the exercise. Dyspnea during exercise is the primary symptom of exercise intolerance with mitral stenosis, and is commonly seen in patients with severe aortic stenosis. A worsening of any of these symptoms over time may indicate worsening valve disease and should be closely monitored. Absolute contraindications for resistance training include Marfan syndrome and severe, symptomatic aortic stenosis.[18]

Dysrhythmias

Although cardiac dysrhythmias are not uncommon in CR/SP participants, the majority of these occurrences are not life threatening, and some are associated with varying levels of symptoms.

Nonetheless, cardiac dysrhythmias may result in significant and life-threatening occurrences.[1-4] The following are commonly encountered cardiac dysrhythmias and associated symptomatology.

Cardiac Dysrhythmias in CR/SP

Generally Benign

- Premature atrial complexes (PACs) and premature ventricular complexes (PVCs)
- Atrial fibrillation (Afib) or atrial flutter with controlled ventricular rate
- Paroxysmal supraventricular tachycardia (PSVT)
- Mild bradycardia (50-60 bpm)
- First-degree AV block and asymptomatic type I second-degree AV block (Wenckebach)

Potentially Malignant

- Atrial fibrillation or atrial flutter with a rapid rate
- Symptomatic or severe bradycardia
- Symptomatic or advanced AV block
- Ventricular tachycardia
- Ventricular fibrillation

Symptoms Associated With Cardiac Dysrhythmias

Stable Symptoms Without Hemodynamic Compromise

- Palpitations
- Dizziness or light-headedness
- Shortness of breath
- Chest pain or discomfort
- Nonspecific or associated symptoms:
  - Weakness or fatigue
  - Sweating
  - Blurred vision
  - Nausea
  - Anxiety
  - Edema

Unstable Symptoms

- Hypotension
- Near-syncope or loss of consciousness
- Heart failure
- Unstable angina or myocardial infarction
- Cardiac arrest

Although most of these dysrhythmias are unremarkable, it should be remembered that exercise potentially exerts a multitude of metabolic, hemodynamic, and electrophysiologic effects, all of which can be arrhythmogenic and independent of induced ischemia. In addition, the occurrence of dysrhythmias may be, but is not always, related to exercise intensity; that is, dysrhythmias can be associated with mild activity, disappear with increasing intensity, or not be reproducible regardless of the intensity. However, in addition to exercise intensity, other factors can be associated with dysrhythmias, including autonomic nervous system variability, medications with proarrhythmic side effects, electrolyte imbalance, dehydration, and certain environmental factors (figure 9.2).

Although there are risks associated with exercise, one of which is dysrhythmia, the benefit generally outweighs the risks if the exercise prescription is tailored to individual cardiac status. Patients with known dysrhythmias in CR/SP programs should have predetermined goals, should be monitored during activity for some defined period of time, and should have predetermined criteria for exercise termination.

Atrial Fibrillation

Light-to-moderate physical activities, particularly leisure-time activity and walking, are associated with a significantly lower incidence of atrial fibrillation in older adults.[5] Recent evidence indicates that chronic high-intensity or high-volume endurance training may be associated with an increased incidence of atrial fibrillation.[6,7] For those already diagnosed with atrial fibrillation, regular moderate physical activity is known to increase exercise capacity and control ventricular rate during atrial fibrillation.[8,9] Patients without structural disease and in the absence of Wolff–Parkinson–White (WPW) syndrome can safely perform moderate-intensity isometric and isotonic exercises, depending in part on the presence and severity of underlying CVD.

Pacemakers

Cardiac pacemaker technologies have advanced substantially in recent years. As a result, the physiological response to exercise for patients with pacemakers can be essentially the same as for other patients. Increasing heart rate (HR)

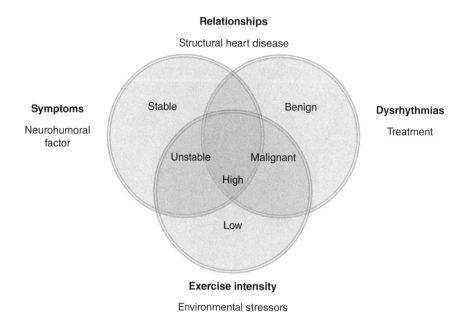

Figure 9.2 Factors associated with the occurrence of dysrhythmias.

during exercise is the single most important factor with respect to increasing cardiac output and oxygen uptake. For patients who cannot provide an appropriate intrinsic HR response to exercise, a cardiac pacemaker, programmed in a rate-responsive mode, can increase HR and thus cardiac output to meet the changing physiological demands of increased activity.

Atrioventricular (AV) (dual chamber) pacing is common and allows for physiological pacing, which refers to the maintenance of the normal sequence and timing of the contractions of the upper and lower chambers of the heart. AV synchrony provides a higher cardiac output without dramatically increasing myocardial oxygen uptake. A dual-chamber pacemaker senses the sinus node and, if intrinsic AV block exists, sends an impulse to the ventricle following a programmed AV timing interval.

The development of rate-responsive pacing (also called rate-adaptive or rate-modulated pacing) has markedly changed the application of pacing with regard to exercise. The adaptive rate function is applied when the native sinus node cannot increase HR to meet metabolic demands. Rate-responsive pacemakers can use different types of sensors to adjust the pacing rate to produce an appropriate cardiac rate in patients with chronotropic incompetence. Sen-

sors have been developed to detect motion and physiological and metabolic changes that occur with increased exercise. Based on computer algorithms, the sensors drive the pacemaker to generate electrical impulses that appropriately pace the heart to meet energy demands. The most common rate-responsive pacemakers detect motion in response to physical activity using a piezoelectric crystal located in the pacemaker device. Other functions that are monitored are minute ventilation, body temperature, and ECG waveform intervals. Advances in pacemaker technology have allowed the use of combined or blended sensors and advanced algorithms to improve rate performance over that with a single-sensor system.[10] Blended sensors measure patient workload through respiration and motion, providing optimal rate response during changing levels of activity. Nevertheless, definitive clinical benefits from blended sensors have yet to be fully established.[11,12]

Implantable Cardioverter-Defibrillators

Evidence suggests that exercise training in patients with an implantable cardioverter-defibrillator (ICD) is safe.[13] Reports have also indicated that it results in increases in peak $\dot{V}O_2$ similar to those in control patients,[13-15] without serious complications,[16] and that patients who participated in an exercise-based CR/SP program received fewer total and exercise-related shocks compared to those who did not participate.[17] In addition, low-intensity competitive sports that do not constitute a significant risk of trauma to the defibrillator are permissible if 6 months have passed since the last ventricular dysrhythmia requiring intervention.[18]

Personnel working with patients with implanted defibrillators should know the device-programmed ventricular tachycardia/ventricular fibrillation (VT/VF) detection HR for delivery of therapy, although newer devices have better supraventricular tachycardia discrimination algorithms using QRS morphology to reduce the threat of ICD discharge simply with elevated HR. Baseline exercise testing can help determine whether exercise is likely to cause a discharge and assists in determining whether exercise brings on ventricular dysrhythmias. Subsequent adjustments of antiarrhythmic medications may be necessary. In any case, exercise prescription HR should be set at least 10 to 15 beats below the ICD VT/VF detection HR. If pacing rate does not increase appropriately with exercise, physical activity intensity must be gauged by a method other than pulse count, for example rating of perceived exertion or systolic blood pressure response to a quantifiable or objectively measured workload.

Cardiac Resynchronization Therapy

Cardiac resynchronization therapy (CRT) or biventricular pacing is an adjunctive therapy for patients with advanced heart failure.[19,20] These patients commonly have left bundle branch block or an intraventricular conduction delay, resulting in left ventricular dyssynchrony and a high mortality rate. The benefit of CRT is based on the reduction in the conduction delay between the right and left ventricles. CRT functions to maintain right and left ventricular synchrony by regulating the electrical impulses to each ventricle. CRT contributes to the optimization of the ejection fraction, decrement in mitral regurgitation, and left ventricular remodeling, thus resulting in symptom improvement and enhanced quality of life. Several studies have shown the efficacy of CRT in patients with heart failure and conduction delays.[21-24] Improvements have been

demonstrated in the mean distance walked in 6 min, quality of life, New York Heart Association functional class, peak $\dot{V}O_2$, total exercise time, reduction of hospitalization, left ventricular (LV) function, and the LV end-diastolic diameter. Data suggest that improvements in functional capacity with CRT can be maintained long-term.[25] In addition, ventricular–arterial coupling, mechanical efficiency, and chronotropic responses are improved after CRT. These findings may explain the improved functional status and exercise tolerance in patients treated with CRT.[26]

In appropriate patients, exercise training may be used as an adjunct to CRT for improving cardiac and peripheral muscle function. Exercise training after CRT helps to improve exercise tolerance, hemodynamic measures, and quality of life.[27,28] Recommended typical precautions regarding exercise participation should be applied to this patient population.

Practice Considerations

The goals of exercise for patients with atrial fibrillation, pacemakers, ICDs, and CRT vary widely. Therefore, baseline evaluation and treatment plans must be individualized. As an example, in some cases, patients with nonsustained ventricular dysrhythmias and normal myocardial function may require only a limited number of sessions of ECG-monitored exercise with subsequent serial assessments before embarking on a nonmonitored or home exercise program. In other cases, some patients with ICDs have limited functional capacity because of severe myocardial dysfunction and may also be psychologically disabled by a history of sudden cardiac death and the potential for conscious defibrillation. These patients often require more formal and prolonged ECG-supervised exercise programs.

Baseline evaluation at program entry should include a clear description of the dysrhythmias, the hemodynamic consequences of the dysrhythmias, possible inciting factors such as exercise or cardiac ischemia, and potential therapies should the dysrhythmia recur.[29,30] Before exercise is prescribed, the presence and severity of underlying heart disease should be evaluated, including the severity of CAD and LV function (ejection fraction). Details about programmed pacemaker or ICD rates, detection parameters, and algorithms should also be obtained. The results of Holter monitoring or electrophysiological stimulation studies, exercise testing results, and the most current medical regimen should be reviewed with the patient. Exercise testing has been shown to be helpful in identifying the presence and thresholds of myocardial ischemia and angina. For patients with a cardiac pacemaker, exercise testing can be used to guide the adjustment of the pacemaker settings and is particularly useful in active patients with rate-responsive pacemakers to ensure appropriate rate responses. Exercise testing is also helpful for ICD patients to evaluate any overlap of intrinsic HR and programmed ventricular tachycardia (VT) detection rate.

A common goal in the management of patients with dysrhythmias and devices is the early recognition of change of rhythm or signs and symptoms associated with dysrhythmias in order to prevent and treat these disorders. CR/SP professionals are frequently the first to identify rest- or exercise-related dysrhythmias. Any new cardiac dysrhythmia or change in severity of a cardiac arrhythmia should be brought to the attention of the program physician and referring physician for evaluation and management.

CR/SP professionals can play an important role in the overall evaluation of the patient with an implanted device by providing feedback to the physician about HR, blood pressure, and symptomatic responses to exercise. This information allows the device to be programmed to more closely match the needs of the patient. In many cases, adjustments can improve exercise capacity and reduce symptoms. Because the type and potential consequences of rhythm disturbances vary among patients, the CR/SP specialist is faced with the challenge of understanding the significance of the dysrhythmias, the corresponding hemodynamic consequences, and the resulting impact on the exercise physiology. Additionally, staff must have a clear knowledge of the various rhythm management devices, including pacemakers, ICDs, and CRTs, in order to work with these and teach patients effectively. Standing orders should provide direction to individual staff members for responding to various rhythm disturbances and for providing limits to exercise levels in those patients whose dysrhythmias are exercise related or who have ICDs. Table 9.9 lists common dysrhythmias, including atrial fibrillation, and their corresponding implications for exercise and education.

Heart Failure and Left Ventricular Assist Devices

The purpose of this section is to provide an overview of patient evaluation considerations and strategies for successfully implementing secondary preventive services for patients with chronic

Table 9.9 Dysrhythmias and Their Corresponding Recommendations for Evaluation, Exercise, and Education

Dysrhythmias	Clinical status	CR/SP program recommendations
Premature atrial complexes	Asymptomatic	No restrictions
Sick sinus syndrome	Asymptomatic, pauses <3 s; heart rate (HR) ≥ 50 and increases with activity	No restrictions
	Syncope	Needs evaluation and physician recommendation
	Pacemaker	May participate with physician approval
Atrial flutter	Asymptomatic, <10 s duration with exercise	May participate with physician approval
	Asymptomatic with good rate control	May participate with physician approval
	Anticoagulation	May participate with physician approval
	Postcardioversion or postablation	After 1 to 4 weeks, may participate with physician approval
Atrial fibrillation	Preexisting, asymptomatic, good rate control; HR increases and decreases appropriately in response to level of activity	May participate with physician approval
	Anticoagulation	May participate with physician approval
	Postcardioversion or postablation	After 1 to 6 weeks, may participate with physician approval

Dysrhythmias	Clinical status	CR/SP program recommendations
Supraventricular tachycardia (SVT)	Asymptomatic, <10 s duration with exercise	May participate with physician approval
	Syncope	Needs evaluation and physician recommendation
	Postcardioversion or postablation	After 1 to 6 weeks, may participate with physician approval
Frequent complex premature ventricular complexes (PVCs)	Chronic, asymptomatic	Physician recommendation regarding restrictions
	First detected	Needs evaluation and physician recommendation
Ventricular tachycardia	Stable, asymptomatic, <10 beats duration, monomorphic, HR <150 bpm, no cardiac disease	May participate with physician approval
	First detected	Needs evaluation and physician recommendation
	Postablation	After 1 to 6 weeks, may participate with physician approval
	Medical therapy or postcardioversion	After 1 to 3 months, may participate with physician approval
	Post-ICD placement	After 1 to 3 months, may participate with physician approval
Ventricular fibrillation	Post-ICD	After 1 to 3 months, may participate with physician approval
First-degree atrioventricular (AV) block	Asymptomatic, normal QRS complex, PR interval <300 ms, no worsening with exercise	No restrictions
Type I second-degree AV block (Wenckebach)	Asymptomatic, normal QRS, no worsening or conduction improves with exercise	No restrictions
	Asymptomatic, but worsens with activity	Needs evaluation and physician recommendation
	Pacemaker	May participate with physician approval
Complete right bundle branch block (CRBBB)	Asymptomatic, no AV block with exercise, no ventricular arrhythmia	May participate with physician approval
Complete left bundle branch block (CLBBB)	Asymptomatic, no AV block with exercise, no ventricular arrhythmia	May participate with physician approval

Based on Pescatello et al. 2004; Appel et al. 1997.

heart failure (HF) or for patients who have received a left ventricular assist device (LVAD). Special emphasis is placed on practices that

- maximize patient safety,
- individualize rehabilitation services, and
- optimize patient outcomes.

Recent statistics on the incidence and prevalence of HF indicate that more than 5.7 million Americans are affected, with 670,000 new cases diagnosed each year. Additionally, more than 990,000 hospitalizations each year are caused by HF and mortality remains high; ~50% of people diagnosed with HF die within 5 years.[1] HF will likely continue to be a major health concern in the future, and managing the clinical manifestations is often associated with repeated hospitalizations and numerous physician visits. The estimated annual expenditure for the management of HF exceeds $39 billion.[2] Therefore, therapies and methods aimed at decreasing the clinical manifestations and disability associated with HF remain areas of great interest.

Heart failure is a condition characterized by a reduction in cardiac output such that it is insufficient to meet the metabolic demands of vital organs and physiological systems. The pathophysiology of HF involves an impairment in the ability of the ventricles to either sufficiently contract (HF due to reduced ejection fraction, HFREF) or relax (HF with preserved ejection fraction, HFPEF). Inadequate delivery of blood to specific areas is associated with a variety of pathophysiological sequelae (table 9.10), many of which develop as compensatory mechanisms aimed at maintaining adequate cardiac output. However, these mechanisms may improve or maintain heart function for only a temporary period, after which HF usually progresses. The pharmacologic management of patients with HF currently targets these compensatory mechanisms through the routine use of a combination of beta-blocker, angiotensin-converting enzyme (ACE) inhibitor or angiotensin-receptor blocker (ARB), and a diuretic as indicated.[3]

Clinical Manifestations of Heart Failure

The following are the clinical manifestations of HF:

- Dyspnea and fatigue
- Tachypnea
- Paroxysmal nocturnal dyspnea
- Orthopnea
- Peripheral edema
- Cold, pale, and possibly cyanotic extremities
- Weight gain
- Hepatomegaly
- Jugular venous distension
- Crackles (rales)
- Tubular breath sounds and consolidation

- Presence of a third (S3) or fourth (S4) heart sound
- Sinus tachycardia[4]

Among those listed, two key characteristics are

- Exercise intolerance as manifested by fatigue or dyspnea on exertion; and
- Fluid retention as evidenced by pulmonary or peripheral edema, recent weight gain, or a combination of these factors.

Importantly, the CR/SP professional working in a preventive cardiology or CR/SP clinic needs to evaluate changes in clinical status routinely to ensure that the patient can safely engage in exercise.

Although clinicians often use New York Heart Association (NYHA) function class to describe clinical status or severity of illness, use of that system has limitations in that it does not fully reflect the breadth of the disorder. Table 9.11 shows the stages in the development of HF as designated by the ACC and AHA.[3] This staging system covers all patients with left ventricular dysfunction, regardless of the presence or absence of symptoms. Note that patients experiencing symptoms (NYHA classes II-IV) fall only within stage C and stage D.

Table 9.10 Physiological Consequences of Congestive Heart Failure

Pathology	Effects
Cardiovascular	Decreased myocardial performance, with subsequent peripheral vascular constriction to increase venous return (attempting to increase stroke volume and cardiac output)
Pulmonary	Pulmonary edema because of elevated cardiac filling pressures resulting from poor myocardial performance and fluid overload
Renal	Fluid retention resulting from decreased cardiac output
Neurohumoral	Increased sympathetic stimulation that eventually desensitizes the heart to beta-1 adrenergic receptor stimulation, thus decreasing the cardiac inotropic effect
Musculoskeletal	Skeletal muscle wasting and possible skeletal muscle myopathies as well as osteoporosis resulting from inactivity or other accompanying diseases
Hematologic	Possible polycythemia, anemia, and hemostatic abnormalities resulting from a reduction in oxygen transport, accompanying liver disease, or stagnant blood flow in the heart chambers caused by poor cardiac contraction
Hepatic	Possible cardiac cirrhosis from hypoperfusion resulting from an inadequate cardiac output or hepatic venous congestion
Pancreatic	Possible impaired insulin secretion and impaired glucose intolerance as well as the source of a possible myocardial depressant factor
Nutritional/ biochemical	Anorexia that leads to malnutrition (protein, calorie, and vitamin deficiencies) and cachexia

Adapted from *Essentials of cardiopulmonary physical therapy*, L.P. Cahalin, "Cardiac muscle dysfunction," pg. 132, Copyright 1994, with permission from Elsevier.

Determining the disability caused by HF involves assessing and tracking changes in signs and symptoms (e.g., dyspnea, fatigue), functional status (e.g., walking, stair climbing, activities of daily living), and health-related quality of life.[4] Evaluating response of functional capacity or exercise tolerance before, during, and after CR/SP can be accomplished using a 6-minute walk test, measuring exercise duration from a regular exercise test, or measuring peak $\dot{V}O_2$ during a cardiopulmonary exercise test. Other exercise test–related parameters to help determine response to CR/SP can include change in HR or systolic blood pressure at a standardized or fixed workload and change in the magnitude of symptoms (e.g., dyspnea, angina) at submaximal and peak effort.

Changes in quality of life and health status before, during, and after CR/SP can be evaluated using disease-specific questionnaires such as the Minnesota Living with Heart Failure Questionnaire,[5] the Chronic Heart Failure Questionnaire, or the Kansas City Cardiomyopathy Questionnaire,[6] as well as general health status questionnaires such as the Medical Outcomes Short Form (SF-36).[7]

The objective documentation of progress can (1) alert a rehabilitation specialist to maintain or modify the current regimen and (2) serve as a basis for database development either in an individual program or on a larger scale through local, regional, or national oversight.

CR/SP

The efficacy of CR/SP in patients with NYHA class II to III heart failure has been previously described.[8,9] The major areas briefly addressed in this section are the physiological and clinical effects of cardiorespiratory exercise training, strength or resistance training, and breathing exercises. Since little formal exercise-related rehabilitation usually occurs in the United States while patients are hospitalized for new-onset or exacerbation of HF, this section summarizes studies involving patients engaged in home-based or supervised outpatient exercise programs. The ideal scenario for both the patient and the rehabilitation professional might be to provide exercise first in a supervised setting, then begin to incorporate some home-based sessions, and finally progress to an all home-based program. Due to travel distance this approach may not be possible for all patients, so an entirely home-based program may be required.

Cardiorespiratory Training

The reduced exercise capacity in patients with HFREF[10,11] is caused by abnormalities in cardiac, pulmonary, peripheral vascular, and skeletal and respiratory muscle function[12-18] and can be quantified by measuring peak $\dot{V}O_2$. Of the more than two dozen single-site randomized clinical exercise training trials that evaluated change in peak $\dot{V}O_2$ due to moderate-to-vigorous cardiovascular

Table 9.11 Stages in the Development of Heart Failure: ACC/AHA Guidelines[3]

Stage	Description	Example	New York Heart Association functional class
A (patient at risk)	High risk for heart failure; no anatomic or functional abnormalities; no signs or symptoms	Hypertension, coronary artery disease, diabetes, alcohol abuse, family history	
B (patient at risk)	Structural abnormalities associated with heart failure but no symptoms	Left ventricular hypertrophy, prior myocardial infarction, asymptomatic valvular disease, low ejection fraction	
C (heart failure present)	Current or prior signs or symptoms and structural abnormalities	Left ventricular systolic dysfunction with or without dyspnea on exertion or fatigue, reduced exercise tolerance	II or III
D (heart failure present)	Advanced structural heart failure with symptoms at rest despite maximal medical therapy	Frequent hospitalizations, awaiting transplant, intravenous support	III or IV

Abbreviations; ACC, American College of Cardiology; AHA, American Heart Association.

Adapted from Jessup et al. 2009.

endurance exercise, most demonstrated improved peak $\dot{V}O_2$ of 1 mL · kg^{-1} · min^{-1} or more,[19] equating to an approximate 10% to 25% increase in exercise tolerance.[20] In the multicenter randomized HF-ACTION trial, the median increase in peak $\dot{V}O_2$ after 3 months of combined supervised and home-based exercise was 0.6 mL · kg^{-1} · min^{-1} among patients in the exercise arm of the trial (vs. 0.2 mL · kg^{-1} · min^{-1} change for patients in the usual-care group).[21] In addition to improvement in exercise tolerance, several important central and peripheral physiological adaptations occur as well, including an increase in peak HR, an increase in nutritive blood flow to the active skeletal muscle due to improved endothelial function, improved skeletal muscle function (e.g., oxidative capacity), and a downregulation of neurohormonal activity with exercise training.[19]

Interestingly, over the past decade, several authors have used intermittent high-intensity aerobic interval training (vs. continuous moderate-intensity exercise) to improve exercise capacity. This method of training yields higher-intensity training levels (i.e., up to 95% of peak HR vs. 75% of peak HR) and more total work during a single training session. Wisloff and coauthors[22] showed that aerobic interval training improved peak $\dot{V}O_2$ by 6 mL · kg^{-1} · min^{-1} (+46%); however, an adequately powered investigation evaluating the safety of such training has not yet been performed.

It is important for the CR/SP professional to note that responses to exercise training do vary in patients with HFREF. For example, Tabet and colleagues[23] demonstrated significant increases in both mean peak $\dot{V}O_2$ (14%) and mean percent predicted $\dot{V}O_2$ (13%) with exercise training; however, 50% of their subjects were classified as nonresponders, based on achieving a less than 6% increase in percent predicted peak $\dot{V}O_2$. As with other treatments, the response of individuals to exercise training varies, likely due to biologic factors, etiology of disease, and other clinical factors. CR/SP clinicians should be prepared to identify and appropriately modify the exercise regimen of patients experiencing less than satisfactory improvement in fatigue and well-being.

With respect to regular exercise and clinical events, several meta-analyses and the multicenter HF-ACTION trial have shown beneficial effects, including a 39% relative reduction in risk for mortality,[24] an 11% reduction in the adjusted risk for all-cause mortality or hospitalization, a 15% reduction in adjusted risk for the combined end point of cardiovascular mortality or HF hospitalization,[21] and a 28% decrease in hospitalization for HF.[9] Importantly, a recent study demonstrated that, among elderly Medicare beneficiaries with a diagnosis of HF, mortality and MI were reduced by approximately 19% and 18%, over 4 years, respectively, in patients who attended 36 CR/SP sessions (vs. those patients who attended 12 sessions).[25]

Data on exercise training and health status reveal a favorable effect of training on health-related quality of life as measured by the Minnesota Living with Heart Failure Questionnaire (−9.7 points, $P < .001$).[26] Using the Kansas City Cardiomyopathy Questionnaire, the HF-ACTION trial examined the effects of exercise training on self-reported health status and showed a modest improvement in the total score at 3 months, which was maintained over 2 years.[27]

Exercise Prescription

With respect to prescribing aerobic-type exercise, the parameters pertaining to intensity, duration, and frequency of exercise must be considered (see table 9.12). In all patients, the clinician responsible for writing the exercise prescription and monitoring progress should adjust these parameters such that the total volume of exercise is gradually, safely, and consistently increased to 180-360 MET-min/wk. For most patients, increasing to this level of exercise should require no more than 3 to 4 weeks.

In general, the target levels for duration and frequency of exercise should be 20-60 min per bout or more and three (preferably most days of the week) bouts per week, respectively. For patients with an initially very poor exercise tolerance it may be helpful to begin with intermittent instead of continuous exercise, such that one continuous 30 minute bout of exercise is broken up into three or four separate bouts interspersed with brief rest periods. Over several weeks, the length of the rest periods is decreased while the exercise period is extended until 30 continuous minutes can be completed. Regardless of which approach is chosen, both exercise duration and frequency should be increased to target levels before intensity of effort is increased.

Table 9.12 Summary of Exercise Prescription for Patients With Heart Failure

Type of training	Description	Intensity	Frequency	Duration
Cardiorespiratory endurance	Dynamic activities involving large muscle groups	40% to 80% of HRR RPE 11 to 14 (where HRR is not appropriate)	Minimum of 3 days per week, but preferably on most days of the week	20 to 60 min/session
Resistance training	8 to 10 muscle-specific exercises involving resistance bands, weight machines, handheld weights, or combination; begin with one set of 10 to 15 repetitions	50% to 70% 1RM for lifts involving the hips and lower body; 40% to 70% 1RM for lifts involving the upper body	2 or 3 days a week	20 to 30 min/session; contraction should be performed in a rhythmical manner at a moderate to slow controlled speed

Abbreviations: HRR, heart rate reserve, computed as (peak HR − seated resting HR) × training level expressed as a percent + seated resting HR; RM, repetition maximum; RPE, rating of perceived exertion.

With respect to guiding exercise training intensity, the most common approach involves progressively increasing effort to a training range between 40% and 80% of heart rate reserve.[28] Intensity is then modified as needed to achieve a rating of perceived exertion (RPE, scale range = 6 to 20) between 12 and 14. The measurement of peak HR is required for this method and can be safely obtained from a symptom-limited maximal exercise test.[29] As mentioned previously, higher-intensity aerobic interval training may represent an effective alternate method for improving exercise tolerance.[22] For patients with atrial fibrillation or those with frequent ectopic beats that interfere with the accurate measurement of HR during exercise, training intensity can be guided by RPE alone.

Resistance Training

Although resistance or strength training is not included as a component of the recommended exercise guidelines for patients with HFREF,[30,31] such training should be considered in selected patients. Regular resistance training improves both muscle strength and endurance, without adverse effects on hemodynamics[32] or left ventricular characteristics (i.e., left ventricular ejection fraction, left ventricular end-diastolic volume).[33-35] The increases in both muscle strength and endurance often exceed 20% to 30%;[34-37] however, whether or not resistance training improves aerobic exercise capacity in patients with HFREF requires further investigation.[33,34,36] Before the start of a resistance training program, it is important that patients first demonstrate that they can tolerate the aerobic training component, which usually requires about 3 to 4 weeks.

Exercise prescription. Similarly to the prescription for cardiorespiratory training, the prescription for resistance training needs to be increased in a progressive manner. For example, the intensity for upper body lifts should be progressively increased over several weeks, from 40% of 1RM to 70% of 1RM. Lower body lifts can begin at 50% of 1RM. Table 9.12 also outlines the components of a resistance training regimen for patients with HF.[36,38]

Breathing Exercises or Training

Several studies have investigated the effects of breathing exercises on the clinical manifestations of HF;[39-42] most used an inspiratory muscle training device. Inspiratory muscle training was performed daily for an average of 15 to 30 min at 15% to 60% of maximal inspiratory mouth pressure for 2 to 3 months.[42] Threshold inspiratory muscle training appears to consistently improve ventilatory muscle strength and endurance and dyspnea.

Practice Considerations

Following hospital discharge, all-cause 30-day rehospitalization remains quite high (~25%) in patients with HF; because of this and disease-related comorbidities, CR/SP programs are becoming increasingly involved in the comprehensive care of patients with HF. CR/SP represents an ideal setting to address disease-specific education and medication reconciliation, as well as to provide clinical surveillance aimed at preventing rehospitalization by identifying signs and symptoms of cardiac decompensation and referring for treatment. To help fulfill this role, the CR/SP professional must work with physicians to report patient progress and help monitor the overall medical plan, including compliance with diet and medications and self-monitoring weights, edema, and symptoms. To ensure that the CR/SP services are delivered appropriately, staff should consult a detailed history, results of medical and psychological tests, and results from disease-specific and general health status questionnaires.[43] Exercise test results can also provide important information about the severity of HF and the safety of exercise training, and can help guide the development of a correct exercise prescription. Patients with a peak $\dot{V}O_2$ less than 10 to 14 mL · kg^{-1} · min^{-1} may have a poorer prognosis and are often considered candidates for cardiac transplantation or a left ventricular assist device (LVAD).

Table 9.13 summarizes several common safety, exercise, and educational strategies for patients with HF. In addition to expanding their education and exercise strategies, CR/SP professionals who work with the HF population need expanded assessment and communication skills. It is essential that CR/SP professionals become expert in assessing patients for early signs of HF, including auscultation of heart and lung sounds, assessing for peripheral and central edema, and monitoring weight gain. They must establish strong communication links with attending physicians, home health nurses, specialty clinics, and other health care providers with a role in managing patient care. Clear communication on how secondary prevention achieves goals and contributes to successful patient outcomes can help set the stage for future referrals.

Left Ventricular Assist Devices

Historically, heart transplantation was the only viable option for patients with end-stage HF on optimal drug therapy. However, due to both the limited availability of donor hearts and advances in technology, mechanical LVADs have become a standard therapeutic option as either a bridge to transplant or a destination therapy for patients who do not qualify for transplant. The REMATCH trial was the first to demonstrate superior survival following LVAD implantation in patients with NYHA class IV heart failure (48% survival at 2 years) when compared to standard medical therapy.[46]

Table 9.13 Safety, Exercise, and Educational Strategies for Patients With Heart Failure[44,45]

Safety	Exercise	Education
• Uncompensated HF is a contraindication to starting an exercise program; decompensation is reason to discontinue the exercise program • A thorough patient assessment should be part of preexercise assessment of vital signs with each CR/SP visit • As part of the initial evaluation, patients should be asked about advance directives; copies of such decisions should be placed in the patient's chart	• Exercise stress tests should include, where possible, metabolic assessment using a carefully progressing protocol (e.g., 1 MET per stage) • Patients are at high risk for ventricular arrhythmias and decompensation • Exercise protocol: longer warm-up and cool-down; use interval exercise (1-6 min) as needed; encourage weight bearing for ADL • Use ECG and BP monitoring during exercise, as needed; use subjective RPE and dyspnea scales • Common side effect: fatigue for rest of the day • Due to slow progression in exercise program and high-risk nature of patients, the supervised exercise may need to be extended	• Priority: sign and symptom recognition and response, including fatigue, weakness, dyspnea, orthopnea, edema, weight gain • Nutrition consult: low-sodium diet (e.g., 1500 mg), heart-healthy diet • Drug regimen: medication education and compliance monitoring, diuretics, digitalis, ACE inhibitors, beta-blockers • Psychosocial consult for depression symptomatology; HF support group and individual counseling • Basic information regarding disease processes

ACE, angiotensin-converting enzyme; ADL, activities of daily living; BP, blood pressure; HF, heart failure; ECG, electrocardiogram; MET, metabolic equivalent; RPE, rating of perceived exertion.

There are several different types of LVADs that provide circulatory or hemodynamic support to underperfused organs and reverse the pathophysiological sequelae of HF.[47] In brief, the LVAD pump is implanted intra-abdominally or in a preperitoneal pocket external to the abdominal viscera. The left ventricle is cannulated at the apex of the heart for inflow to the pump, which then sends blood into the ascending aorta distal to the aortic valve (figure 9.3). The technology of LVADs has evolved dramatically over the past 20 years. First-generation LVADs used in the early 1990s tethered patients to hospital floors for months awaiting transplant. These were quickly replaced by battery-powered portable models, allowing patients the freedom to return to normal daily activities.[48] Current-generation LVADs have smaller internal components, due to the use of continuous- versus pulsatile-flow pumps, and have resulted in fewer mechanical device failures and a longer life span for the device.[49]

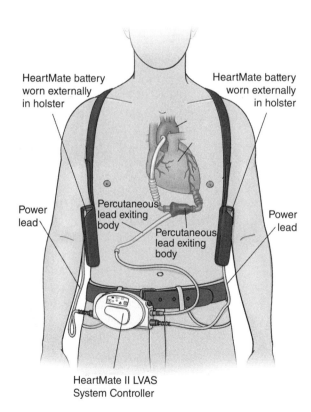

HeartMate battery worn externally in holster

HeartMate battery worn externally in holster

Power lead

Percutaneous lead exiting body

Percutaneous lead exiting body

Power lead

HeartMate II LVAS System Controller

Figure 9.3 HeartMate II left ventricular assist system (LVAS). LVAD, left ventricular assist device.

Reprinted with permission from Thoratec Corporation.

Considerations for Exercise

Participation in traditional aerobic-based exercise, including symptom-limited exercise testing, appears to be safe and well tolerated in patients with LVADs.[50-56] The LVAD has the capacity to increase cardiac output during exercise, with contemporary continuous-flow models able to increase flow up to approximately 10 L/min.[53] Functional capacity 3 to 6 months following LVAD implantation is significantly improved, and in some patients the increase is comparable to changes observed following heart transplantation.[57,58] In a cohort of 281 patients with NYHA functional class IV, 83% of patients receiving LVADs were reclassified as NYHA class I or II at 6 months following implantation, with a >70% increase in 6-minute walk distances.[59] In addition, improvements in functional status have been associated with increased quality of life and higher self-reported exercise ability.[57,60] In short, patients with an LVAD feel better and may be more willing to participate in a structured exercise program.

Cardiac Rehabilitation and Secondary Prevention

An obvious benefit of CR/SP with this patient population is reversal of the skeletal muscle atrophy that occurs through extended periods of poor peripheral perfusion (i.e., before implantation) and prolonged sedentary behaviors. Although patients receiving an LVAD may be more functional than patients with severe HF, those with a recently (i.e., <3 months) implanted device are still likely to be extremely deconditioned and have unique medical concerns requiring attention from the CR/SP staff. Additionally, CR/SP staff can play an important role in a multidisciplinary LVAD team by providing feedback to other clinicians regarding signs or symptoms. For example, staff might report a paroxysmal dysrhythmia detected using ECG telemetry monitoring that otherwise could go undetected and possibly lead to the development of right-sided HF.

Exercise prescription. To date, there are no large prospective exercise trials on the effects of exercise training in patients with LVADs; thus the optimal training prescription has not yet been established. Additionally, it is not known if exercise can be guided by the patient's intrinsic HR in this population. While the intrinsic HR does

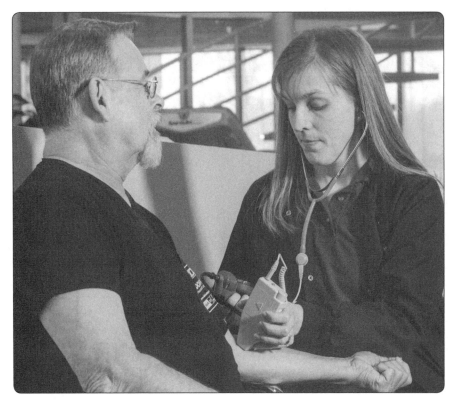

Participation in traditional aerobic-based exercise is beneficial for patients with LVADs and can lead to increased quality of life.

increase with exercise, it is uncertain whether discordance exists between intrinsic HR response and the cardiac output of continuous-flow devices during exercise as seen in studies involving the pulsatile-flow LVADs.[50,54]

Similar to the situation in transplant patients, maintaining a moderate level of perceived exertion (RPE scale 11-13) while gradually increasing exercise intensity represents a plausible and appropriate method for progressing the exercise prescription. An initial exercise workload of 2.5 METs or below is appropriate in most individuals, with modification guided by perceived exertion and symptomatic response to the workload. Factors that can influence the overall functional capacity of a patient and initial workloads chosen for rehabilitation include time from LVAD implantation, current activity habits, comorbidities, and age. Response to training can be safely evaluated with the 6-minute walk test.[61]

The safety and efficacy of resistance training in LVAD patients is another area void of research. As is advised with postthoracotomy patients, CR/SP staff should wait >12 weeks after device implant before beginning a light resistance training pro-gram. Other considerations include avoiding any exercises that may dramatically increase intra-abdominal pressure (e.g., sit-ups) or that have the potential for physical trauma (i.e., contact sports); the latter could cause a fracture of the drive line or potentially create damage to the LVAD itself.

Special Considerations

Extensive education is required for the LVAD patient; this includes knowledge of signs and symptoms of exercise intolerance and how to modify exercise, device console alarms (e.g., low battery, low flow), duration of the power supply, and who to contact during a medical emergency. CR/SP staff should also be familiar with the LVAD device and should work with the patient and LVAD coordinator at their institution regarding emergency procedures and complications common with the device:

Differential Diagnosis for a Low Flow Alarm on the Left Ventricular Assist Device

- Obstruction
- Right ventricular failure

- Pulmonary embolism
- Hypovolemia
- Pump failure
- Bleeding cardiac tamponade
- Arrhythmias
- Systemic hypertension

As with other participants in CR/SP, a brief review of any clinical changes and assessment of vital signs should be performed before exercise, along with the patient's subjective response to exercise. However, due to the nonpulsatile flow of blood in the newer LVAD models, auscultatory blood pressure assessment may be difficult and may not be reliable. Instead, the clinician might want to consider measuring mean arterial blood pressure via Doppler ultrasound.[62]

Special considerations regarding exercise are similar to those for other CR/SP participants, with particular attention to exercise tolerance. Additionally, exercise is contraindicated if mean arterial pressure is less than 70 mmHg, if the low flow device alarm is activated, or if the patient exhibits intolerance to the workload, regardless of objective normal blood pressure findings.[59] Should an LVAD patient lose consciousness, it is important to remember not to perform chest compressions, as this may damage the LVAD and dislodge the lines attached to the heart. Emergency defibrillation for lethal arrhythmias may be performed; however, most LVAD patients have an implantable cardioverter defibrillator (ICD).

The number of patients who have received an LVAD has grown exponentially over the last few years, and the restoration of exercise tolerance and clinical surveillance represent a new opportunity and responsibility for the CR/SP professional. Many patients and their families need counseling for home exercise parameters given the approval of LVADs as destination therapy. While parallels can be drawn with other types of patients who benefit from CR/SP, additional research is needed to help define and describe how patients with LVADs benefit from exercise and the procedures associated with ensuring a safe exercise prescription.

Cardiac Transplantation

The first successful human heart transplantation (HT) was performed by Christian Barnard in Cape Town, South Africa, in 1967.[1] Despite only a brief period of survival in this patient, enthusiasm among the medical community spurred a number of surgical centers to perform the operation. Developments at Stanford University, including improved techniques for preservation of the donor organ, the transvenous right ventricular endomyocardial biopsy technique for early detection of acute rejection, and the introduction of the powerful immunosuppressant cyclosporine in the 1980s, resulted in marked improvement in survival.[2] These important advances, as well as eventual insurance funding of the operation and aftercare in the United States, made the procedure an attractive treatment for patients with terminal HF.

The 2010 report of the Registry of the International Society for Heart and Lung Transplantation listed 225 transplant centers worldwide, the majority located in North America, performing approximately 3,000 HT procedures annually.[3] The most common reasons for HT are nonischemic cardiomyopathy, ischemic cardiomyopathy, retransplantation, adult congenital heart disease, and VHD.[3]

Immunosuppression is achieved with a variety of drugs, including combinations of tacrolimus, sirolimus, mycophenolate mofetil, mycophenolic acid, and prednisone.[3,4] The goals of immunosuppression are the prevention of acute rejection and also minimizing the risks of infection and malignancy. Common comorbidities associated with immunosuppressant use include hypertension, obesity, diabetes mellitus, and hyperlipidemia.[3]

Median survival is approximately 10 years after HT.[3] Survival at 1 and 5 years averages 90% and 70%, respectively.[5] The highest mortality occurs in the first 6 months after surgery, with a fairly constant annual mortality rate of 3% to 4% after the first year.[3] Antibody-mediated acute rejection is characterized by T-lymphocyte infiltration of the myocardium, which may result in myocyte injury and necrosis. Patients are most susceptible to acute rejection during the first several months after transplantation. Periodic endomyocardial biopsies are performed to detect rejection. Treatment includes increased amounts of immunosuppressants and may require hospitalization. Allograft vasculopathy, an unusually accelerated form of coronary disease with a poorly understood pathophysiology, is a major limiting factor in long-term survival.[3]

In general, most patients report a favorable quality of life after HT.[3] It is not uncommon for patients to return to work, school, and their usual avocational activities, although exercise capacity remains below normal for most.[6]

Psychological Factors

The psychological response to the transplant process is understandably intense for most patients.[7] During the waiting period for the operation after acceptance as a transplant candidate, emotions range from relief and happiness to anxiety (indefinite waiting time, lack of absolute assurance that the transplant will occur) and thoughts of death. Postsurgery, as the period of convalescence continues, patients must adjust to the tedium of medical appointments and procedures. The immunosuppressant prednisone may cause mood swings and personality change. The first episode of acute rejection may result in heightened feelings of anxiety and transient depression. As the recovery from surgery progresses and the degree of medical surveillance decreases, patients generally shift their attention from transplant-related activities to becoming more independent, resuming family roles, and engaging in occupational and avocational pursuits. The readjustment to life after transplantation requires months, and the 1-year anniversary is an important milestone in this process. Following the acute phase of recovery, most patients are able to return to productive and meaningful lives.

Noncompliance with medications, skipping clinic appointments, smoking recidivism, lack of regular exercise or failure to participate in CR/SP, and dietary lapses are common.[8] Predictors of noncompliance include young age at transplant, lower educational level, depression, anxiety, hostility, substance abuse, and poor social support.

Responses to Exercise

The responses of HT recipients to acute exercise are unique and are related, in part, to the following factors: [9-11]

- The transplanted heart is surgically denervated. A minority of patients demonstrate evidence of partial sympathetic reinnervation months after transplantation (discussed later in this section).[12]
- The donor heart has experienced ischemic time and reperfusion.

- There is no intact pericardium.
- Diastolic dysfunction (elevated filling pressures at rest and with exercise) is common.
- Abnormal skeletal muscle histology and energy metabolism, developed during the course of chronic HF, may continue after HT.[13]
- Peripheral and coronary vasodilatory capacity may be impaired, in part due to endothelial dysfunction.

Heart Rate and Exercise

The loss of parasympathetic innervation of the donor heart causes an elevated resting HR (95 to 115 bpm).[14] With graded exercise, the HR typically does not increase initially due to sympathetic nervous system denervation but then gradually rises. Peak HRs are only slightly lower than expected (approximately 150 bpm). The highest exercise-related HRs usually occur during the first few minutes of recovery. Heart rate may remain near peak values for several minutes during recovery before gradually returning to resting levels. The chronotropic reserve is less than normal. Regulation of HR during exercise is dependent on circulating catecholamines, especially during the first few months after transplantation.[15]

Blood, Intracardiac, and Vascular Pressures

Blood pressure at rest is often mildly elevated, even though most patients receive antihypertensive medications. Exercise blood pressure generally increases appropriately, although the peak is slightly lower than expected.[16] Vascular resistance is elevated along with intracardiac and pulmonary vascular pressures (particularly right-sided pressures).[17]

Left Ventricular Function

For most HT patients, left ventricular ejection fraction is normal at rest and during exercise.[17] However, as mentioned previously, left ventricular diastolic function is often impaired, as evidenced by an elevated filling pressure for a given end-diastolic volume.[17] This impairment results in a below-normal increase in stroke volume during exercise.

Exercise Cardiac Output

At the onset of exercise, cardiac output in HT recipients with complete cardiac denervation increases due to augmentation of stroke volume via the Frank-Starling mechanism. Subsequently, increased HR also contributes to augmentation of cardiac output.[18]

Skeletal Muscle Structure and Biochemistry

During the clinical course of chronic HF, several skeletal muscle structural and biochemical abnormalities develop; these include reduced aerobic metabolic enzyme activity, lower capillary density, endothelial dysfunction with impaired vasodilation during exercise, and conversion of some slow-twitch motor units to fast-twitch motor units with greater reliance on anaerobic than on aerobic energy production. These abnormalities generally persist after HT, with partial improvement after several months for some patients.[19-21]

Pulmonary Function and Arterial Oxygenation

The efficiency of pulmonary ventilation during exercise may be below normal (increased ventilatory equivalent for CO_2 [$\dot{V}E/\dot{V}CO_2$]) during the first several months after HT.[9,22] The normal increase in exercise tidal volume is blunted.[23] Alveolar gas diffusion impairment is present in approximately 40% of patients. However, arterial oxygen saturation at rest and during exercise is normal for most patients.[24] A minority of patients with pre-HT diffusion abnormalities experience mild arterial desaturation (to approximately 90%) with exercise.[25]

Oxygen Extraction by Exercising Skeletal Muscle

Extraction of oxygen at rest is normal after HT. However, during exercise the arterial–mixed venous oxygen difference does not increase in a normal manner. This reflects abnormalities with the delivery of capillary blood to the exercising skeletal muscle and impairment of the oxidative capacity of the muscle.[17]

Oxygen Uptake Kinetics, Peak Oxygen Uptake ($\dot{V}O_2$)

With the onset of exercise, the rate of increase in $\dot{V}O_2$ (oxygen uptake kinetics) is slower than normal because of the impaired rise in cardiac output and a diminished oxidative capacity of the skeletal muscle.[26] Because of these abnormalities (impaired exercise cardiac output and reduced arterial–mixed venous oxygen difference), peak $\dot{V}O_2$ is usually below normal for HT patients. In

a series of 95 patients with a mean age of 49 years who performed a cardiopulmonary exercise test approximately 1 year after HT, the mean peak $\dot{V}O_2$ was 20 mL · kg^{-1} · min^{-1} (range, 11 to 38 mL · kg^{-1} · min^{-1}).[27] Selected highly trained HT patients may achieve much higher values.[28,29]

Rarely, highly motivated and well-trained transplant recipients are able to perform impressive athletic feats.[30,31] The upper limit of endurance exercise performance after HT is probably that reported for a 49-year-old man, 22 years after surgery, who completed an Ironman triathlon (3.8 km swim, 180 km cycle, 42.2 km run) in 15.6 h, finishing 1881st out of 2067 athletes.[32]

The Impact of Partial Cardiac Reinnervation

Occasionally, HT patients with allograft vasculopathy resulting in myocardial ischemia report typical anginal symptoms, suggesting at least partial afferent cardiac reinnervation.[33] Additionally, sympathetic efferent reinnervation may occur in many patients during the first several months to years after surgery as evidenced by neurochemical evaluation of autonomic nervous system activity in the heart and the observation of improved chronotropic responsiveness during exercise.[34,35] The heart rate reserve (also called chronotropic response) increases during the first 6 weeks after surgery in many patients, and there are continuing increases in a subset of patients.[35] A more rapid decline in HR from peak exercise to baseline is observed in some patients at 1 to 2 years after HT.

Heart rate responsiveness to maximal graded exercise was assessed in a group of 95 HT recipients at 1 year after surgery.[27] Partial normalization of the HR response to exercise was demonstrated in 33.7% of the group. Maximal HR ($P < .008$) and exercise test duration ($P < .05$) increased significantly, although peak $\dot{V}O_2$ did not. Other investigators, using fewer subjects than in the study just mentioned, have reported either no effect of partial reinnervation on aerobic capacity[36] or a prominent improvement.[37]

Responses to Exercise Training

HT recipients are excellent candidates for progressive exercise training (ET) for several reasons: pre-HT syndrome of chronic HF with poor exercise capacity due to central and peripheral circulatory abnormalities, skeletal muscle pathology, deconditioning, the healing process with open heart surgery (similar to that observed with coronary or valvular surgery), and post-HT use of corticosteroid medications with resultant skeletal muscle atrophy and weakness.

Aerobic Exercise Training

The literature contains multiple reports demonstrating the benefits of aerobic ET for patients after HT.[38-45] In general, HT recipients respond to training similarly to other cardiac patients. Peak $\dot{V}O_2$ improves by an average of 24% after 2 to 6 months of ET; this training improves mitochondrial oxidative capacity but apparently does not increase skeletal muscle capillary density as it does in healthy subjects.[46] Potential additional benefits of regular ET for HT recipients include the following:

- Improved submaximal exercise endurance
- Increased peak treadmill exercise workload or peak cycle power output
- Increased maximal heart rate
- Decreased exercise heart rate at the same absolute submaximal workload
- Increased ventilatory (anaerobic) threshold
- Decreased submaximal exercise minute ventilation
- Reduced exercise ventilatory equivalent for CO_2
- Lessened symptoms of fatigue, dyspnea, or both
- Reduced rest and submaximal exercise systolic and diastolic blood pressure
- Decreased peak exercise diastolic blood pressure
- Reduced submaximal exercise ratings of perceived exertion
- Improved psychosocial function
- Increased lean body mass
- Reduced body fat mass
- Increased bone mineral content

Two of the early, larger group studies were published in 1988. Niset and coauthors[40] studied 62 patients at approximately 1 month after HT and again at 1 year. Kavanagh and colleagues[42] reported results of 16 months of training in 36 HT recipients. Neither study used a control group. Niset found that directly measured peak

$\dot{V}O_2$ increased by 33% ($P < .01$), and Kavanagh reported a 27% increase in peak $\dot{V}O_2$. Some limitations of these earlier investigations were overcome in a 6-month-long study reported by Kobashigawa and colleagues in 1999.[45] Twenty-seven HT patients were randomized to an ET or control group early after surgery. The ET group underwent supervised ET (aerobic and strengthening exercises), whereas the control group performed an unstructured home walking program. Peak $\dot{V}O_2$ improved more in the supervised ET group (+4.4 vs. +1.9 mL · kg^{-1} · min^{-1}, $P < .01$). There were no differences between the two groups in number of episodes of acute rejection or infection. Supervised ET programs appear to improve fitness to a greater extent than less structured approaches.

Resistance Exercise

Most HT patients require prednisone, at least during the first several months after surgery, for immunosuppression. Skeletal muscle atrophy and weakness are common side effects related to prednisone. Resistance ET partially reverses corticosteroid-related myopathy and improves skeletal muscle strength. Horber and coauthors[47] found definite evidence of skeletal muscle wasting and weakness in the lower extremities of renal transplant patients who received prednisone. Fifty days of isokinetic strength training substantially increased muscle mass and strength in these patients. In addition, strength training has been shown to improve bone density and to reduce the potential development of osteoporosis (also caused by prednisone) in HT recipients.[48]

Effect of Exercise Training on Immune Function and Longevity

An obvious and important question concerning ET in immunosuppressed HT recipients is the effects of training on immune function. Traditional, moderate ET does not increase or decrease the number or severity of episodes of rejection.[45,49] In addition, ET does not require changes in immunosuppressant dosage or treatment. Infection risk is not changed by ET. There are no data regarding the effect of ET on survival after HT.

Interventions in CR/SP Programs

The types of interventions provided to HT patients are similar to those provided for more typical CR/SP patients: patient and family counseling and education, psychosocial evaluation and counseling, early mobilization, outpatient ET, and CVD risk factor management. One difference is the longer inpatient stay after transplantation, which provides the opportunity for inpatient ET.

Specific education topics for patients and families include the following:

- Medications: purposes, potential side effects, importance of strict compliance with recommended dosing
- Risk of rejection, infection, and allograft vasculopathy
- Postoperative management schedule: tests, appointments
- Nutrition: reduced fat, caloric intake, and sodium to help prevent weight gain related to prednisone use and to help control blood pressure

Considerations for psychosocial intervention include providing ongoing emotional support and encouragement. Group interactions or support sessions that include the patient, family members, and group facilitators are useful in assisting patients in rebuilding family relationships and responsibilities as well as with interactions with friends and business or professional contacts. Specific goals of such interventions include the development of coping skills, stress management techniques, and practical skills to deal with the multiple issues involved in posttransplant life. The relationship of standard coronary risk factors such as tobacco use, dyslipidemia, hypertension, obesity, and sedentary living to allograft vasculopathy is not well established. However, most transplant programs seek to optimally control all modifiable risk factors.

Exercise Testing and Training in Heart Transplantation Patients

Exercise testing is an important part of the evaluation process for HT and subsequently, after HT, for determining recommendations for the patient's return to appropriate levels of physical activity. The following section provides the basis for exercise testing, recommendations for performing the exercise test, and considerations for exercise training early mobilization, and inpatient and outpatient training.

Pretransplant Graded Exercise Testing and Training

As part of the evaluation process for HT, many ambulatory patients undergo cardiopulmonary exercise testing. Peak $\dot{V}O_2$ is a powerful prognostic indicator: Patients with an aerobic capacity of 10 to 14 mL · kg^{-1} · min^{-1} (3-4 METs) or below experience a markedly reduced 1-year survival, independent of left ventricular ejection fraction.[50]

Based on the results of the exercise test, an ET prescription may be developed with the goal of maintaining or even improving cardiorespiratory fitness. Ideally, the exercise program should be carried out under medical supervision, although many patients have performed home-based, independent exercise successfully.

Posttransplant Graded Exercise Testing

Exercise testing after HT is helpful in determining exercise capacity post-transplantation, thus facilitating the prescription of ET, and counseling of patients regarding the timing of return to work or school or resumption of avocational pursuits. In addition, exercise testing provides a mechanism for the evaluation of patient's response to exercise, including ECG findings which frequently demonstrate right bundle branch block and nonspecific repolarization abnormalities at rest. However, the sensitivity of the exercise ECG in detecting ischemia due to the presence of allograft vasculopathy is poor (<25%) unless combined with myocardial imaging.[51]

Due to the healing and recovery process after surgery, and the usual deconditioned state before surgery, it is best to wait 6 to 8 weeks after surgery before performing graded exercise testing to maximal effort. For patients with more complicated postoperative courses, an even longer period of recovery is recommended before performance of an exercise test.

Treadmill or cycle ergometer protocols with continuous exercise (2 or 3 min stages or ramp tests) may be used. Arm cranking protocols may also be employed, after adequate sternal healing, for a specific upper extremity fitness evaluation or an arm cranking exercise prescription.[52] The initial exercise intensity during the test should be approximately 2 METs, with 1 or 2 MET increments in intensity per stage.[33,52] Continuous multilead ECG monitoring with assessment of blood pressure and rating of perceived exertion for each stage is recommended. For precise determination of aerobic capacity, direct measurement of $\dot{V}O_2$ and associated variables is highly desirable. The end points of the graded exercise test should be maximal effort (symptom-limited maximum) or standard signs of exertional intolerance.[53]

Early Mobilization and Inpatient Exercise Training

After surgery, patients are extubated expeditiously, usually within 24 h. Passive range of motion exercises for both the upper and lower extremities, sitting up in a chair, and slow ambulation may begin and progress gradually after extubation.[54] Walking or cycle ergometry for up to 20 to 30 min may be implemented as tolerated. Exercise intensity is guided using the ratings of perceived exertion 11 to 13 ("fairly light" to "somewhat hard") while maintaining a respiratory rate below 30 breaths per minute and arterial oxygen saturation above 90%. Exercise frequency is two or three sessions per day.[9] Patients whose postoperative courses are uncomplicated remain hospitalized for 7 to 10 days.

During inpatient rehabilitation, as well as during the outpatient phase, episodes of rejection of a moderate or greater severity may require alteration of the ET plan. If the rejection episode is graded as moderate, activity may be continued at the current level but should not progress until after the rejection has been adequately treated. Severe rejection necessitates suspension of all physical activity with the exception of passive range of motion exercises.

Outpatient Exercise Training

The Centers for Medicare and Medicaid Services (CMS) recognizes cardiac transplantation as a diagnosis that is eligible for CR/SP coverage, removing barriers for HT recipients to enter an outpatient CR/SP program upon discharge from the hospital.[9,55] Patients are generally required to remain near the transplant center for approximately 3 months for close follow-up. Ideally, they should exercise both in a supervised environment and independently.

Continuous monitoring of the ECG during the first few supervised ET sessions is standard practice, although many weeks of ECG-monitored ET is seldom useful. It is not necessary to perform graded exercise testing before beginning the outpatient exercise program; however, performance of a 6-minute walk test is helpful in assessing functional capacity. Graded exercise testing should be performed 6 to 8 weeks after surgery for patients without complicated recoveries as discussed previously.

Exercise prescription for HT patients is similar to that used with patients who have undergone other cardiothoracic surgery. The one exception is that a target HR is not used unless the patient exhibits a partially normalized HR response to exercise, as discussed previously. The typical denervated heart increases in rate slowly during submaximal exercise, and the HR may either drift gradually higher during steady-state exercise or plateau after several minutes.[26] The rating of perceived exertion scale is useful for prescription of exercise intensity. Table 9.14 provides specific suggestions for exercise prescription.

At the aforementioned 6-8 weeks of sternal recovery following surgery, aerobic activities including arm involvement may be introduced. The sternal incision requires special emphasis on upper extremity active range of motion exercises. More vigorous upper body physical activity or sports such as tennis and golf may be considered as the patient becomes fully recovered and level of fitness is adequate (≥5 METs).

Skeletal muscle weakness in HT recipients is common and is related to skeletal muscle atrophy due to advanced HF, pre-HT deconditioning, and corticosteroid use post-HT as part of the immunosuppressant regimen. Resistance ET should be incorporated into the ET program to counteract these factors. For the first 6 weeks after surgery, bilateral arm lifting is restricted to less than 10 lb (4.5 kg) to avoid sternal nonunion. Strength gains of 25% to 50% or greater commonly occur after 8 weeks of resistance ET in these patients.[9,48] Performance of the strengthening exercises immediately following the aerobic portion of the exercise prescription (after the cool-down) is recommended. Because HT recipients are likely to require antihypertensive medications, periodic blood pressure measurement during both aerobic and strengthening ET is recommended.

Conclusion

Both exercise testing and exercise training including aerobic and strength training are critical com-

Table 9.14 Exercise Prescription Suggestions for Outpatients After Cardiac Transplantation

Mode	Frequency	Intensity	Duration
1. Warm-up, cool-down (stretching, range of motion, low-intensity aerobic exercise)	Each session	RPE <11	10+ min
2. Aerobic First 6 weeks after surgery: walking (treadmill, indoors, outdoors), cycle ergometer (upright, recumbent) At 6 weeks, include combination arm and leg ergometer, elliptical, rower, arm ergometer, jogging (treadmill, track, outdoors), water-based exercise	Five to seven sessions per week (three supervised, two or more independent)	RPE 12 to 16 (if HR response to exercise has normalized, 50% to 80% of HRR)	Begin with 5 to 10+ min per session; increase to 5 min per session; progress to 30 to 60 min per session; may use intermittent, continuous, or interval approaches
3. Strength (e.g., free weights, weight machines, elastic bands; include exercises for major muscle groups)	Two or three sessions per week on nonconsecutive days	First 6 to 8 weeks after surgery: <10 lb for upper extremities, otherwise RPE 12 to 16	One to three sets, 8 to 15 slow repetitions per set

RPE, rating of perceived exertion (scale 6-20); HR, heart rate; HRR, heart rate reserve technique.

ponents of care for HT patients. Encouragement to continue a lifelong exercise program should be a consistent message from the HT team and the primary health care provider. Patients should continue in a supervised ET program indefinitely, exercise independently, or use a combination of supervised and unsupervised ET.

Peripheral Arterial Disease

Peripheral arterial disease (PAD) is the result of systemic atherosclerosis. The underlying disease process that affects the blood vessels is common to patients with CAD and stroke. The risk factors for these atherosclerotic conditions are essentially the same; diabetes is an exceptionally strong risk factor for PAD. People with PAD may be asymptomatic or may experience exertional leg discomfort. Some present with the classic symptom of intermittent claudication (IC), which most commonly manifests as leg pain during walking. IC limits exercise tolerance and presents a unique challenge to CR/SP specialists in that it potentially requires modification to the rehabilitative process, including the exercise prescription, which is typically used in CR/SP.

Evaluation of Claudication

Because leg discomfort is not an uncommon complaint, particularly among older patients, it is helpful to identify some of the characteristics of claudication that differentiate it from other causes of leg pain. By definition, IC is pain or profound fatigue in a muscle brought on by exertion and relieved by a few minutes of rest. Typically, a patient with PAD experiences pain in the calf, thigh, or buttocks, which is exacerbated by walking. The distance to onset of claudication usually depends on the severity of the disease. The pain subsides after a variable period of rest, and the patient may resume walking, often for the same distance. The symptom is consistent and reproducible and is associated with a *chronic* arterial occlusive disease process. It should not be confused with the severe pain due to a sudden occlusion or thrombosis of an artery in the lower extremity. *Acute* occlusion of an artery causes pain that is severe, constant (even at rest), and associated with other exaggerated signs of obstructed blood flow such as a cold, pale, or bluish extremity without pulses below the area of obstruction.

Claudication should also be differentiated from other frequent causes of leg aches and pains in the older population such as arthritis and chronic venous insufficiency. Arthritis differs from claudication in that it causes pain in the joints, may vary from day to day or with changes in the weather, and may occur with or without activity. Chronic venous insufficiency in the lower extremities results in blood pooling in the extremities and is associated with leg or ankle edema. The symptom is aggravated by standing or sitting for long periods. It is described as an ache or full sensation in the legs and may include sciatic pain; it is typically worse at the end of the day and is relieved by resting with the legs elevated.

Specific findings on physical assessment help confirm the diagnosis of PAD and claudication. Peripheral pulses are diminished or absent by palpation. Color changes include pallor of the extremity, especially if elevated above heart level, or dependent rubor, a bright reddish color occurring in the affected limb when it is placed in the dependent (dangling) position. Diminished arterial flow results in a cooler extremity compared to the unaffected leg. Mild to moderate claudication is not a limb-threatening condition. The goal of treatment is the relief of symptoms and risk factor modification. If claudication becomes severely limiting and interferes with the ability to work, revascularization may be necessary.

When PAD becomes severe, it is referred to as critical limb ischemia, and patients may develop rest pain. The patient experiences this symptom as a burning pain in the toes, and it occurs most often when the patient is in bed or has the affected limb elevated. Patients may get some relief by hanging the foot over the side of the bed or by sitting up in a chair. Even narcotics may provide only minimal relief. Ischemic pain may progress to paresthesia and paralysis of the toes and foot. Rest pain is a limb-threatening symptom, and the patient must be referred immediately for further evaluation and revascularization.

Diagnosing Peripheral Arterial Disease

Lower extremity PAD can be readily diagnosed using the ankle–brachial index (ABI), which is a ratio of systolic blood pressure measured in the ankle and brachial arteries. Specific peripheral arterial blood flow and anatomic evaluation is often done with other tests such as ultrasonography, computed tomographic angiography (CTA),

magnetic resonance angiography (MRA), or conventional angiography. Postexercise ABIs, measured immediately after walking on the treadmill, can also be used to confirm the diagnosis. A common initial procedure after the diagnosis is established by the ABI is noninvasive Doppler arterial testing of the lower extremities. A complete study begins with segmental systolic arterial pressures. These are obtained using BP cuffs placed in four locations on the leg: the upper thigh, above the knee, below the knee, and at the ankle. A Doppler ultrasound stethoscope is used to measure systolic pressures at all four levels. Generally, these pressures should be equal to, or slightly higher than, the brachial systolic pressure. Leg pressures that are lower than brachial pressures by 20 mmHg or more indicate arterial insufficiency.

Evaluation of Functional Status

The comprehensive assessment of the PAD patient should focus on the impact of claudication on activities of daily living (ADL). Improving the functional capacity of the patient becomes a central goal of the exercise rehabilitation for PAD. A baseline of functional disability documented at the beginning of the program can then be used to measure therapeutic outcomes. Disease-specific questionnaires, such as the Walking Impairment Questionnaire and the PAD Physical Activity Recall Questionnaire, have been found to be beneficial in documenting the functional status of patients before and after participation in an exercise rehabilitation program.[1]

Assessing Cardiac Status in the PAD Patient

The risk of CVD is markedly increased in patients with PAD,[2] and more than 95% of persons with PAD have one or more CVD risk factors.[3] Because claudication limits their activity, many patients may not experience any cardiac symptoms. Before beginning any cardiovascular exercise program, these patients should undergo appropriate cardiac stress evaluation. A cycle ergometer, instead of a treadmill, may permit increased myocardial work before leg symptoms occur and therefore allow more accurate assessment of cardiac risk. Pharmacologic stress testing such as dobutamine stress echocardiography and sestamibi or thallium scintigraphy with adenosine may be considered for the patient with claudication and thus limited ability to achieve adequate physiological stress. However, an exercise evaluation before beginning exercise training is helpful to specifically describe exercise limitations resulting from PAD as well as associated symptomatic responses, including time of onset of pain, pain level, HR, blood pressure, and workload at exercise cessation, all of which are helpful in defining an exercise prescription.[1,4-6]

Walking Capacity

Once cardiac risk has been determined, the effects of claudication on walking capacity should be assessed. A treadmill is useful for evaluating the extent of claudication, as well as the effectiveness of any treatment. Historically, claudication distance and maximum walking distance were evaluated using a fixed speed and grade. Two graded protocols are suggested for use with claudication patients. The same speed, 2 mph (3.2 kph), is used in both protocols. The Gardner-Skinner protocol increases the grade by 2% every 2 min.[4] The Hiatt protocol increases the grade by 3.5% every 3 min.[5] Both protocols are widely accepted and have proven effective and accurate in evaluating onset of claudication and maximum walking distance.

Following a preexercise measurement of ankle pressures, the patient is asked to walk on a treadmill until the claudication forces cessation of exercise. Immediately after the patient stops, ankle pressures are recorded again. In the absence of PAD, ankle pressures do not decrease with exercise. A postexercise drop in ankle systolic pressure confirms the diagnosis of arterial disease. Subsequent ankle pressures are recorded at 1 min intervals for 10 min or until the return to preexercise levels. In addition to estimating the location and severity of the disease, this testing provides baseline information for subsequent progress evaluations. Follow-up testing should be performed upon completion of exercise rehabilitation and should include a resting ABI calculation, a treadmill walk at the same settings as at the baseline evaluation, and postexercise ankle pressures with recovery time. Though the ABI may actually change very little in response to exercise training, improvement is noted by a delayed onset of claudication, increased maximum walking distance, and shorter recovery time of ankle pressures.

Cardiovascular Disease Risk Factors

The same risk factors that contribute to cardiac disease also cause PAD and should be treated aggressively. Strong evidence indicates that smoking is the most significant controllable risk factor for PAD. Aside from its contribution to the development and progression of atherosclerosis, cigarette smoking increases the severity of claudication pain, reduces peripheral circulation, and negatively affects cardiopulmonary responses with exercise.[7] These effects further reduce the exercise capacity of patients with claudication. Strict adherence to an exercise program is of marginal benefit if patients, particularly those who have undergone revascularization procedures, continue to smoke. Refer to the section "Tobacco Use" in chapter 8 for information related to this intervention.

Skin and Foot Assessment

Impaired arterial flow to the extremities contributes to poor skin perfusion, making skin more fragile and susceptible to injury and infection. Many patients with PAD also have diabetes and suffer from neuropathy, which decreases their ability to feel pain or irritations to the feet until damage is severe. When the protective barrier of the skin is broken, the arterial system is unable to meet the extra demands required for healing. Unfortunately, specialized wound care treatment or revascularization may be the only alternative. In more severe cases, if infections cannot be controlled, amputation may be required. Foot care should follow the recommendations described in the "Diabetes" section of chapter 8 ("Instructions for Foot Care for Patients With Diabetes"). If ulcers are present on the extremity, boots or casts that keep pressure off of the ulcer or alterations in the rehabilitation program such as arm exercise are required until the ulcers are healed.

Practice Considerations

Efforts to provide greater structure to rehabilitation of the vascular patient have increased since the mid-1980s. These efforts have taken two directions: (1) the development of dedicated exercise rehabilitation programs for PAD and (2) the incorporation of PAD care within existing CR/SP programs to accommodate the patient with both cardiac disease and PAD. In January 2001, the current procedural terminology (CPT) editorial board of the American Medical Association approved a code for PAD rehabilitation. This code, 93668, is a major step toward providing structured vascular rehabilitation to patients with PAD. Unfortunately, reimbursement remains inconsistent. In 2010, the AACVPR in conjunction with the Vascular Disease Foundation published *PAD Exercise Training Toolkit: A Guide for Health Care Professionals*. The toolkit was developed to allow CR/SP and other exercise and rehabilitation health care professionals to work within their communities to improve access to supervised exercise programs for people with IC. It includes information to help exercise and rehabilitation professionals implement appropriate and safe supervised exercise programs. It also includes practical tools such as sample brochures plus participant and staff education materials. The toolkit can be found at www.vasculardisease.org/files/pad-exercise-training-toolkit.pdf.

Exercise Prescription

A program of supervised exercise rehabilitation is considered a primary treatment for people with PAD and IC. The ACC/AHA clinical practice guideline for treatment of PAD rated exercise therapy for IC as a Class I, Level of Evidence A, recommendation, which compares very favorably to levels of recommendation for medications or some revascularization procedures.[6] This is the highest recommendation that is given to a treatment. Because of the efficacy of exercise rehabilitation, in 2010 the ACC and AHA Task Force on Performance Measures recommended that health care providers either refer a patient to a program or discuss exercise rehabilitation as a treatment option for appropriate patients with PAD.[8]

For the patient with PAD, supervised exercise is performed three times per week, generally in a CR/SP or wellness program setting, usually for 12 to 24 weeks for 1 h per session. The 60 min exercise session includes a 5 min warm-up and 5 min cool-down period. The initial exercise training intensity is established using a graded treadmill test or a functional evaluation during the first exercise session, and is defined as the grade (% incline) that brings on the onset of claudication pain (i.e., level 2 of 5 on the claudication scale; see the "Intermittent Claudication Rating Scale" in chapter 6, with the initial speed set at 2.0 mph

(3.2 kph). Some patients may not be able to tolerate a treadmill speed of 2 mph and may need to start the exercise program at a slower speed and progress as tolerated. Participants are asked to walk to a mild to moderate pain level (3-4 on a scale of 5), stop and sit down and rest until the claudication pain has completely abated, and then resume walking. The initial goal of the early training sessions is to have the participants accumulate 15 min or more of total treadmill time, excluding warm-up and cool-down, with the eventual goal to progress to a cumulative exercise session of 50 min including rest periods and warm-up and cool-down periods of 5 min.

The following is one example of an exercise session for patients with PAD.[1,4-6] (Patients walk at a constant speed throughout each session without change. Note that the claudication pain scale is an important tool for monitoring symptomatic improvements in exercise performance and resulting increases in exercise intensity.) If the participant is able to walk at a workload for 8 min or more before experiencing moderate claudication pain (3-4/5), the grade is increased by a 1% or 2% increment for the following training session. Once the participant is able to walk at a 10% grade for 8 min or more, the speed is increased by 0.1 to 0.2 mph (0.16 to 0.32 kph) increments at the next session, up to 3.0 mph (4.8 kph). If the participant is able to walk for 8 min or more at 3.0 mph and 10% grade, the grade is once more increased by 1% or 2% increments at the next training session up to 15% grade (i.e., last increase is 1% increment). This is followed by increases in speed by 0.1 to 0.2 mph increments for the subsequent training session as tolerated.

Alternative Modes of Exercise

Treadmill walking is the cornerstone of rehabilitation exercise for people with IC. There is some evidence that other modalities of aerobic training may also be beneficial in improving symptoms. These modes of exercise may be useful if the patient cannot or will not tolerate walking. In addition, because these exercises largely avoid leg pain, they may be useful to achieve higher exercise intensity in the presence of IC that markedly limits exercise capacity. These alternatives include pole striding, experimental pain-free treadmill training where possible, leg cycle ergometry, lower extremity resistance training, and arm ergometry.[9-15] However, the studies are relatively few, and further study with larger samples is needed to warrant changes in PAD exercise rehabilitation guidelines. Though resistance training has been shown to provide some benefits in terms of functional capacity[11], the existing data are too limited to support a recommendation for resistance training as a primary mode of exercise rehabilitation for reducing claudication symptoms. Thus, resistance training for a total of 60 minutes per session can be performed as tolerated, as a supplement to, but not as a substitute for walking.

Postrevascularization Considerations

The length of time after surgery until it is permissible to begin rehabilitation depends on the procedure and the overall condition of the patient. Generally, patients who have a minimally invasive procedure, such as peripheral angioplasty, are ready for a rehabilitation program relatively quickly, within a week or two. Conversely, abdominal aortic surgery carries a much longer recovery period (generally 6-8 weeks). Lower extremity bypass procedure patients may recover more quickly but are limited more by groin and knee incision soreness. Any graft placement that crosses the knee joint requires the avoidance of any prolonged, sharp flexion of that joint, which could cause a kink in the graft. Cycle ergometers are usually permissible with proper seat height adjustment, but these patients should probably avoid rowing machines.

Pharmacologic Treatment

Medications used to control atherosclerotic risk factors (e.g., lipid-lowering agents, antihypertensives, nicotine replacement therapy) are part of the regimen for patients with PAD. Patients who have thromboembolic disease may also benefit from antithrombotic agents such as anticoagulants, antiplatelet medications, or thrombolytic therapy. Medications specifically targeted at treating the symptoms of claudication are very few. Pentoxifylline has been used for the treatment of claudication. This agent is said to increase red cell flexibility and reduce blood viscosity, thereby increasing the delivery of oxygenated blood to ischemic extremities. Some patients have noted improved walking tolerance, whereas others have not. Cilostazol has been shown to improve pain-free walking distance and increase maximum walking distance in claudication patients.[16] The exact mechanism of action is unclear, though it seems to have a peripheral vasodilating effect. Other beneficial effects are decreased triglycerides and increased high-density lipoprotein cholesterol. Several other drugs are currently under investigation. When using any medication for claudication, it is important to inform patients that it does not cure atherosclerosis and should not be used as a substitute for a regular walking program. Perhaps the greatest role of these medications is as an adjunct to CR/SP, because they lessen the severity of claudication symptoms and enable patients to comply with the all-important daily exercise regimen that helps them achieve and maintain cardiovascular health.

Chronic Lung Disease

Many people who have significant CVD, such as CHD, cerebrovascular disease, or peripheral vascular disease, also have significant chronic lung disease; and in many instances, it is the latter that limits exercise ability. Given the prevalence of cigarette smoking and the significant lag time (often several decades) leading up to the development of symptoms and disability related to the effects of cigarette smoke on the lungs, it is not surprising that many patients have both cardiac and lung disease. Additionally, chronic lung disease such as chronic obstructive pulmonary disease (COPD) often goes undetected until it is moderately to severely advanced. It is thus very important to consider the possibility of the presence of chronic lung disease for all patients who are entering a CR/SP program, particularly in those with a smoking history (greater than 20 pack-years) or symptoms of dyspnea, cough, or mucus production. As many as 20% of patients entering a CR/SP program have symptoms related to underlying lung disease.[1]

Patients with comorbid pulmonary impairment are likely to have shortness of breath (either at rest or with exercise) and may have cough or sputum production or both. Increases in respiratory rate, wheezing, hyperinflated chest, muscle wasting, or more than one of these may be noted on examination. For patients who may have underlying chronic lung disease, a few diagnostic tests can help to determine its presence or absence. Pulmonary function testing (e.g., spirometry) is the diagnostic tool of choice to diagnose COPD. Pulmonary function testing can help to determine the presence, type, and severity of disease, for example obstructive (e.g., COPD or asthma) versus restrictive lung disease (interstitial lung disease such as pulmonary fibrosis). Arterial blood gases are helpful to determine the presence of underlying hypoxemia, hypercapnia, or both. Arterial oxygen saturation, as measured by pulse oximetry, is helpful to determine whether oxygen desaturation (at rest or with exercise) may be present. A chest x-ray may indicate the presence of lung hyperinflation or diaphragmatic flattening, in the case of COPD, and chest wall abnormalities such as kyphosis or scoliosis. A chest computed tomograpghy (CT) scan can be used to diagnose interstitial lung disease, including pulmonary fibrosis as well as bronchiectasis. Pulmonary hypertension may be suspected from elevated right heart pressures on echocardiogram, which is the noninvasive screening test of choice.[2] However, a right heart catheterization is the gold standard for accurate diagnosis. Several questionnaires have been developed that can help determine whether or not a patient is at risk for the presence of COPD and are helpful in the initial assessment of patients undergoing CR.[3,4]

Cardiopulmonary exercise testing with the measurement of expired gases is helpful in the evaluation of a patient undergoing CR/SP who is suspected to have underlying chronic lung disease. For a patient with chronic lung disease, decreased ventilatory reserve, increased dead space ventilation, hypoxemia, and increased respiratory rate at isotime (a standardized exercise period of time) may be noted. In some instances the pulmonary impairment is the limiting factor to exercise before significant cardiac abnormalities (e.g., angina) manifest. Although such exercise testing need not be performed in every patient who is entering a CR/SP program, it can be very helpful for patients who have both cardiac and pulmonary disease to help determine the principal cause for the exercise limitation and to determine an effective exercise prescription. If a field test such as the 6-minute walk or shuttle walk test is used, continuous oxygen saturation monitoring during testing can uncover desaturation during activity. A finger oximeter may be used. If a handheld oximeter is used, it should be placed in a pouch or fanny pack to avoid the evaluator's influencing patient walk stride.

COPD is the most common type of chronic lung disease in patients with CVD. COPD includes both emphysema and chronic bronchitis and is characterized by the inability to exhale air fully or by chronic airflow obstruction. Shortness of breath and exercise intolerance may subsequently develop given the effects of the disease process on the lung parenchyma, dynamic hyperinflation, and skeletal muscle dysfunction. Hypoxemia can also develop and further limit exercise tolerance. Asthma, another type of chronic lung disease, is characterized by variable airflow obstruction that is often reversible either spontaneously or with treatment. Asthma is characterized by airway inflammation causing airway hyperresponsiveness, airflow limitation, dyspnea, and chronic disease. Patients often have a sensitivity to aeroallergens and worsening of symptoms due to viral respiratory infections. Other types of lung disease may be present in patients with CVD, including interstitial fibrosis or pulmonary hypertension. Exercise limitation occurs due to the effects of the disease process on the mechanics of the lung, hypoxemia, and skeletal muscle dysfunction.

Optimal management for a patient with chronic lung disease includes both pharmacologic and nonpharmacologic therapy. For patients who continue to smoke, smoking cessation should be undertaken as a first step in the management process. For a patient with COPD, optimal management of pharmacologic therapy is an important cornerstone of treatment. Appropriate use of inhaled bronchodilator should be addressed. Patients are usually managed with one or more long-acting agents, including a beta agonist or long-acting anticholinergic agent. Short-acting bronchodilators are normally used for rescue or during exacerbations. Inhaled corticosteroid therapy is normally reserved for severe COPD with frequent exacerbations or for patients with persistent asthma. In some instances, medications used in the treatment of COPD are associated with side effects for patients with cardiac disease. For example, theophylline (though rarely used today in clinical practice) and beta agonists (in some patients) may aggravate underlying cardiac dysrhythmias.

Some patients with chronic lung disease have associated hypoxemia (either at rest or with exercise) requiring supplemental oxygen. Oxygen therapy should be administered to those who have oxygen desaturation to below 90% (either at rest or with exercise). Titration of supplemental oxygen to maintain an oxygen saturation measure above 90% should be performed and can be easily assessed during the exercise sessions with the use of pulse oximetry.

Nonpharmacologic therapy for every patient with chronic lung disease must be considered. Breathing retraining techniques (e.g., pursed-lip breathing; for some, diaphragmatic breathing), energy conservation measures such as pacing, and self-management techniques such as prevention and early management of exacerbations should be discussed with the individual patient. Bronchial hygiene techniques (e.g., postural drainage, chest physical therapy, secretion clearance devices) should be included for patients who have chronic sputum production and retained secretions. Influenza and pneumococcal vaccination should be a standard part of the treatment regimen.

Standard exercise prescription regimens (see the section on physical inactivity in chapter 8) can be used for most patients, although ongoing consideration of the evidence base for this process is strongly encouraged. Both lower extremity and upper extremity training should be included. For patients who have exercise limitation primarily related to the underlying chronic lung disease, an exercise prescription based on symptom-limited end points can be used. For patients who have undergone cardiopulmonary exercise testing, an exercise prescription can be developed based on the findings from that testing. While weakness of the upper extremities is less frequently noted in patients with isolated CHD, it is frequently noted in patients with chronic lung disease. Specific upper body exercises including resistance training should be included in the exercise regimen for these patients. Upper extremity training has been shown to improve functional ability during activities of daily living.[5,6]

Summary

Underlying lung disease may well be present in patients undergoing CR/SP, particularly in persons with long-standing, habitual smoking. In patients with a high index of suspicion of comorbid chronic lung disease, an important first step in the management process is an accurate diagnosis through pulmonary function testing and evidence-based management. Strategies for developing an effective CR/SP program should address not only the cardiovascular component of the disease process but also the pulmonary component in order to optimize the effects of the program.

Program Administration

Providing excellent service to patients requires effective leadership to develop programs that foster continuous patient service and quality improvement. The application of standards and guidelines to improve both clinical efficacy and cost-effectiveness requires a sophisticated approach to management and administration (see the "AACVPR Resources for Professionals" www.aacvpr.org/Resources/ResourcesforProfessionals/tabid/531/Default.aspx)

Effective administration requires knowledge of

- performance measures,
- core competencies,
- data collection and analysis of patient-centered outcomes,
- clinical practice guidelines and position statements,
- budget,
- policy and procedure formation and implementation,
- productivity and utilization,
- insurance and managed-care contracting, and
- quality and performance improvement issues.

OBJECTIVES

This chapter reviews the following administrative considerations for program operation:

- Program priorities
- Facilities and equipment
- Organizational policies and procedures
- Insurance and reimbursement
- Documentation
- Personnel
- Continuum of care and services

Program Priorities

The AACVPR has emphasized several important program priorities over the past few years. Performance measures based on outcomes measures were one of the first initiatives, as was increasing referral rates. The Core Components addressed the need for a comprehensive program for all patients. The Core Competencies for program professionals were developed to integrate specific knowledge and skills into the implementation of the Performance Measures as well as the Core Components. Lastly, AACVPR Program Certification embraces these priorities to which programs and personnel aspire to. This chapter deals with the administrative issues that programs must address and contend with in order to be efficacious and, in fact true secondary prevention programs.

Applying CR/SP Performance Measures

The emergence of performance measures in all areas of health care has been embraced by governmental entities and providers seeking to promote and deliver both efficacious and cost-effective services. Scientific research demonstrating significant underutilization of cardiac rehabilitation/secondary prevention (CR/SP)[1] led to the development of performance measures by the American Association of Cardiovascular and Pulmonary Rehabilitation (AACVPR), American College of Cardiology (ACC), and American Heart Association (AHA) that promote physician referral to early outpatient CR/SP.[2,3] The inclusion of the measures discussed in chapter 2 for appropriate patient populations has served to reduce the underutilization barrier and is an example of clinical actions taken as a result of scientific evidence. The integration of the CR/SP performance measures into program operation should be a goal of the program director.

Maximizing Program Utilization

The application of referral performance measures in an early outpatient CR program is one strategy that will enhance program enrollment. Automation of the referral process results in significant improvement in referral patterns.[4] Taking an active role in facilitating referrals and beginning the early outpatient CR program within 1 to 3 weeks after hospital discharge are other effective strategies to address underutilization of the service.[5,6] Barriers to utilization due to capacity restraints may be addressed through various methods, including expanding days of operation, adding more sessions at more convenient times, relocating to a larger space, adding a satellite site, or changing the program model to an open gym design rather than limited class slots. The program director and staff must consider many factors and continually assess for optimal utilization and program growth opportunities.

Outcomes-Based Programming

There is increasing focus on clinical outcomes of procedures and treatments on the part of health care providers, payers, and consumers. While the reasons for this shift are multifactorial, the result has been heightened emphasis on scientific research and evidence-based guidelines to justify medical interventions. This transition has occurred in the field of CR/SP as well. One illustration is the Medicare-added designation of Intensive Cardiac Rehabilitation (ICR), which is reimbursed for significantly more CR sessions.[7] This designation was developed by the Centers for Medicare and Medicaid Services based on identified clinical outcomes demonstrated by these ICR programs.[8] Measurement and attainment of significant clinical patient outcomes upon completion of CR/SP should be a top priority for all programs. Emerging meaningful evidence-based patient and program outcomes are addressed in chapter 11.

Ensuring Program Comprehensiveness

CR/SP is typically provided by a multidisciplinary team of health professionals. This model has served the profession well by providing a broad spectrum of expertise through the combined use of various disciplines. Familiarity with the AACVPR Core Competencies assists a program director in building a comprehensive team (see table 10.1).[9] Mastery of core competencies by individual CR/SP staff members enables the team to be successful in meeting the scientifically documented AACVPR Core Components of a comprehensive CR program (see chapter 2, tables 2.1 and 2.2).[10]

Alternative Models of CR/SP Delivery

A changing clinical profile of patients entering cardiac rehabilitation over recent years has significant implications for contemporary CR/SP programs. CR/SP patients are older, more overweight, and more likely to have diabetes mellitus and hypertension, and to be relatively less fit than their predecessors.[11] For the majority of modern-day CR/SP patients, the focus may need to shift to behavioral weight loss counseling and more effective exercise training strategies, such as high-intensity exercise or long-duration training, to achieve desired clinical outcomes.[12] Attention

Table 10.1 Core Competencies for Cardiac Rehabilitation and Secondary Prevention Professionals

Competency	Knowledge	Skills
Patient assessment	Demonstrate an understanding of: • Cardiovascular anatomy, physiology, and pathophysiology • Process of arteriolosclerosis and pathogenesis of cardiovascular risk factors • Cardiac arrhythmias (e.g., complex PVCs, atrial fibrillation, SVT) and their influence on physical activity and symptoms • Cardiac device therapies (e.g., pacemakers, defibrillators, and left ventricular assist devices) • Cardiovascular assessments, diagnostic tests, and procedures • Signs and symptoms of CVD • Appropriate emergency responses to changing signs and symptoms • Effective lifestyle management of CVD and associated risk factors • Pharmacologic approaches for CVD and risk factor management • Comorbidities limiting or otherwise influencing function or treatment strategies • Side effects from pharmacologic therapies • Psychosocial factors related to CVD • Adult learning principles, theoretical models for behavior change, adherence, coping, disease management strategies • Compliance and adherence to therapeutic regimens • Effective communication to referral sources and the interdisciplinary team to promote care coordination • Principles and methods for outcome assessment and reporting	Ability to perform the following: • Obtain a comprehensive medical, social, and family history through interview, review of medical records, and questionnaires • Physical examination of cardiovascular system (e.g., measure HR, BP; auscultate heart and lung sounds; palpate and inspect extremities for edema, pulses, signs of DVT and PAD; inspect surgical wound) • Develop risk factor profile and CVD risk reduction strategies • Basic tests and assessments: 12-lead ECG, oximetry, blood glucose, and blood lipids • Obtain information on patient preferences and goals • Interactive communication and counseling with patient and family on treatment plan through shared decision making • Develop an ITP • Document and communicate ITP and progress reports to physicians and interdisciplinary team • Quantify patient outcome assessment through pre- and postprogram assessment
Nutritional counseling	Demonstrate an understanding of: • Role and impact of diet on CVD progression and risk factor management • Analysis of diet composition with specific emphasis on total caloric intake and dietary content that influences risk factors (e.g., total fats, cholesterol, refined and processed carbohydrates, sodium) • Potential risks and benefits of nonprescription nutritional supplements and alcohol intake • Target goals for dietary modification and nutrition interventions for identified risk factors and comorbidities (e.g., dyslipidemia, hypertension, diabetes, obesity, heart failure, kidney disease) • Effective behavior change strategies based on common theoretical models and adult learning strategies	Ability to perform the following: • Dietary intake assessment to estimate total calories; amounts of saturated fat, trans fat, cholesterol, sodium, fruits and vegetables, whole grains, fiber, and fish; number of meals and snacks; portion sizes; frequency of eating out; alcohol consumption • Education and counseling on specific dietary modifications needed to achieve target goals • Behavioral interventions to promote adherence and self-management skills in dietary habits • Measure and report outcomes of nutritional management goals at the conclusion of the program

(continued)

Competency	Knowledge	Skills
Weight management	Demonstrate an understanding of: • Physiological and pathological effects of overweight and obesity and those of low body weight • Principles of weight management through the balance of caloric intake and caloric expenditure • Awareness of fad diets and possible risks to CVD patients • Current guidelines and recommendations for healthy body weight and secondary prevention • Weight loss interventions that promote gradual, sustainable weight loss (5-10%) over 3 to 6 months • Medications and surgeries for weight loss • Nutritional and medical risks associated with rapid weight loss and cyclical weight gain and weight loss • Recognition that weight loss and weight maintenance is often complex and difficult and requires ongoing dietary management, physical activity, and behavioral management • Importance and efficacy of regular physical activity, modification of dietary patterns, changes in caloric balance, and drug therapy in weight management • Effective behavior change strategies based on common theoretical models and adult learning strategies	Ability to perform the following: Measure body weight, height, and waist circumference Calculate body mass index and determine proper category: normal, overweight, or obese Develop short- and long-term weight loss goals for those in overweight or obese categories Assess nutritional and dietary habits as well as daily energy intake and expenditure to help guide individualized education and counseling for weight management Behavioral interventions to promote adherence and self-management skills in weight management Measure and report outcomes of weight management at the conclusion of the program
Blood pressure management	Demonstrate an understanding of: • Hypertension as a risk factor for atherosclerotic vascular disease and potential end-organ damage • Signs and symptoms of hypotension and hypertension • Normal range of BP at rest and during exercise • Current BP targets for secondary prevention • Role of home BP monitoring in BP management • Actions of classes of antihypertensive medications and common side effects • Postural and postexercise hypotension • Elements of the DASH diet for treating hypertension • Principles of measurement and operation for different devices used to measure BP • Recognition that BP control is often complex and difficult and may require ongoing medication adjustments, dietary management, physical activity, and behavioral management • Importance and efficacy of sodium restriction, weight management, physical activity and exercise, smoking cessation, alcohol moderation, and drug therapy in the control of BP	Ability to perform the following: • Accurate BP determinations at rest (seated, supine, and standing) and during exercise • Recognize significant BP deviations from the expected range or targeted outcome • Assess compliance with BP medications and management plan • Measure and report outcomes for BP management at the conclusion of the rehabilitation program
Lipid management	Demonstrate an understanding of: • Definitions of LDL-C, HDL-C, VLDL-C, TG, non-HDL-C • Physiological role of lipids in the atherosclerotic disease process • Elements of the Therapeutic Lifestyle Change Diet and the Mediterranean diet • Actions of classes of antihyperlipidemic medications, including nonprescription, and side effects • Types of dietary fats and simple carbohydrates and their effect on serum lipid levels • Current serum lipid target values for secondary prevention • Importance and efficacy of weight management, physical activity and exercise, smoking cessation, alcohol moderation, and drug therapy in the control of serum lipids	Ability to perform the following: • Interpret LDL-C, HDL-C, non-HDL-C, VLDL-C, and TG values in light of secondary prevention target values • Assess compliance with antihyperlipidemic medications and management plan • Assess compliance with lifestyle interventions for the management of serum lipid values • Provide patient education information concerning serum lipids • Develop a risk reduction plan for abnormal serum lipids and communicate the plan to the patient and family • Measure and report outcomes for serum lipids at the conclusion of rehabilitation

Competency	Knowledge	Skills
Diabetes management	Demonstrate an understanding of: • Type 1 and type 2 diabetes • Fasting and casual blood glucose values that define hypoglycemia and hyperglycemia • Importance of and recommended target value for HbA1c • Complications related to diabetes: micro- and macrovascular; autonomic and peripheral neuropathy; nephropathy; and retinopathy • Signs and symptoms related to hypoglycemia and hyperglycemia • Use of carbohydrates for hypoglycemia • Actions of glucose-lowering medications and insulin • Importance of monitoring blood glucose values, especially before and after exercise • Contraindications to exercise based on blood glucose values • Importance of compliance with diabetic medications and dietary, body weight, and exercise recommendations • Importance of recognizing and managing the metabolic syndrome and the associated CVD risk factors • Importance and efficacy of weight management, physical activity and exercise, alcohol moderation, and drug therapy in the control of blood glucose	Ability to perform the following: • History of complications related to diabetes, including frequency and triggers of hyperglycemia and hypoglycemia • Calibration and proper use of glucometers • Assess signs and symptoms of hyperglycemia and hypoglycemia and take appropriate actions • Provide patient education concerning the effects of lifestyle and medications on glycemic control • Referral of the patient to a diabetic educator or clinical dietitian, as needed • Measure and report outcomes for glucose control at the conclusion of rehabilitation, including episodes of hyperglycemia and hypoglycemia during and after exercise
Tobacco cessation	Demonstrate an understanding of: • Current guidelines for treating tobacco use and secondary prevention goal • Biochemical and physiological consequences of smoking on CVD • Exposure to secondhand smoke as a risk factor for cardiovascular events • Effective behavior change strategies based on common theoretical models • Available services to support smoking cessation (e.g., community smoking cessation programs, counselors, psychologists) • Physiological and psychological aspects of tobacco addiction • Efficacy of pharmacologic interventions, including risks and benefits	Ability to perform the following: • Assessment of use and categories of tobacco use: never, former, recent, or current • Behavioral interventions to promote tobacco cessation and long-term tobacco-free adherence • Measure and report outcomes of tobacco cessation at the conclusion of the program
Psychosocial management	Demonstrate an understanding of: • Influence of psychosocial factors on the pathophysiology of CVD and adherence to treatment • Depression and its major association with recurrent CAD events, poorer outcomes, and adherence to treatment • Other psychological indicators that may affect treatment response, such as anxiety, anger or hostility, and social isolation • Actions of pharmacologic and lifestyle interventions for psychological distress • Socioeconomic factors that may serve as barriers to treatment adherence, such as educational or income level, lack of resources or support • Available support services to augment psychological interventions (e.g., psychologists, counselors, social workers, clergy) • Effective behavior change strategies based on common theoretical models and adult learning strategies[17]	Ability to perform the following: • Screening and assessment for psychological distress, especially depression, anxiety, anger or hostility; social isolation; marital or family distress; sexual dysfunction; and substance abuse • Appropriate referrals for psychiatric or psychological care when needs are recognized as beyond the scope of usual care • Individual and group education and counseling interventions that address stress management and coping strategies • Measure and report outcomes of psychosocial management at the conclusion of the program[7,18]

(continued)

(continued)

Competency	Knowledge	Skills
Physical activity counseling	Demonstrate an understanding of: • Lack of regular physical activity and sedentary behavior as a risk factor for CAD • Negative health consequences of time spent being sedentary • Current recommendations for intensity, frequency, and duration for regular physical activity in persons with CVD • Preexisting musculoskeletal and neuromuscular conditions that may affect physical activity • Identifying physical activities that may increase the risk for an untoward cardiovascular event and environmental conditions that may also increase the risk • Barriers to increasing physical activity • Metabolic requirements for recreational, occupational, and sexual activities • Recommendations to avoid musculoskeletal injury related to physical activity • Effective behavior change strategies based on common theoretical models and adult learning strategies	Ability to perform the following: • Assess current physical activity level using both questionnaires and available activity-monitoring devices • Assist patients in setting realistic incremental goals for future physical activity • Recommendations for increasing the level of safe and appropriate daily physical activity and structured exercise • Assess physical and metabolic requirements for activities of daily living and occupational and recreational activities • Communication and behavioral strategies that will improve compliance with regular physical activity recommendations • Measure and report outcomes for physical activity at the conclusion of rehabilitation
Exercise training evaluation	Demonstrate an understanding of: • Normal and abnormal responses to exercise including signs and symptoms of exercise intolerance, myocardial ischemia, acute coronary syndrome, and ventricular arrhythmias • Physiological responses to acute exercise and adaptations to chronic exercise • Risk stratification according to patient assessment and exercise test results • Exercise prescription methodology for cardiovascular endurance exercise and resistance training in a broad range of patients with heart disease • Absolute and relative contraindications for exercise • Absolute and relative indications to terminate an exercise session	Ability to perform the following: • Recognize life-threatening cardiac arrhythmias, myocardial ischemia or infarction, hypoxemia, hypotension, hypoglycemia, and other signs and symptoms of exercise intolerance • Risk stratify each patient according to AHA and AACVPR criteria • Develop an individualized, safe, and effective cardiovascular endurance exercise prescription, including modes, intensity, duration, frequency, and progression • Develop an individualized, safe, and effective exercise prescription for resistance training, including load, number of repetitions, frequency, and progression for appropriate muscle groups • Include warm-up, cool-down, and exercises for flexibility and balance in the exercise prescription • As needed, accommodate existing comorbidities within the exercise prescription • Skin preparation and electrode placement for exercise ECG telemetry monitoring • Measure and report outcomes for exercise training at the conclusion of rehabilitation

Abbreviations: AACVPR, American Association of Cardiovascular and Pulmonary Rehabilitation; AHA, American Heart Association; BP, blood pressure; CAD, coronary artery disease; CVD, cardiovascular disease; DASH, Dietary Approaches to Stop Hypertension; DVT, deep vein thrombosis; ECG, electrocardiogram; HbA1c, glycosylated hemoglobin; HDL-C, high-density lipoprotein cholesterol; HR, heart rate; ITP, individual treatment plan; LDL-C, low-density lipoprotein cholesterol; PAD, peripheral artery disease; PVCs, premature ventricular contractions; SVT, supraventricular tachycardia; TG, triglycerides; VLDL-C, very low-density lipoprotein cholesterol.

Reprinted, by permission, from L.F. Hamm et al., 2011, "Core competencies for cardiac rehabilitation/secondary prevention professionals: 2010 Update. Position statement of the American Association of Cardiovascular and Pulmonary Rehabilitation," *Journal of Cardiopulmonary Rehabilitation and Prevention* 31: 2–10.

should be paid to applying current principles of exercise physiology in the early outpatient and maintenance CR/SP settings. Strategies may need to move beyond an early outpatient CR model established in the 1970s to one that is more effective given the present-day cardiovascular patient population.

Current knowledge of adult learning and behavior change theory as discussed in chapter 3 suggests that an individualized approach to education is more effective than the historical approach in CR using preselected topics delivered in a set number of educational classes for all CR/SP participants. A CR/SP program can provide critical tools and support in fostering self-efficacy and behavior change if these concepts are understood, supported, and put into practice by the entire CR/SP staff.

The longstanding paradigm for early outpatient CR patients has been 1 h sessions of primarily cardiovascular exercise, two or three times per week. If this is not provided in combination with an emphasis on a concurrent progressive home exercise prescription, it fails to successfully integrate science into practice. The evidence that a dose greater than 250 min/week of physical activity is most effective in eliciting clinically significant weight loss should be considered in the development and progression of the exercise prescription.[13] Most participants in early outpatient and maintenance CR/SP programs fail to perform significant amounts of activity on non-CR/SP exercise days.[14-16] These findings reinforce the importance of the CR/SP team in providing exercise, physical activity, and educational components that will assist in achieving the best possible outcomes for each patient. In addition, the importance of resistance training, as well as its safety and efficacy for patients with cardiovascular disease, is well substantiated.[17] For that reason, it is one of the fundamental interventions included in the exercise training core component for CR/SP programs.[10] A delivery model for exercise prescription that provides for individualized exercise components—that is, exercise frequency, intensity, duration, and modality—promotes increased physical activity consistent with evidence-based recommendations.

Since the inception of CR, improved cardiovascular fitness through exercise training has been a principal goal. This is based on strong scientific evidence that the level of peak aerobic capacity is a very strong predictor of the risk of death among subjects with or without cardiovascular disease.[18]

On an ongoing basis, program directors should critically evaluate program delivery models in order to provide those clinical outcomes that are the foundation of CR/SP and are based on the science of exercise physiology and behavior change.[19]

Lastly, quality improvement is advantageous only if it is more than a perfunctory process to satisfy regulatory, accreditation, and internal institutional requirements. The AACVPR program certification process is a useful examination of program quality. It is the obligation of the program director to maintain an atmosphere of continuous quality improvement (guideline 10.1) through continuous oversight of operations relative to objectives in striving to consistently elevate program quality and ultimately add value to the patient experience.

Fiscal Accountability

Operating a fiscally sound CR/SP program requires analysis of utilization barriers and opportunities to increase utilization, innovative programming, strategic hiring, prudent control of costs, and maximizing use of space. In the past, Medicare regulations restricted varied program paradigms, but today early outpatient CR/SP programs are able to offer flexible participation as the importance of identifying individual patient needs has been emphasized by both regulating bodies and payers.[20,21] Continuous analysis of referral and enrollment rates to track program utilization and removing barriers to program participation increase utilization.[22] It is essential to maintain good communication with the business office and upper-level administration to ensure accurate assessment of program performance by all decision makers and to ensure full awareness of administrative expectations. Hospital and facility

---

 Guideline 10.1 Continuous Quality Improvement

Program staff should develop a process for ongoing

- review of policy and procedure manuals to ensure that they are current, comprehensive, and accurate;
- evaluation of performance dimensions, such as timeliness, effectiveness, continuity, safety, and efficiency;
- evaluation of client satisfaction; and
- continued scrutiny of related research to compare outcomes with national, regional, and local programs.

administrators should be regularly provided with evidence-based summaries of the value of CR with respect to program outcomes, as well as mortality, morbidity, and cost-effectiveness analyses.[23,24]

Facilities and Equipment

Policies and procedures regarding the management of the facility are aimed at providing a safe, functional, and effective environment. Many of the requirements for services provided within institutions are regulated by federal, state, and local agencies. The components of these policies should include

- planning of space utilization,
- maintenance of equipment,
- reduction and control of environmental hazards and risks,
- maintenance of safe conditions, and
- climate control.

Specific AACVPR delineations are provided here to better ensure safe and effective CR/SP programming, facilities, and equipment. These guidelines are organized into four areas:

- General—apply to all CR/SP service facilities and equipment

- Inpatient—specifically address the needs of inpatient services
- Outpatient—specifically address the needs of outpatient CR/SP, both early and long-term services
- Stress testing specific to programs that provide stress testing services

Inpatient Exercise Facilities and Equipment

In the current era of short hospital stays and very limited time for the patient to receive even a basic evaluation of cardiovascular disease (CVD) risk, initiation of preventive therapies, and referral to outpatient CR/SP, specific inpatient exercise facilities and equipment are not necessary components to inpatient CR program services. Nonetheless, the environment for such services should allow safe and easy patient movement. Exercise services may be conducted in patient rooms, hospital hallways, and stairwells. Where used, hallways should be free of obstruction, with access to handrails, and distances should be measured. Equipment needs depend on the services provided but might include 1 to 3 lb (.45 to 1.3 kg) dumbbell weights or low-level resistance bands, cycle ergometers, and treadmills with low-speed capabilities. Inpatient and outpatient program areas should comply with guidelines 10.2 and 10.3.

Guideline 10.2 General Facility Considerations

- Space must meet the requirements for the activities and services provided and the unique needs of patients. There must be emergency access to all patient areas, and floor space must allow easy access of personnel and equipment. Floor space should be approximately 40 to 45 sq ft (3.7-4.2 sq m) per patient.

- All areas should provide temperature and humidity control that allow for a comfortable environment. Humidity should be at or below 60%, temperature 68 to 72 °F.

- Sound levels should be kept at a level comfortable for all participants.

- Ceiling height in exercise areas must allow for full, unrestricted activity with a minimum height of 10 ft (3 m).

- A water source should be immediately available to all exercise areas. Food and drink should not be allowed on or near exercise or monitoring equipment.

- All facilities must provide for confidentiality of patient records and patient privacy.

- A regularly tested telephone and emergency call system should be available in all exercise areas and an emergency phone list available at all phones. Emergency delivery system guidelines are discussed in chapter 12. Basic first aid should be available to all exercise areas.

Guideline 10.3 General Equipment Considerations

- Equipment requirements may vary depending on the patient population and the staff training.
- All equipment should be commercial grade, with stringent maintenance guidelines to ensure patient safety.
- Scheduled maintenance, preventive maintenance, and cleaning programs for all exercise equipment must be documented.
- Equipment that is not functioning properly or that is damaged and may cause a hazard should be designated as out of service until repairs are complete.
- Equipment such as treadmills or cycle ergometers should be regularly calibrated and maintained as recommended by the manufacturer.

- Staff should be thoroughly trained in the use of all equipment, and manufacturer information for correct use, calibration, and troubleshooting should be readily available.
- A chair and an exam table or a cart suitable for supine and recumbent positions should be available in the area.
- Equipment for patient assessment including a quality stethoscope, portable sphygmomanometer, electrocardiogram (ECG) monitors, pulse oximeter, portable oxygen, and a posted and clearly visible rating of perceived exertion (RPE) scale should be available to all exercise areas.

Outpatient Facilities and Equipment

Facilities should provide separate space for patient reception and waiting, patient consultation and education; exercise; confidential chart storage; safekeeping of valuables; and easily available rest rooms, which may include showering facilities. Outdoor exercise areas may also be included. Participants with disabilities should have full access to all CR/SP facilities in adherence with requirements of the Americans with Disabilities Act (ADA). Outpatient facilities should provide for the following[25]:

- Program and safety information that is accessible and prominently posted
- Open-access circulation, avoiding blind corners, unnecessary doors, pointless partitions, and other hazards that present a safety risk to users
- Space for program operation, storage, and maintenance that is separate from that used for physical activity; floor surfaces in physical activity areas should provide the proper level of absorption and slip resistance to minimize the risk of impact- or fall-related injuries
- Exercise floor space between 25 and 50 sq ft (2.3 and 4.6 sq m) per piece of equipment for aerobic conditioning and resistance training, as well as adequate floor space for stretching activities

- Physical activity spaces with sufficient air circulation and outside air to maintain air quality, room temperatures, and humidity at safe and comfortable levels during times of physical activity
- A patient consultation area with adequate space, privacy, and amenities for interviewing, counseling, teaching, and physical examination
- Separate rest rooms, which may include showering facilities; showers should be equipped with nonslip surfaces that are cleaned and disinfected regularly
- A regularly tested emergency call system in locker rooms and shower rooms

Specific equipment selection depends on individual program preference, available space, and budget. Exercise equipment should provide multiple modalities for safe and effective aerobic conditioning. Examples of such equipment are motorized treadmills with speed and grade control; calibrated upright or supine cycle ergometers; and calibrated upper body ergometers, rowers, or elliptical trainers that display accurate ergonomic work units. Other potential exercise equipment includes resistance training equipment with adjustable benches; individual dumbbell weights, in pairs, that are easily accessible and safely stored; and elastic bands. Individual step benches, floor mats, and sport balls provide for an increased variety of activities, and an outdoor or indoor walking track (or other space) free of obstruction and wide enough for easy passage is attractive and effective in exercise programs. Additional facility and equipment (materials) recommendations for program operations include the following:

- Emergency equipment (see chapter 12)
- Clearly visible rating scales for perceived exertion, angina and other pain, and dyspnea
- Heart rate monitoring technology or a clock with a sweep secondhand, easy to read from all exercise areas
- Blood glucose meter and glucose supplements (e.g., fruit juice and crackers) in programs that include persons with diabetes
- Calibrated weight scale and protocols for determining body composition (e.g., body mass index) or other necessary equipment (e.g., automated body fat calculating devices, skinfold calipers, or circumference measuring tapes)
- Education area with comfortable chairs and, ideally, access to computers with Internet, audiovisual equipment, a resource library, and anatomical models or diagrams

Stress Testing Facility and Equipment

Areas used for exercise testing should comply with guidelines 10.2 and 10.3. A treadmill and leg-alone or arm–leg cycle ergometer with measurable, calibrated workload are most often the equipment used in a testing facility.

Patient selection, safety, and financial considerations should influence decisions concerning facilities and equipment for programming. The selection of equipment that patients will most likely need in a maintenance or fitness setting should be considered. Given that long-term adherence is a primary goal of early outpatient CR/SP, familiarity with such exercise equipment facilitates a smoother transition to a new setting.

Organizational Policies and Procedures

All health care providers come under the purview of regulatory bodies, including federal and state regulatory boards. In Medicare terminology, *providers* include patient care institutions such as hospitals, critical access hospitals, hospices, nursing homes, and home health agencies. The Social Security Act (SSA) mandates the establishment of minimum health and safety standards that must be met by providers participating in the Medicare and Medicaid programs. These standards are published in Title 42 Code of Federal Regulations (CFR) Part 482.[26] The U.S. Department of Health and Human Services (HHS) has designated the Centers for Medicare and Medicaid Services (CMS) to administer the standards compliance process. State survey agencies carry out the Medicare certification process on a contractual basis. Title XVIII of the SSA, Section 1861, contains Conditions of Participation (CoP) and Conditions for Coverage (CfC) that health care organizations must meet in order to participate in the Medicare and Medicaid programs. CMS ensures that the standards of accrediting organizations recognized by CMS meet or exceed the Medicare standards in the CoP and CfC. All accrediting entities must have first completed a CMS application process to obtain "deemed status." For example, a hospital accredited by the Joint Commission (TJC) is deemed to meet all Medicare requirements for hospitals (excluding special conditions for psychiatric hospitals and other specified services). Most accrediting entities are independent and hold nonprofit status. Other examples are the Commission on Accreditation of Rehabilitation Facilities (CARF) and the National Committee for Quality Assurance (NCQA). Hospital-affiliated programs must meet Occupational Safety and Health Administration (OSHA) regulations for safety of personnel. National Patient Safety Goals (NPSG) is an important component of TJC accreditation that is periodically reviewed and revised. See "Websites for Regulatory and Accrediting Organizations and Information" for a list of these websites.

Policies and Procedures

Institutional policies and procedures must conform to these regulatory standards in addressing such topics as infection control and hazardous waste, human resource management, nursing practice, performance improvement, emergency and disaster response, administrative policy and procedures, and safety.

Departmental policies and procedures are subordinate to institutional policies and func-

Websites for Regulatory and Accrediting Organizations and Information

- American Association of Cardiovascular and Pulmonary Rehabilitation (AACVPR), www.aacvpr.org
- American Board of Physical Therapy Specialists (ABPTS), www.abpts.org/home.aspx
- American Physical Therapy Association (APTA), www.apta.org
- Centers for Medicare and Medicaid Services (CMS), www.cms.gov
- Commission on Accreditation of Rehabilitation Facilities, www.carf.org
- Health Insurance Portability and Accountability Act of 1996—HIPAA "Privacy Rule," www.hhs.gov/ocr/hipaa
- National Commission for Quality Assurance, www.ncqa.org
- Occupational Safety and Health Administration, www.osha.gov
- Medicare Conditions of Coverage for Cardiac Rehabilitation Program and Intensive Cardiac Rehabilitation Program, http://edocket.access.gpo.gov/cfr_2010/octqtr/pdf/42cfr410.49.pdf
- Medicare Hospital Conditions of Participation[27], www.cms.gov/medicare-coverage-database/details/ncd-details.aspx?NCDId=36&ncdver=1&NCAId=241&NcaName=Cardiac+Rehabilitation+Programs&ISPopup=y&bc=AAAAAAAAAQAAAA%3D%3D&
- Medicare Coverage Center, www.cms.gov/center/coverage.asp
- National Patient Safety Goals (NPGS), www.jointcommission.org/standards_information/npsgs.aspx
- The Joint Commission (TJC), www.jointcommission.org
- Social Security Act, www.ssa.gov/OP_Home/ssact/title18/1861.htm

tion to define numerous aspects of the CR/SP program philosophy, processes, and plans of action. These are living documents that should be reviewed annually and revised as frequently as is necessary to maintain relevancy. Policies and procedures are helpful resources for new staff members and are useful in fostering consistency of care provided in the CR/SP program. Policies, procedures, and professional guideline references should be easily accessible and familiar to all CR staff.

Information Management

Information management involves oversight of the storage, transmission, use, and tracking of patient information. The passage of the Health Insurance Portability and Accountability Act of 1996 (HIPAA) led to the development of the Privacy Rule in 2000 (www.hhs.gov/ocr/hipaa). This established a set of national standards for the protection, use, and disclosure of certain health information by organizations subject to the Privacy Rule and standards for the privacy rights of individuals. Policies and procedures related to information management should include storage and access to

- patient records, patient privacy and confidentiality, and outcome data;
- financial records and analysis, budget allocation, capital and operational expenses;
- insurance billing, precertification, and reimbursement;
- provision of charity and scaled remunerative services; and
- patient registration and procedure scheduling.

The policies for management of information are usually developed and implemented by the institutional management team in a centralized area or department.

Insurance and Reimbursement

Continuous change in health care management and reimbursement patterns for CR/SP is evident in nearly all markets across the United States. Advances in technology will continue to affect all areas of medicine through

- proliferation of electronic medical records (EMR) and consequent enhanced health information communication between health care providers;

- use of telemedicine in the treatment of chronic disease and targeted patient populations; and
- growth of evidence-based treatment decisions through greater integration of endorsed performance measures, appropriateness criteria, and guidelines.

The escalating cost of health care in the United States is one of the major driving forces behind the direction of these advances. Demonstration projects funded and implemented by government and private insurance companies seek treatments that result in effective patient outcomes and cost savings. Payers and providers recognize that these technological changes in medicine have begun to demonstrate improved patient care.

Health Insurance Companies

Health insurance companies can be divided into two distinct sectors, private and public. The private sector contracts with individuals or groups to offer a variety of plans that provide no coverage or minimum coverage with copays and deductibles through a continuum to 100% coverage with no copays or deductibles. The enrollee may make these contracts directly with an independent insurance company or through the employer. Managed-care plans may be promulgated by integrated delivery systems, hospital systems, insurance companies, and private for-profit companies. Public sector insurance is administered under a government-sponsored program. Examples of public sector entities are Medicare and Medicaid, TRICARE for military and public health service workers, and the Bureau of Vocational Rehabilitation (BVR).

Medicare

The Centers for Medicare and Medicaid Services (CMS) is the governing body within Health and Human Services (HHS) responsible for the enactment of congressional laws that oversee the government public medical insurance plan. CMS administers coverage and payment guidelines for the following categories of Americans who qualify for Medicare:

- People age 65 or older
- People under age 65 with certain disabilities

- People of all ages with end-stage renal disease (permanent kidney failure requiring dialysis or a kidney transplant)

Medicare is relatively comprehensive in its coverage for hospital inpatient, outpatient, and physician services. Outpatient benefits for CR/SP are summarized here:

- **Part A, Hospital Insurance.** Most people do not pay a premium for Part A because they or a spouse already paid for it through their payroll taxes while working. Medicare Part A (Hospital Insurance) helps cover inpatient care in hospitals, including critical access hospitals, inpatient rehabilitation facilities, and skilled nursing facilities (not custodial or long-term care). Beneficiaries must meet certain conditions to qualify for these benefits.

- **Part B, Medical Insurance.** Most people pay a monthly premium for Part B. Medicare Part B (Medical Insurance) assists with physician services and hospital outpatient care when medically necessary.

CMS has established geographical jurisdictions and currently awards Medicare contracts to insurance companies through competitive procedures. Medicare Administrative Contractors (MACs) for Parts A and B Medicare jurisdictions administer Medicare services and process Medicare claims for the jurisdictions. Although MACs may not deny coverage of services covered by CMS, latitude is allowed in the interpretation of these rules. As a result, local coverage rules for CR may vary among local Medicare contractors. MAC instructions to providers are typically issued via bulletins and articles and for some services through local coverage determinations (LCD), although LCDs are not required. It is therefore imperative that each program be familiar with both federal and local policies that govern CR/SP.

Medicare Provision for Cardiac Rehabilitation and Intensive Cardiac Rehabilitation Services

In 2008, the U.S. Congress passed Public Law 110-275, which included the addition of coverage for cardiac rehabilitation and intensive cardiac rehabilitation services in the SSA, Title XVIII, Section 1861 (eee). From that mandate, CMS promulgated provisions for early outpatient CR services, headed "Cardiac rehabilitation program and intensive cardiac rehabilitation program: Conditions of coverage."[28]

The CMS definition of early outpatient CR is "a physician-supervised program that furnishes physician-prescribed exercise, cardiac risk factor modification, psychosocial assessment, and outcomes assessment." Medicare provisions are subject to modification and shifting interpretation by CMS. Therefore, it is important to remain current on regulatory aspects of program delivery. This is most successfully accomplished through active participation in local, state, and national professional organizations. Networking at this level ensures that accurate and timely information is received. Erroneous information can lead to detrimental consequences. Two settings are designated by CMS as appropriate for delivery of CR and ICR services:

1. Physician office
2. Hospital outpatient setting

"Medicare Requirements for Early Outpatient Cardiac Rehabilitation" lists required components of a CR program. Eligible diagnoses are subject to change; therefore these should be obtained from current CMS regulations. Medical emergencies and equipment necessary for appropriate preparedness are discussed in chapter 12.

Documentation

The requirements for documentation of program services specify uniform standards for evaluation, intervention, and outcomes measurement. A properly documented program record shows a clear, concise, logical, and organized evaluation and intervention plan. This is essential for capturing the comprehensive components provided by the program. Relevant documentation includes subjective and objective information and measurable indices for describing outcomes (see chapter 11). For Medicare beneficiaries, outcomes assessment evaluates progress related to the CR treatment and includes the following:

- Assessments based on patient-centered outcomes measured from entry to completion of CR/SP

- Objective clinical measures of exercise performance and self-reported measures of exertion and behavior[28]

The following considerations should influence the design and selection of documentation format and the use of terminology:

- Clarity of information—information should be accessible and understandable to all staff using the document.
- Consistency of information—the type and extent of information should be consistent from patient to patient and staff member to staff member.
- Efficiency of information—essential information should be recorded accurately, without redundancies, using acceptable abbreviations and terminology.
- Electronic medical records, computerized documentation methods, or both should be a goal that all programs work toward.

An individualized treatment plan (ITP) tailored to each individual patient should be developed at the initial CR session(s). Information that should be included in the ITP is listed in guideline 10.4. The ITP is developed by a physician in conjunction with the interdisciplinary team. It is important that all members of the team be familiar with and able to provide input on the ITP as the patient progresses through early outpatient CR.[29] The ITP is CMS-required documentation that must be completed or revised at program entry, every 30 days, and upon program completion. Programs should determine which outcomes are most effectively measured at program entry and completion and which will be collected on a more frequent basis, for example on a weekly or monthly schedule.

All communications with physicians, other health care professionals, and families that may affect patient outcomes must be documented in compliance with general guidelines. This includes telephone conversations with physicians or physician extenders regarding adverse reactions to exercise therapy, progress on risk factor modification, and formal physician communications. Any occurrences related to clinical status, including those away from the program, should be documented; examples include changes in medical therapy, new signs or symptoms, physician

Medicare Requirements for Early Outpatient Cardiac Rehabilitation

The Medicare provisions for CR require the following components:

- Physician referral with Medicare-eligible diagnosis identified
  - Medical documentation to support the diagnosis—should be available to the CR program upon request
- The following diagnoses are accepted by Medicare (Medicare regulations may change, so periodic review of the regulations is essential):
  - Acute myocardial infarction within the preceding 12 months*
  - Coronary artery bypass surgery
  - Current stable angina pectoris
  - Heart valve repair or replacement
  - Percutaneous transluminal coronary angioplasty (PTCA) or coronary stenting
  - Heart or heart–lung transplant
  - Other cardiac conditions that would require specification through a national coverage determination
- Individualized treatment plan:
  - Details on how components of CR are provided for each patient
  - Description of the diagnosis
  - Type, amount, frequency, and duration of services furnished under the plan
  - Agreed-upon goals and outcomes
  - Should be established, reviewed, and signed by a physician at program entry, every 30 days, and upon program completion
- Outcomes assessment that evaluates progress from entry to completion of the CR/SP course:
  - Includes objective clinical measures of exercise performance
  - Includes self-reported measures of exertion and behavior
- Physician-prescribed (aerobic, strength, stretching) exercise as appropriate, provided each day the patient receives CR services
- Cardiac risk factor modification, tailored to individual needs, that includes education, counseling, and behavioral intervention
- Psychosocial assessment
- One or more medical directors who are responsible for the program and are involved, in consultation with staff, in directing the progress of individuals in the program
- Physician supervision that is immediately available and accessible for medical consultations and medical emergencies at all times during which CR is being furnished.
  - See Medicare policies for interpretation and requirements for compliance with this standard

*12-month window applies only to postacute myocardial infarction in the federal regulation. Other diagnoses have no time window *unless additional requirements are stipulated in local Medicare policies,* which is the case for some.

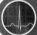 **Guideline 10.4   Individualized Treatment Plan (ITP)**

The initial, periodic, and discharge ITP should include the following:

- A description of the diagnosis
- Type, amount, frequency, and duration of the items and services furnished under the plan
- Individual goals for the patient
- Development and progression of ITP by all members of the CR/SP staff with direction, review, and signature of the medical director

visits, or other information that may affect patient progress or outcome.

The program director should be aware of the processes for determining the rules and regulations regarding reimbursement. Before enrollment, it is particularly important to verify the insurance coverage for CR/SP services, including billing codes, reimbursement amounts, copayments, and specific plan limitations and requirements. Variations in coverage plans are numerous and may call for CR/SP staff or clinician intervention in situations in which the rules are a barrier to participation or are clinically inappropriate. It is important to maintain a list of the names and telephone numbers of health plan intermediaries, case managers, and precertification officers to ascertain the extent of coverage for services before enrollment and application. It may also be beneficial to identify the top private insurance plans in the geographical location and provide them information on program operations and goals, as well as patient outcomes. Ultimately, the insurance verification process requires close oversight by the program director and thorough training of CR/SP staff if this process falls within the departmental responsibilities.

Personnel

Qualified health care personnel, including the program medical director, provide the services for a successful program. The collective knowledge, skills, and clinical experience of the professional staff must reflect the multidisciplinary competencies necessary to affect the desired treatment outcomes (see guideline 10.5). The clinical skills and medico-legal authority required for patient safety must be ensured by appropriate requirements for individual staff positions.

The knowledge and technical skills required for optimal care are derived from several disciplines and health care professions. No particular combination of staffing defines a minimum guideline for program competence. Given the multidisciplinary nature of the program, applying these staffing principles allows enough flexibility for even small clinical facilities to meet program competency guidelines. Each program and facility should select personnel with professional specialties that fit the model and policies of the institution and the human resource department. Additionally, title and level of positions are a function of the institution and program. Nevertheless, the collective knowledge base of the staff should include a comprehensive understanding of CVD, cardiovascular emergency procedures, nutrition, exercise physiology, pharmacology, behavior change strategies, health psychology, and medical and educational strategies for CAD risk factor management. Both licensed and nonlicensed health care professionals may be included on the CR/SP team. The professions most frequently represented in the essential staff positions include specially trained registered nurses, exercise physiologists, dietitians, health educators, health psychologists, vocational rehabilitation counselors, physical therapists, occupational therapists, pharmacists, and physicians. It is important for staff to participate in multidisciplinary patient care continuing educational activities. Ongoing education and certification of staff also ensures the maintenance of competence.

The competency guidelines for program personnel specified here agree with standards published in the AACVPR Core Competencies

---

Guideline 10.5 Medical Director Qualifications

- Every early outpatient CR/SP program shall have a medical director or team of medical directors who share the responsibility.
- Standards for the physician(s) responsible for a CR/SP program are
  - expertise in the management of individuals with cardiac pathophysiology,

- cardiopulmonary training in basic life support or advanced cardiac life support, and
- license to practice medicine in the state in which the CR/SP program is offered.

document[9] (see table 10.1). In addition, guidelines for professional education and minimum competencies for certification of Clinical Exercise Specialist (CES) and Registered Clinical Exercise Physiologist (RCEP) have been developed by the American College of Sports Medicine (ACSM).[30] The American Board of Physical Therapy Specialists (ABPTS) offers a Cardiovascular and Pulmonary Specialist certification.[31]

Core Functions

Core functions for secondary prevention programs include the provision and coordination of a broad range of services and adequate emergency response capability. In addition, each program professional should possess a common core of professional and clinical competencies regardless of academic discipline. The following are recommended minimum qualifications for all CR/SP staff:

- Bachelor's degree in a health field such as exercise science or licensure in the jurisdiction, for example for a registered nurse or physical therapist
- Experience or specialty training in CR/SP as outlined in the AACVPR Core Competencies document
- Successful completion of basic life support (BLS) course with training in advanced cardiac life support (ACLS) preferred

Staff recommendations and core competencies specific to emergency services in the CR/SP setting are discussed in chapter 12.

Program Staff

Outlined here are specific personnel and associated core competencies typically found in program settings for the purpose of effectively meeting AACVPR Core Components.[10]

Medical Director

Guideline 10.5 presents qualifications mandated by CMS for medical directors. The primary responsibilities are as follows[32]:

- Ensuring that the CR/SP program is safe, comprehensive, cost-effective, and medically appropriate for individual patients
- Ensuring that policies and procedures are consistent with evidence-based guidelines
- Ensuring that the program complies with regulatory standards

The interactive role of multiple physicians and team members involved in patient care is strengthened by active leadership of the medical director.

Program Director: Preferred Qualifications

1. Master's degree in an allied health field, such as exercise physiology, or licensure as a health care practitioner in a related health care discipline such as a registered nurse or physical therapist (or both master's degree and licensure)
2. Mastery of the AACVPR Core Competencies,[9] which include advanced knowledge of exercise physiology, nutrition, risk factor modification strategies, counseling techniques, and uses of behavioral change programs and technologies as applied to CR/SP services
3. Experience in staff coordination and delivery of CR/SP services to patients
4. Successful completion of AHA Basic Life Support (BLS) and, where applicable, Advanced Cardiac Life Support (ACLS) courses
5. Where applicable, certification as a Clinical Exercise Specialist (CES) or Registered Clinical Exercise Physiologist (RCEP) by the American College of Sports Medicine (ACSM) or the Cardiovascular and Pulmonary Specialist certification of the American Physical Therapy Association (APTA)

Registered Nurse: Preferred Qualifications

1. License to practice as a registered nurse in the jurisdiction
2. Successful completion of an ACLS course
3. Advanced knowledge of exercise physiology, nutrition, risk factor modification strategies, counseling techniques, and uses of behavioral change programs and technologies in CR/SP services, as defined in the AACVPR Core Competencies position statement

Exercise Specialist: Preferred Qualifications

1. Bachelor's in exercise science or related field.
2. Where applicable, successful completion of an ACLS course.

3. Certification, experience, or training equivalent to that specified for an ACSM Clinical Exercise Specialist (CES). This would include advanced knowledge of exercise physiology, nutrition, risk factor modification strategies, counseling techniques, and uses of behavioral change programs and technologies as applied to CR/SP services and defined in the AACVPR Core Competencies position statement.

Exercise Physiologist: Preferred Qualifications

1. Master's degree in exercise science or related field.
2. Where applicable, successful completion of an ACLS course.
3. Certification, experience, or training equivalent to that specified for an ACSM Registered Clinical Exercise Physiologist (RCEP). This would include advanced knowledge of exercise physiology, nutrition, risk factor modification strategies, counseling techniques, and uses of behavioral change programs and technologies as applied to CR/SP services and defined in the AACVPR Core Competencies position statement.

Physical Therapist: Preferred Qualifications

1. License to practice physical therapy in the jurisdiction
2. Successful completion of an ACLS course
3. Experience in the identification and physical remediation of various musculoskeletal limitations that may be present in CR/SP patients
4. Advanced knowledge of exercise physiology, nutrition, risk factor modification strategies, counseling techniques, and uses of behavioral change programs and technologies as applied to CR/SP services and defined in the AACVPR Core Competencies position statement
5. American Board of Physical Therapy Specialists (ABPTS) Cardiovascular and Pulmonary Specialist certification, or training equivalent to that specified for the APTA advanced specialty certification

Respiratory Therapist: Preferred Qualifications

1. Licensure or registration (per state law) for practice in the jurisdiction as a respiratory therapist

2. Successful completion of an ACLS course
3. Advanced knowledge of exercise physiology, nutrition, risk factor modification strategies, counseling techniques, and uses of behavioral change programs and technologies as applied to CR/SP services and defined in the AACVPR Core Competencies position statement

Registered Dietitian: Preferred Qualifications

1. Master's degree in nutrition
2. Registered dietitian status with the American Dietetic Association
3. Experience in practicing therapeutic dietetics in a clinical or community setting, particularly in areas of lipid disorders, obesity, diabetes, and hypertension

Mental Health Professional: Preferred Qualifications

1. License for practice in the jurisdiction as a clinical social worker, counselor, psychologist, or psychiatrist
2. Experience in psychological assessment, administration of behavioral health interventions, and counseling with CR/SP or chronic disease

Health Educator: Preferred Qualifications

1. Certification as a health education specialist
2. Master's degree in health education
3. Experience in providing individual and group educational programs for patients and family members to reduce CHD risk factors and promote health self-maintenance
4. Experience in the wide range of available technologies to provide individual health self-monitoring and promote positive health behaviors

Occupational Therapist: Preferred Qualifications

1. Master's degree in occupational therapy
2. License to practice as an occupational therapist in the jurisdiction, if applicable
3. Registration with the American Occupational Therapy Association
4. Experience in providing occupational therapy to CVD patients or related field

Vocational Rehabilitation Counselor: Preferred Qualifications

1. Master's degree in vocational rehabilitation counseling
2. Experience in vocational counseling with CR/SP patients

Staff Education and Performance Review

A requirement of AACVPR program certification and TJC is that staff members receive continuing education. All professional staff should strive for full and independent functioning in the content areas described in the AACVPR Core Competencies document. It is recognized that mastery of all knowledge and skills criteria is an ongoing process. Policies should be in place regarding the number of continuing education hours, in-services, and educational experiences required of staff. TJC and most other surveying organizations require documentation of monthly emergency education and skill in-services, department meetings, agendas, education programs, and completed certifications and certificates. The policies and procedures manual should describe this process.

Continuum of Care and Services

Policies delineating the integration of all activities directly or indirectly related to the continuum of care from entry through exit should be in place. The needs of patients should be matched with the appropriate appraisals, programs, and services. Policies in this section should establish the process by which the patient is able to move through the secondary prevention program, affording a minimum of difficulty and excess time involvement, with a clear understanding of the process and expectations. These policies should address

- appointment scheduling,
- parking,
- registration,
- insurance preauthorization and enrollment,
- informed consent,
- intermittent progress evaluations,
- communication between the program and primary caregiver(s) throughout the CR/SP course, and
- discharge planning and follow-up.

Establishing a program does not require a large facility with state-of-the-art equipment, a large staff, and the most expensive monitoring equipment. Innovative programs could include such designs as these:

- Telephonic health coaching
- Once per week participation with a well-structured home exercise regimen for patients who travel from a farther distance or have other barriers to more frequent weekly participation
- A higher-frequency program, for example 5 days per week, for patients who are able and eager to progress more rapidly or have a short-term window for program participation
- Flexible attendance options for patients with other obligations that prohibit a rigid schedule of attendance

There are opportunities for facilitating a successful transition through partnering early outpatient CR/SP programs with maintenance programs in existing facilities such as high school and elementary school gymnasiums, YMCAs, Jewish Community Centers, and other fitness facilities.

Summary

It is the responsibility of the patient to assume ownership of this chronic disease, but a knowledgeable and well-trained multidisciplinary team can provide guidance and ongoing support that contribute greatly to success in the long-term management of cardiovascular disease. The medical community and health insurance industry recognize CR/SP as a treatment that has demonstrated significant, positive patient outcomes with respect to mortality, morbidity, risk factor reduction and management, and quality of life.

Outcomes Assessment and Utilization

Outcomes reflect program performance, quality, and accountability. Therefore, the process of measuring, collecting, and analyzing patient outcomes is a critical component of the successful provision of health care services. Ideally, outcomes should reflect therapeutic goals and drive tailored approaches to disease management.[1] An outcomes-focused approach to patient care occurs at two levels: (1) measuring clinical variables for individual patients at program entry and at subsequent intervals to assess individual patient outcomes, and (2) evaluating composite patient outcomes at periodic intervals to assess program effectiveness. Health status is assessed at cardiac rehabilitation/secondary prevention (CR/SP) program entry to determine priorities and objectives in order to develop an Individual Treatment Plan (ITP). Formal assessments should be repeated during the program as appropriate and at program exit. Outcomes measured during the program are used to evaluate patient progress and guide discharge and long-term goal planning (guideline 11.1).

OBJECTIVES

The objectives of this chapter are to

- define outcome domains (categories) using the Cardiac Rehabilitation Outcomes Matrix[3] (table 11.1) and provide examples of acceptable tools that can be used to measure outcomes in CR/SP;

- establish recommendations for creating a comprehensive systematic approach for collecting, tracking, analyzing, and reporting outcomes data within routine clinical practice; and

- introduce how outcomes are used to plan and implement quality improvement (QI) projects in CR/SP.

Guideline 11.1 Outcomes Assessment

Program professionals should uniformly measure outcomes in a variety of domains within the core components of care and use these analyses to develop, monitor, and drive quality improvement projects in order to promote effective treatments and outcomes. The resulting data provide valuable information for quality improvement, accreditation, and reimbursement.

Outcomes Matrix

The Cardiac Rehabilitation Outcomes Matrix (see table 11.1) is the model that the American Association of Cardiovascular and Pulmonary Rehabilitation (AACVPR) suggests for classifying and organizing measurable patient outcomes in CR/SP (see guideline 11.2).

The Cardiac Rehabilitation Outcomes Matrix was developed by the AACVPR Outcomes

Table 11.1 AACVPR Cardiac Rehabilitation Outcomes Matrix

Core components of care	Clinical	Behavioral	Health	Service
Overall management	Risk factor profile Evaluation of symptoms Hemodynamic responses Activities of daily living assessment	**Self-efficacy** 1. Improved knowledge and application of self-care actions 2. Return to desired physical activity level 3. Desire to return to work Cardiac disease knowledge score Appropriate response to symptoms and complications Medication adherence, compliance Accessibility to needed resources Session attendance rate	**Morbidity and mortality** Health care utilization: a. Hospitalizations, readmissions b. Emergency room visits c. Physician sick visits Untoward events during supervised sessions Health-related quality of life Return to work, loss of work days	**Patient satisfaction** 1. Satisfaction with the care received 2. Progress toward goals **Performance measures** 1. Cost per patient 2. Program cost 3. Enrollment rate 4. Dropout rate 5. Completion rate 6. Admission rate
Exercise testing and training[2]	**Exercise testing** 1. Maximal exercise test 2. Submaximal exercise test or functional assessment (e.g., 6-minute walk test) **Resting, exercise, and recovery responses** 1. Heart rate and rhythm 2. Blood pressure 3. Rating of perceived effort 4. Peak METs 5. Rating of perceived dyspnea 6. Oxygen saturation level	**Exercise compliance** 1. Supervised sessions 2. Home or outside sessions 3. Adherence to exercise prescription **Energy expenditure** 1. Minutes of physical activity per week 2. Calorie expenditure daily, weekly Physical activity stage of change		

Core components of care	Clinical	Behavioral	Health	Service
Strength and flex-ibility training[2]	Strength measures (e.g., RM, 5RM, grip strength) Flexibility measures (e.g., sit and reach test, goniometer)			
Lipid management[3]	Lipid levels Initiation of or adjust-ment in medication dosage	Adherence to diet, exer-cise, and medications Diet and exercise stage of change		
Hypertension management[3]	Resting blood pressure Exercise and recovery blood pressures Initiation of or adjust-ment in antihypertension medication dosage	Adherence to diet, exer-cise, and medications Diet and exercise stage of change Self-monitoring behav-iors		
Diabetes manage-ment[3]	Blood glucose levels HbA1c Initiation of or adjust-ment in hypoglycemic medication dosage	Adherence to diet, exer-cise, and medications Diet and exercise stage of change Self-monitoring behav-iors		
Nutrition and weight management[3]	**Anthropometric mea-sures** 1. Height, weight, BMI 2. Body fat, lean body weight measures 3. Abdominal circum-ference 4. Sum of skinfolds, girths **Nutritional biochemical markers, bone mineral density test**	Adherence to diet and exercise Diet and exercise stage of change Diet recording logs Physical activity record-ing logs Diet habit scores		
Psychosocial management[3]	**Measurements of mood** Depression, anxiety, hos-tility, emotional distress **Measurements of cog-nitive function** Memory, orientation, judgment	Coping mechanisms Stress management and relaxation skills Social support network Sexual dysfunction		
Smoking cessation[3]	Serum cotinine levels Exhaled carbon mon-oxide Number of cigarettes or cigars smoked per day Duration of smoking habit (pack-years)	Smoking stage of change		

Abbreviations: MET, metabolic equivalent; RM, repetitions maximum; HbA1c, glycosylated hemoglobin; BMI, body mass index

Adapted from Sanderson, Southard and Oldridge 2004.

> ### Guideline 11.2 Cardiac Rehabilitation Outcomes Matrix
>
> AACVPR recommends using the Cardiac Rehabilitation Outcomes Matrix as a guide for a systematic approach to assess patient outcomes. Outcomes should be assessed, at a minimum, at program entry, during participation, at discharge, and at later follow-up, for example, 3 months, 6 months, or 1 year.

Committee and is designed to help link outcomes assessment to the evidence-based core components of CR/SP and provides a standardized method for categorizing outcome data in four domains: clinical, behavioral, health, and service. The clinical, behavioral, and health domains are based on Green's PRECEDE Model.[4,5] The service domain was created by the AACVPR as a category to measure patient satisfaction and service utilization. Within each of the domains are outcome measures related to the core components of care in CR/SP.[6] *Core components* are elements of patient care that have strong scientific evidence of their ability to optimize cardiovascular risk reduction, reduce disability, and promote healthy behaviors.[7] Examples of outcome measures in each domain are shown in "Examples of Clinical Domain Measures and Relevant Instruments," "Behavioral Domain Measures and Relevant Instruments," and "Health Domain Measures and Relevant Instruments."

The basis for the measurement of multiple outcomes from different domains is the inherent value in assessment of effectiveness of patient care and individual progress toward achieving goals. Multiple outcomes used collectively best define success for individuals and programs.[1] For example, if assessment of a clinical outcome related to exercise capacity (e.g., change in metabolic equivalent [MET] level during or following CR/SP) indicates that a patient or program has not achieved the goal, then staff can evaluate the processes of providing physical activity or specific exercise programming to more effectively influence the clinical outcome. When a program consistently meets the threshold of "quality" care, then it is time to move to another outcome or add an outcome to the assessment of program effectiveness. Depending on available program resources, program directors should select from the measures best suited for their population and resources from the Cardiac Rehabilitation Outcomes Matrix.

Clinical Outcomes Domain

This domain includes physical and psychological outcome variables that are objectively measured during the initial assessment, intake history, chart review, and subsequent exercise sessions. These outcomes relate to the detection and evaluation of disease status and the effects of therapy. Clinical outcomes include the results of tests used for the assessment of risk, the diagnosis and prognostic evaluation of the disease and its components, physiological measurements, and laboratory values. Physical or biometric variables such as measured or estimated exercise capacity, blood pressure, heart rate and rhythm, fasting blood lipids, glycosylated hemoglobin (HbA1c), and anthropometric measurements are common clinical measures.[2]

The results of surveys, questionnaires, or other instruments used to assess psychological, emotional, or cognitive function are also included in this domain. Psychological measures include objective assessments of depression, anxiety, and anger. The reliability of these findings increases when scientifically valid and reliable questionnaires and instruments are used. When psychological variables are measured singularly they are considered a clinical outcome measure; however, when combined in a profile with clinical and social measures like sleep, energy, activity, and pain, psychological variables are considered outcomes within the health domain. Clinical outcomes are influenced by individual patient choices and behaviors. Examples of clinical outcomes are shown in "Examples of Clinical Domain Measures and Relevant Instruments."

Behavioral Domain

Outcomes within this domain are individualized and reflect self-reported behaviors, self-efficacy, knowledge, adherence to medical and behavioral therapies, and lifestyle modifications.[15] This includes core components such as indi-

Examples of Clinical Domain Measures and Relevant Instruments

- Anthropometric data:
  - Waist circumference
  - Body mass index
  - Percent body fat
- Functional capacity:
  - Functional MET level in CR/SP
  - Graded exercise test (GXT) MET level
  - One-repetition maximum (1RM) (strength) or equivalent (e.g., 5RM)
  - Joint-specific range of motion
  - 6-minute walk test distance[8]
  - Balance and mobility tests[9]
- Functional status:
  - Duke Activity Status Index (DASI)[10]
  - Dartmouth Primary Care Cooperative (CO-OP) charts (www.dartmouthcoopproject.org/coopcharts.html)[a]
- Smoking:
  - Blood cotinine level
  - Carbon monoxide level
- Blood pressure—resting or peak assessed during exercise
- Heart rate—resting or peak assessed during exercise
- Lipids—for example, total cholesterol, low-density lipoprotein cholesterol, high-density lipoprotein cholesterol, triglycerides
- Diabetes:
  - Blood glucose level
  - HbA1c
- Psychosocial assessments:
  - Beck Depression Inventory (www.pearsonassessments.com/HAIWEB/Cultures/en-us/Productdetail. htm?Pid=015-8018-370)[a]
  - Center for Epidemiologic Studies-Depression[11]
  - Hospital Anxiety and Depression Scale[12]
  - Patient Health Questionnaire-9 (www.depression- primarycare.org/clinicians/toolkits/materials/forms/phq9)[13]
  - Psychosocial Risk Factor Survey (www.deltapsychologycenter.com)[a,14]

[a]Requires licensing or usage fee.

vidual behavioral management of exercise, lipids, hypertension, diabetes, nutrition, and smoking cessation. These measures reveal patient ability to make and maintain recommended lifestyle changes that lead to goal achievement in the clinical and health domains. Behavioral interventions offered to the patient are determined as a result of abnormal or unsatisfactory clinical findings.

For example, if a patient has hyperlipidemia and a BMI of 31.7 kg/m², behavioral interventions such as a dietary consult and weight loss program will be recommended.

Patients should be encouraged to assume increasing responsibility for their own health behaviors while participating in CR/SP. Behavioral measures are typically obtained through

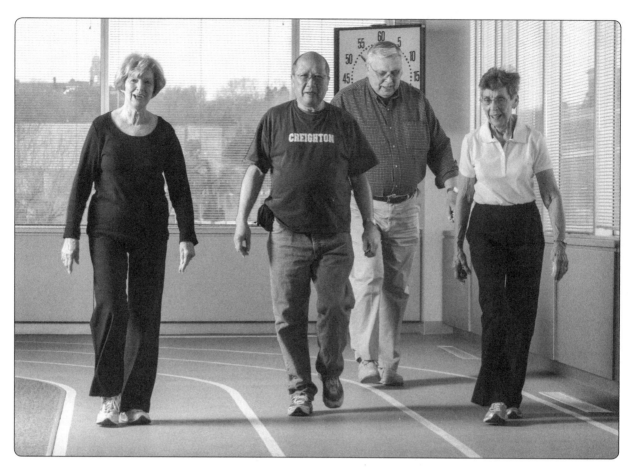

Patients should be encouraged to assume increasing responsibility for their own health behaviors while participating in CR/SP.

the use of standardized questionnaires, surveys, logs, or diaries to characterize adherence to a structured regimen such as physical activity, diet, or medications. It is important to review the ITP with each patient to determine compliance and adherence to the plan. The ITP follow-up is an opportunity for reassessing individual behavioral goals and determining patient progress. Ultimately, when patients adhere to a mutually established ITP, this has a positive impact on health and clinical outcomes. Adherence to healthy lifestyle behaviors and to medication therapies is integral to the attainment of sustained benefits.[5] Examples of additional behavioral outcomes are provided in "Behavioral Domain Measures and Relevant Instruments."

Health Domain

Outcomes related to the overall health of the patient include the occurrence, recurrence, or exacerbations of the primary disease or comorbid conditions, either fatal or nonfatal; the impact of the disease on function or quality of life; and use of health care resources in response to these events. The health domain represents general or primary indicators of health outcomes that include morbidity, mortality, and quality of life. Unfortunately, changes in morbidity and mortality associated with CR/SP participation are generally described in large trials or through meta-analyses, whereas these data are not readily available to most CR/SP programs, particularly once the patient has been discharged from the program.

Health status and health-related quality of life (HRQL) are important to the patient and, unlike morbidity and mortality, can easily be measured to determine personal well-being and overall satisfaction with life; thus, the AACVPR recommends that HRQL be measured by CR/SP

Behavioral Domain Measures and Relevant Instruments

- Step counts per day (log)

- Stress management or coping strategies (log or journal)

- Tobacco use (i.e., number of cigarettes smoked per day, packs per day), frequency of exposure to secondhand smoke

- Medication adherence (logs, pill counts, filled prescriptions)

- Home exercise logs

- Specific instruments to assess adherence and self-efficacy

  - Diet Habit Survey[a,16]

  - MEDFICTS (www.nhlbi.nih.gov/guidelines/cholesterol/dietappx.pdf)

  - Block Food Frequency Questionnaire (www.nutritionquest.com/assessment/)

  - Self-Efficacy for Exercise Scale[17]

  - International Physical Activity Questionnaire (IPAQ) (https://sites.google.com/site/theipaq)[18]

[a]May require a licensing or usage fee.

programs. HRQL tools that measure various aspects of health affected by disease and treatment provide a global health profile.[19] The three main dimensions of HRQL are (1) physical function, (2) psychological well-being, and (3) social functioning. Tools used to measure HRQL may be disease specific or generic. The disease-specific instrument provides an indication of the patient's perception of health with regard to specific disease components such as symptoms. Generic tools can be used when one is comparing patient health status to that of an apparently healthy population. If resources allow, both types of tools should be used. Examples of other common health outcomes are provided in "Health Domain Measures and Relevant Instruments."

Health Domain Measures and Relevant Instruments

- Mortality following hospital discharge and CR/SP enrollment

- Repeat morbidity—emergency department visits and hospital readmissions related to primary diagnosis, all cause, or both[a]

- Health-related quality of life instruments:

  - Dartmouth Primary Care Cooperative (CO-OP) charts (www.dartmouthcoopproject.org/coopcharts.html)

  - EuroQol EQ-5D (www.euroqol.org)[b]

  - Ferrans and Powers Quality of Life Index-Cardiac Version (www.uic.edu/orgs/qli)

  - MacNew Health-Related Quality of Life Instrument[b] (www.macnew.org/wp)

  - Medical Outcomes Study SF-36/12 Health Status Questionnaire (http://www.sf-6.org)[b]

  - Nottingham Health Profile[20]

[a]As program resources allow.
[b]Requires licensing or usage fee.

Service Domain

This domain captures measures related to patient satisfaction, service utilization, cost of providing services, and program performance in meeting evidence-based goals. The most commonly measured outcome in the service domain is patient satisfaction. This measure is inherently subjective and based on personal experience. It should be noted that most programs assess patient satisfaction with care or services received while attending the program. However, there is a significant difference between "I am satisfied with the care I received in the program" and "I am satisfied with the care I received in the program but I am not satisfied with my current level of function or recovery." A patient's satisfaction with his health status is an outcome that merits greater attention in CR/SP programs. Patient satisfaction questionnaires should include questions related to how satisfied patients are with personal progress and gains. When the aggregate of individual service domain outcomes is analyzed, the quality of the services provided can be evaluated and future program needs can be better identified and prioritized. Programs often develop their own patient satisfaction survey to meet their particular needs, since no one instrument has been widely accepted in CR/SP and few have been tested for validity and reliability.

Performance measures (PMs) are measures of overall program performance and are part of the service domain. These measures typically are not patient-specific outcomes, but more properly reflect program structures and processes and measure the performance of the program. To evaluate program performance, individual observations are compiled and aggregated, then evaluated for internal or external benchmarking purposes. Calculations exist for several of the performance-related measures such as CR/SP referral rate, enrollment rate, attendance rate, and completion rate. (See "Examples of Cardiovascular Rehabilitation Measures and Calculations" for sample calculations.) It is important to note that except for referral to CR/SP, standardized definitions for these measures have not yet been agreed upon; therefore, any multiprogram projects involving these measures must arrive at working definitions before valid comparisons can be made between programs. It is also important to specify exclusion criteria for patients who will not be counted in the process because of a defined condition that exempts them, as well as to specify the time interval during which the data are captured.

Outcomes in Contrast to Performance Measures

While closely related and important to the success of health care delivery systems, outcomes and PMs are not identical. Performance measures are not a substitute for measuring outcomes.[1] Generally, CR/SP program *outcomes* reflect the individual consequences of using one or more health-related interventions. Within CR/SP programs, outcomes are used to measure individual success and contribute to the overall evaluation of program effectiveness. Optimal outcome evaluation reflects the ability to (1) assess the individual patient's progress toward health, clinical, and behavioral goals; and (2) assess program effectiveness in providing optimal, individualized patient care. Whenever possible, outcomes should reflect patient experiences and goals with regard to the ITP and should be specific to the disease process.[1]

Performance measures assess the effectiveness of a health care system and are derived from evidence-based practice guidelines.[22-24] Performance measures related to CR/SP focus on program, provider, or health care system performance, while CR/SP outcome measures focus on patients and their goals. Performance measures evaluate whether adequate systems and processes of care are in place. *Systems* include resources such as personnel, training, diagnostic and therapeutic equipment, and policies and procedures, whereas *processes* involve the appropriate use of these resources as they relate to patient care. Highly effective systems and processes ultimately lead to optimal patient care. Inpatient and outpatient CR/SP referrals are PMs defined by the AACVPR, the American College of Cardiology Foundation, and the American Heart Association[23] (see "Performance Measures in Outpatient Cardiac Rehabilitation") and endorsed by the National Quality Forum in 2010.

Purposes for Measuring Outcomes

Measuring, reporting, and comparing outcomes are important steps toward rapidly improving outcomes.[1] Simply providing service to patients at a reasonable cost without assessing the benefit does not describe program efficacy. In addition, measuring various parameters without careful consideration of the outcomes assessment process

Examples of CR/SP Measures and Calculations

Sample Calculation for Patient Referral From Inpatient Setting[21]

$$\text{Referral rate (\%)} = \frac{\text{\# of patients referred to the CR/SP program} \times 100}{\substack{\text{\# of patients in the reporting period hospitalized with a qualifying event or diagnosis} \\ \text{who do not meet any of the exclusion criteria}^{a}}}$$

[a]Exclusion criteria include patient refusal, deemed high risk, barriers to enrollment (e.g., financial, geographical distance from CR/SP program).

Sample Calculation for Enrollment[a]

$$\text{Enrollment rate (\%)} = \frac{\text{\# of patients who enrolled in program} \times 100}{\text{\# of patients referred during specified time interval minus \# of patients excluded}^{b}}$$

[a]Enrollment is defined as having attended at least one billable CR/SP session.

[b]Exclusion criteria include, for example, patient expired, repeat morbidity, deemed high risk, relocated, not interested.

Sample Calculation for Attendance

$$\text{Attendance rate (\%)} = \frac{\text{\# of exercise sessions attended by the patient} \times 100}{\text{\# of exercise sessions prescribed}}$$

Sample Calculation for Completion Rate

$$\text{Completion rate (\%)} = \frac{\text{\# of patients from denominator who completed CR}^{a} \times 100}{\substack{\text{\# of patients enrolled in CR/SP program during specific time frame minus} \\ \text{exclusions}^{b}}}$$

[a]Completion defined as having undergone a final, formal discharge evaluation and review of treatment plan.

[b]Exclusions include patients who were physically unable to complete because of move from vicinity, death, or recurrent event.

Performance Measures in Outpatient Cardiac Rehabilitation[23]

- A-1. CR/SP patient referral from the inpatient setting.
    - All patients hospitalized with a primary diagnosis of an acute myocardial infarction (MI) or chronic stable angina (CSA) or who during hospitalization have undergone coronary artery bypass graft (CABG) surgery, a percutaneous coronary intervention (PCI), cardiac valve surgery, or cardiac transplantation are to be referred to an early outpatient CR/SP program.
- A-2. CR/SP patient referral from outpatient setting.
    - All patients evaluated in an outpatient setting who within the past 12 months have experienced an acute MI, CABG surgery, PCI, cardiac valve surgery, or cardiac transplantation or have CSA and have not already participated in an early outpatient CR/SP program for the qualifying event or diagnosis are to be referred to such a program.

---

can result in misleading conclusions. As stated earlier in this chapter, outcomes are indicators not only of program effectiveness but also of quality of patient care. Outcome indicators offer providers the information needed to develop and implement optimal ITPs. Upon program completion, the referring physician is responsible for supervising and refining patient interventions designed to lower the chance of recurrent heart events.

While reporting outcomes is a requirement for AACVPR program certification and recertification, this should not be the sole purpose for tracking outcomes. Programs are encouraged to benchmark outcome findings externally with comparable programs. The AACVPR offers the CR/SP registry for this purpose, providing a mechanism for evaluating program effectiveness. Once programs have been benchmarked externally or internally, staff is encouraged to use the findings to assess further opportunities for quality assurance.

Emphasizing the importance of program outcome measurement to administrators, medical directors, and clinicians creates "buy-in" at all levels. Securing administrative support for measuring program outcomes increases the likelihood of a successful outcomes tracking program. Value is measured by results; thus, outcomes measurement becomes significant to consumers and payers.

Process for Measuring, Documenting, Analyzing, and Reporting Program Outcomes

An effective program of measuring CR/SP outcomes requires a systematic, coordinated team approach. Ensuring that team members are informed about that process is critical to achieving a quality outcomes program. The process begins with data collection and measurement. Outcome assessments can be documented using customized program spreadsheets, outcome tracking programs, or forms created by the program staff. Following documentation, data analysis provides for interpretation of the results. The final step in the process is the reporting phase, which may vary depending on program structure. Generally, outcomes are reported at staff meetings and cardiology conferences and to QI teams, as well as to various administrative and clinical committees.

Protocols and policies defining the outcome process will increase the likelihood of accurate outcomes reporting. Outcomes should be clinically relevant, simple to measure, patient centered, and consistent with patient care goals as set forth in the ITP. All outcome measures selected for assessment should be within the means of the CR/SP program not only to adequately assess, but also to influence and manage. Program staff should recognize that factors outside of CR/SP, including the recovery process itself and medical oversight, can affect the results.

Data Collection and Measurement

Outcomes measurement is the result of a rigorous and organized effort to understand what is clinically, psychologically, socially, and economically valuable to the patient and to the program. Data collection should not be viewed as an "extra" or laborious task. In fact, many of the data are included in the standard measurements obtained during the patient intake or initial evaluation process. The potential outcomes to be measured should be condensed to the minimum required for tracking program quality while maximizing patient care objectives. Each outcome domain (clinical, behavior, health, and service) should be represented with an appropriate measure or measures as resources allow. The ideal is to use measures that assess all of the core components of care and to measure multiple outcomes per domain.

Several sources for obtaining outcome data exist. These include patient interviews, intake forms, medical records, physician notes, observation, surveys, and questionnaires. Medical records are one of the preferred choices for collecting lab results, weight, blood pressure, cardiac rhythm, oxygen saturation, and perceived dyspnea.

The surveys and questionnaires selected for data collection should (1) be appropriate for the cardiac population, (2) be reliable and valid in the context of CR/SP services, (3) be sensitive to change during the brief course of CR/SP, (4) place minimal burden on the patient, and (5) be easily scored and interpreted. As much as possible, instruments should provide objective end points of the outcome(s) they purport to assess. Questionnaires assessing psychosocial aspects of the clinical domain, such as hostility, anxiety, or depression, are typically self-reported and thus subjective.

Outcomes data collection begins at the time of program referral and progresses through the initial intake and repeated patient encounters. Baseline values measured during the initial assessment phase are documented on the ITP and may be recorded on other program forms as specified in individual program policies. After variables have been assessed at program entry, measurements are reassessed every 30 days as appropriate and at program discharge by the program staff in conjunction with the referring physician(s) or the program medical director, as outlined in the program policies and procedures.

Substantial evidence indicates that postdischarge patient contact promotes sustainability of patient outcomes; therefore, collecting outcome data up to 12 months postdischarge is strongly encouraged. Not only is follow-up desirable; it is also important because adherence to lifestyle behaviors diminishes within the first 3 to 6 months of the start of treatment. Follow-up outcome data can be acquired by clinic visit, phone, or mail; phone calls are the most effective and cost-efficient method.[25]

Documentation

Documentation of the initial assessment and reassessments of patient outcomes throughout the program and at discharge is a requirement set forth by the Centers for Medicare and Medicaid Services.[26] Ideally, CR/SP programs should have written policies describing procedures for gathering, documenting, and tracking outcomes. Ultimately, it is the responsibility of the program director or manager to ensure that team members are properly familiarized with documentation forms, as well as with the process for accurately documenting outcome measures. Direct oversight or audits are recommended to ensure correct outcome documentation and accurate reporting.

To promote accuracy, the implementation of written standards for describing the process of data acquisition cannot be overemphasized. Forms for documenting outcomes are available through position statements such as the papers on performance measures.[21] These forms are intended to simplify outcomes documentation. Assessment forms that make liberal use of check boxes and option lists help to ease the process of recording outcome information. The ITP can serve as a ready guide for outcome documentation and simplifies the process for data entry before analysis of the data. Forms may serve dual roles as data management systems and as reporting tools to health care providers. More powerful tools such as database applications and electronic medical records can use error detection, validation, and reminder algorithms to ensure complete and accurate data entry.

Data Analysis

Outcomes data analysis should take place when sufficient quantities of data have been collected. At a minimum, a review of aggregate program outcome data should take place quarterly. Program staff should review data for completeness and for change in values from entry to discharge to follow-up, as well as for trends in measures over time. To calculate percentage change for an individual patient, the difference between the entry and discharge values is divided by the entry value. Simple outcome calculations provide valuable feedback with regard to patient progress toward individual and program goals. This analytic process highlights patient outcomes at a single point in time; however, the true value of outcomes assessment is in using the data to track changes over time.

After individual change scores are assessed, group data can be analyzed to assess outcomes of the CR/SP group as a whole. Group means can then be compared internally from previous quarters for comparison and used to determine program effectiveness. Aggregated outcome results can also be compared externally, for example when programs participate in regional or national registries. Participation in a registry affords programs the ability to benchmark with others while setting stretch goals. Tracking trends using aggregate outcome measures provides programs with information about specific strengths and opportunities for improvement. Quality improvement efforts can then be implemented based on knowledge derived from outcome analysis. Other measures such as the fiscal value of services provided for CR/SP patients may also be assessed when one is evaluating program outcomes.[1]

Reporting

Results from outcome assessments and patient questionnaires or surveys should be shared with the patient and health care provider(s). For patients, this information must take into account their health information literacy. In addition, opportunities should be sought to communicate outcome findings to program administrators and health care payers to demonstrate program effectiveness or, conversely, treatment gaps that can be improved.

It is preferable to report outcomes for all patients enrolled in CR/SP; separate analysis should also be done on those patients who do not complete the program and the reasons for noncompletion. At a minimum, report values should include sample size (number of patients included in the analysis) and means or percentages, depending on the specific measure. More advanced programs may wish to report standard deviations, median values, or other statistical comparisons as needed to convey the significance of the outcomes.

Clinicians, managers, and administrators understand that it is not sufficient merely to collect outcomes. In order to make positive improvements to systems and processes, it is necessary to analyze outcome findings at the programmatic level; compare findings to those outcomes with selected benchmarks; and, when the findings are suboptimal, to initiate QI projects.[27] The outcomes observed are the result of the way in which programs are designed.[28] Therefore, suboptimal programs lead to suboptimal outcomes; highly effective programs produce optimal outcomes. Measuring and analyzing outcome findings can assist staff in ascertaining the quality of a program.

A program must first establish a benchmark by which to compare the effectiveness of care delivery (see guideline 11.3). Benchmark data can come from a number of sources. Programs can establish a historical baseline by using samples of their data aggregated over a specified length of time. These values then serve as internal benchmark measures from which the effects of any procedural changes can be compared. Outcomes from published studies may also be used as a benchmark. However, it is important to first evaluate whether results of a study can be generalized to a specific program population.

National and regional registries provide alternative, real-world benchmarks. Registries attempt to capture demographic, clinical, and treatment data on individual patients in a standardized fashion over time. Data elements and time frames for measurement are strictly defined and consistently adhered to. Data from the registries are combined across numerous participating sites in order to develop aggregated mean values for each demographic, clinical, behavioral, and health outcome measured. Subsets of data can be created within the registry for further analysis of various demographic and clinical characteristics within specific populations. These data can be helpful when one is evaluating the effects of treatments and disparities observed based on differences in gender, age, and race. The advantage of participating in a registry is that questions about program processes and structure can be proposed using the registries' aggregated data as a benchmark for comparative purposes.

Quality Improvement Using Program Outcomes

Following the analysis and reporting of outcome findings, team members should identify opportunities for program improvement based on the lowest-performing outcome scores. Once a system or process of care has been targeted for change, programs may select one of many QI models. The following discussion highlights the use of Deming's Plan-Do-Study-Act (PDSA) model for planning and implementing a QI project.[29]

Once program outcomes have been analyzed, the planning for the QI project begins. The *planning* phase involves targeting an outcome for improvement and studying aspects of the system or process leading to that outcome. The specific goal of the QI project, its duration, the data required to assess change, how the data will be measured, and those responsible for collecting the data are considered during this stage. It is crucial to note that a "perfect" project is not the goal. Many projects suffer from inertia and delay and ultimately failure because of a perceived need to create an ideal project at the outset. Measurement of outcomes is a learning process that helps a program understand what can be improved and clarifies the reasons for improvement. The aim of QI should be learning about a process and should not be about passing judgment.[28]

The QI project moves from the "planning" phase to the "do" phase when the plan has been developed. It is in the "do" phase that the "experiment" is performed and data of interest are gathered. When the planned duration of the

---

Guideline 11.3 Benchmarking Program Outcomes

Program outcomes should be benchmarked to published studies, regional outcomes projects, or national registries.

study has been reached, the "do" phase ends and the "study" phase begins, at which time the data are analyzed and results summarized. Lastly, the outcome of the QI project is used to refine the system or procedure (the "act" phase). Lessons can be learned from adopting promising changes and rejecting others. The process of QI is not a singular occurrence but is instead a continuous cycle of study, change, and refinement until the most effective process is formed, resulting in the best outcome for the patient or program.

When the QI study is evaluated, questions like these are addressed:

- To what extent were strategies employed and adhered to in the project?
- To what extent did program processes change as a result of the QI project?
- What processes were kept or discarded as a result?
- What is the next structure or process that can be evaluated or improved?

Resources

The AACVPR has developed a national CR/SP registry that is available to programs to assist in outcome evaluation. Detailed information about the CR/SP registry, including data elements, frequently asked questions, and directions for participation, can be found at www.aacvpr.org/CRRegistry. While the actual surveys and questionnaires for the domains are not provided within the Cardiac Rehabilitation Outcomes Matrix, recommendations for valid and reliable surveys or questionnaires are identified and listed according to individual outcome domains, which are discussed earlier in this chapter. Additional tools include publications regarding outcome calculations.[15,21]

Summary

While the processes and structure for outcome data collection, measurement, and reporting will continue to evolve, outcomes measurement and assessment will continue to be an important component of CR/SP performance assessment. Programs should have written policies in place for systematic outcomes assessment and management and should regularly use data for quality assurance and improvement projects. As a result of outcome tracking and reporting, the value of CR/SP programs becomes transparent to patients, physicians, and health care payers.

Management of Medical Problems and Emergencies

A critical responsibility of the cardiac rehabilitation/secondary prevention (CR/SP) service is to offer patients a safe environment in which to exercise while anticipating and preparing to provide patient care in situations involving medical complications and emergencies. This responsibility is critically important regardless of whether the site of service is a hospital, freestanding center, community-based facility, or home. It is imperative that the management plan for medical problems and emergencies be individualized to the particular site where the care is being delivered.

OBJECTIVES

The purpose of this chapter is to

- describe the potential risks of medical emergencies in secondary prevention programming;
- identify procedures for assessment and screening for potential problems;
- identify procedures for medical intervention for emergencies, including the use of emergency equipment and standing orders;
- delineate staff training requirements;
- describe documentation procedure; and
- identify considerations for alternatives for service delivery including home health, community-based, or unsupervised home programming.

Potential Risks in Outpatient CR/SP

The safety of CR/SP exercise programs is well established, with very low mortality and myocardial infarction rates during exercise training. An analysis of four reports of exercise-related cardiovascular complications reveals 1 cardiac arrest per 116,906 patient-hours, 1 myocardial infarction per 219,970 patient-hours, and 1 fatality per 752,365 patient-hours. This low fatality rate can be attributed to medically supervised programs that are equipped and prepared to manage adverse events and emergencies.[1] However, even when patients are thoroughly screened at program entry and on each day before beginning exercise participation, the potential for the unpredictable occurrence of complications before, during, or after exercise is ever present, particularly as more patients at increased risk of events are entering programs. In 2008, CR/SP participants as a whole were found to be older and less fit than in previous decades, as well presenting more frequently with features of the metabolic syndrome.[2]

Services offered in hospitals and other facilities that have been accredited by the Joint Commission (TJC) must meet the quality and safety standards established by the accrediting organization.[3-6] Minimum guidelines described in this chapter for the management of medical problems and emergencies do not supersede TJC standards but rather complement and further detail the preparation for and delivery of care in cardiac rehabilitation programs at various locations.

Advance Directives

Health care advance directives are documents that patients prepare to direct their future health care should they become unable to make such decisions. The most common types of advance directives are living wills and durable power of attorney or health care proxy. When a patient enrolls in CR/SP, the staff should ascertain if advance directives exist; if so, these should be documented and communicated to all staff members. In accordance with the Patient Self-Determination Act, all institutions serving Medicare and Medicaid patients are required to provide information to patients and train health care providers about advance directives and to facilitate the completion of the advance directives

if a patient desires them. The outpatient CR/SP setting provides an opportunity for offering this education. Discussions between patients and health care providers regarding patient wishes and desires may lead to a higher prevalence of completion of advance directives.[7,8]

Patient Assessment and Screening

Although patients have been evaluated before entering the CR/SP program, the clinical status of a patient may change. In addition, risk stratification models and routine diagnostic procedures, such as exercise or pharmacological stress testing, may not identify all patients at risk for exercise training–related events, particularly when they use modes of exercise training other than treadmill walking, such as arm or resistance training. Consequently, it is important to observe patients carefully during a variety of exercise situations and modes.

The staff must be prepared to anticipate and recognize impending problems by evaluating a change in patient condition and providing appropriate intervention. In many cases of impending emergency, patients exhibit warning signs and symptoms. A change in the usual clinical status of a patient with otherwise stable disease can alert the staff to the possibility of a developing medical problem (guideline 12.1). The best approach to managing clinical emergencies is through the early recognition of these signs and symptoms that prompt intervention and treatment.

Guideline 12.2 lists clinical problems CR/SP professionals should recognize and for which they should be prepared to provide immediate intervention. CR/SP program policies and procedures and standing orders should describe specific treatment guidelines (see appendixes N and O for examples). New or changing patterns of signs and symptoms should be reported to the supervising physician, the referring physician, or both.

Angina and Ischemia

Both quality and quantity of chest discomfort or angina equivalent (e.g., atypical chest discomfort, shortness of breath), as well as frequency, duration, and triggers for angina (e.g., physical exertion, exposure to cold, the postprandial period, emotional stressors), should be noted. If angina or ischemic changes occur during supervised exercise, the exercise workload and rate–pressure

Guideline 12.1 Routine Patient Assessment and Documentation

All patients should be routinely screened before each exercise session for changes in clinical status including, but not limited to,

- recent medical history and symptoms since the last patient visit,
- heart rate and rhythm,
- electrocardiogram (ECG) when indicated,

- blood pressure (BP),
- body weight, and
- medication compliance and changes in medication regimen.

All screening must be documented regardless of the findings.

Guideline 12.2 Clinical Problems Requiring Intervention

Guidelines for managing the following conditions, including standing orders for emergency interventions where appropriate, should be included in program policies and procedures:

- New or changing pattern of angina
- New or changing patterns of dysrhythmia
- Decompensated heart failure
- Hypoglycemia or hyperglycemia

- Syncopal or near-syncopal episodes
- Hypotension or hypertension
- Dyspnea
- Decreased exercise tolerance
- Claudication
- Depression
- Cardiac or respiratory arrest

product (RPP) at which the signs and symptoms appeared should be documented, as well as associated signs or symptoms (e.g., light-headedness, diaphoresis, decreased BP). Ischemia may also create electrical instability resulting in increased dysrhythmias.

Dysrhythmias

Frequency, duration, and type of dysrhythmia(s), including accompanying signs and symptoms, should be noted (e.g., ECG findings of ischemia, light-headedness, dyspnea, poor perfusion). Dysrhythmias to be documented include, but are not limited to, resting and exercise-induced atrial or ventricular ectopy, and tachyarrhythmias, as well as atrioventricular block, symptomatic bradycardia, and intraventricular conduction delays (see "Dysrhythmias" section in chapter 9).

Heart Failure

Despite having higher overall morbidity and mortality rates, the event rates in exercise training studies in patients with chronic heart failure

have been low. The most common events are postexercise hypotension, atrial and ventricular dysrhythmias, and worsening of heart failure symptoms.[9] Signs and symptoms such as shortness of breath at rest or with usual activity, weight gain, edema, or decreased exercise tolerance may indicate worsening heart failure and should be noted. Patients with decompensated heart failure should not exercise and should be referred back to their physician or health care provider for evaluation and treatment.

Hypoglycemia or Hyperglycemia

Note pre- or postexercise hypoglycemia or hyperglycemia (in patients with type 1 or type 2 diabetes or insulin-resistant patients), as well as whether it is symptomatic or asymptomatic. Glucose monitoring equipment should be available as well as glucose tablets or gel or other source of carbohydrate. Patients using oral agents, insulin, or both should have a blood glucose of 100 mg/dL or higher during the pre- and postexercise period and should maintain that level during exercise. Patients with hypoglycemia unawareness or frequent hypoglycemia episodes may require a higher blood glucose target or more frequent testing. Avoid exercise in type 1 diabetics with a blood glucose of >300 mg/dL, and use caution in type 2 diabetes.[10]

Episodes of Syncope or Near-Syncope

Documentation should include the onset, duration, and severity of the episode, along with BP and cardiac rhythm.

Hypotension or Hypertension

Note pre- or postexercise hypotension that is associated with signs or symptoms, persistent resting hypertension, or excessively high exercise BP.

Dyspnea

Feelings of dyspnea or shortness of breath can be an angina equivalent or a symptom of respiratory distress. Note the level of activity when symptoms occur as well as lung sounds and oxygen saturation.

Exercise Intolerance

Increasing fatigue or level of rating of perceived exertion (RPE) at similar exercise workload and inability to tolerate usual level of activity, as well as abnormal hemodynamic responses to exertion, should be noted.

Intermittent Claudication

Patients with new symptoms of claudication should be evaluated by their physician (see chapter 9). A vascular physical examination and ankle–brachial index are recommended. Note onset, duration, and severity of claudication as well as the exercise workload at which symptoms occur. Evaluated patients with intermittent claudication should exercise until they experience moderate to severe discomfort, followed by a brief period of rest allowing symptoms to resolve. Repeat the exercise, rest, exercise pattern throughout the exercise session. Symptoms of critical limb ischemia include resting limb pain, ulceration, or gangrene; these patients should undergo expedited evaluation and should not exercise.[11]

Depression

Depression screening upon entry to the CR/SP program is recommended since depression is often associated with adverse events, increased mortality, and a worse prognosis in cardiac patients. It may double the risk of cardiac events during the first 2 years after myocardial infarction. Although elevated depressive symptoms are relatively common in hospitalized cardiac patients, as many as 15% to 20% of hospitalized cardiac patients meet criteria for major depression, and women and patients with heart failure may have even higher rates.[12] Patients who have abnormal initial screenings, persistent depression, or changes in affect should be further assessed to determine necessity for treatment and to rule out risk of suicide. Immediate or elective referral to the primary care physician and a professional qualified in the diagnosis and treatment of depression may be indicated.

Cardiac or Respiratory Arrest

Medical evaluation and risk stratification before starting the CR/SP program and a thorough assessment and screening before each rehabilitation exercise session can assist with identifying unstable patients who should not be allowed to exercise at that time. Prompt recognition of adverse signs and symptoms during the exercise session is essential for the CR/SP staff to be able to either modify or terminate the session before more serious events occur. Quarterly emergency drills are required to ensure that the staff will be able to respond efficiently and effectively if a cardiac or respiratory arrest occurs.

Intervention Summary

For each of these occurrences, follow-up should include documentation verifying interventions or changes in medical therapy. Patients involved should be educated about the warning signs and symptoms of these clinical findings. During assessment of a clinical problem or emergency situation and for the general purposes of patient evaluation, CR/SP staff should describe and document measurements of the clinical status of the patient. Appropriate interventions may then be applied. Where appropriate, assessment of clinical status should include the following:

- Self-reported history describing symptoms—the degree and type, precipitating and relieving factors, and any change in pattern
- Heart rate (HR)
- BP

- ECG monitoring (preferably diagnostic quality and more than one lead)
- 12-lead ECG if diagnostic-quality ECG monitoring is not available
- Results of the most recent exercise test or pharmacological stress test
- Auscultation of the heart and lungs
- Assessment of peripheral pulses and perfusion
- Pulse oximetry for oxygen saturation
- Assessment of level of consciousness
- Blood glucose level

Based on these assessments, interventions may include the following, as appropriate:

- Not initiating, altering, or terminating the exercise session
- Assisting the patient to a comfortable sitting or lying position
- Comforting the patient
- Monitoring BP and HR-ECG
- Administering supplemental oxygen
- Administering sublingual nitroglycerin
- Administering glucose orally or intravenously per institutional policy
- Establishing intravenous (IV) access and administering IV fluids
- Administering basic life support (BLS)[13]
- Administering advanced cardiac life support (ACLS)[14]
- Transferring to cardiac catheterization laboratory, intensive care unit, emergency department, or, for freestanding center, transporting to a hospital or providing emergency services for immediate care
- Notifying the supervising physician, program medical director, and the referring physician
- Notifying family

Documentation of Emergencies

Emergencies must be documented according to the standards set forth by the agency risk management or legal department. All incidents must be documented in the patient chart. Other documentation may include an incident or adverse event form (see appendix P). The American Heart Association (AHA) recommends that community- and hospital-based programs sys-

tematically monitor cardiac arrests to improve performance and outcomes using a cycle of evaluation, benchmarking, and developing strategies to address identified deficiencies (see appendix Q). Benchmarking can be facilitated by existing cardiac arrest registries such as the AHA Get With the Guidelines (www.heart.org/HEARTORG/ HealthcareResearch/GetWithTheGuidelines-Resuscitation/Get-With-The-Guidelines-Resuscitation_UCM_314496_SubHomePage. jsp), formerly known as the National Registry of Cardiopulmonary Resuscitation, for in-hospital cardiac arrests, and the Cardiac Arrest Registry to Enhance Survival (https://mycares.net), for out-of-hospital cardiac arrest. The Utstein guidelines are a useful template for measuring key aspects of the resuscitation process and outcome that can be used for quality improvement processes.[15,16]

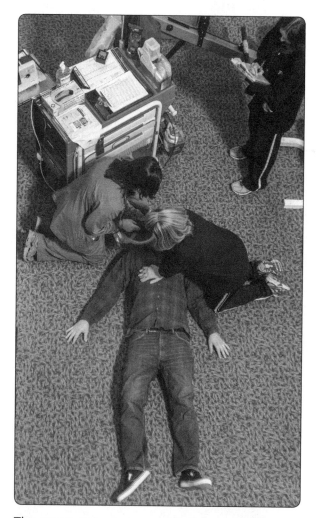

The emergency cart, resuscitation equipment, and medications must be checked regularly.

Guideline 12.3 Emergency Equipment and Maintenance

Emergency equipment should be immediately available to all exercise areas and should include the following:

- Telephone, medical alert signal, or other emergency signal system to call for paramedics or code team as applicable.
- Portable battery-operated defibrillator with ECG printout and monitor that may have external pacemaker capability should be available for programs with moderate- to high-risk patients participating. Direct current (DC) capability in case of battery failure should be available for the defibrillator, monitor, and ECG printout.
- Depending on the individual facility's policies, an automatic external defibrillator (AED) may be used in place of a manual defibrillator. The availability of an AED is especially useful for programs serving low-risk participants, and is strongly recommended when ACLS personnel are not immediately available or in areas of the hospital or in facilities where this will facilitate early defibrillation with the goal of shock delivery <3 min from collapse. However, "the AHA does not recommend continued use of an AED (or the automatic mode) when a manual defibrillator is available and the provider skills are adequate for rhythm interpretation. Rhythm analysis and shock administration with an AED may result in prolonged interruptions in chest compressions."[14]
- Portable oxygen and tubing, with nasal cannula, and face masks.
- Adult oral and nasopharyngeal airways in various sizes should be standard equipment on all emergency carts as well as bag valve mask and pocket face masks.
- Intubation equipment including air adjuncts such as Combitube or laryngeal mask airway. If intuba-

tion equipment is available for use, personnel who are certified and licensed to perform intubation and continuous quantitative waveform capnography should be accessible.

- Additional equipment for medical emergencies and maintenance policies should include:
  - Portable suction equipment.
  - Intravenous access and administration equipment and fluids.
  - Sharps container.
  - ACLS medications as noted in the AHA standards and based on community standards and medical advisory committee recommendations.
  - BP measurement equipment (sphygmomanometer and stethoscope[s]).
  - Cardiac board.
  - Personal protective equipment—gloves, masks, gowns, face shields.
  - General medical supplies.
  - Emergency documentation forms.
- Cart or mobile storage unit for emergency equipment and medications. The emergency equipment and medications should be appropriately stored, locked, and secured out of reach of the general public when not in use.
- Biomedical engineering check of equipment for maintenance and performance should be performed every 6 months, or as TJC standards or state regulations require. Documentation of such maintenance is required.
- Defibrillators should be checked daily for discharge capability.
- Medications should be checked per agency policy by designated professional staff for outdates.

Emergency Equipment

Emergency equipment availability for program services is dependent on the particular site at which care is being delivered. The emergency equipment for CR/SP is presented in guideline 12.3. The emergency cart, resuscitation equipment, and medications must be checked regularly. Examples of forms in appendixes R, S, and T may be used to document equipment checks and maintenance.

Staff Training and Site Preparation

The AHA provides the recommended training courses for emergency cardiac care (ECC) for CR/SP personnel. ECC includes treatments for sudden and often life-threatening events affecting the cardiovascular and pulmonary systems. The 2010 AHA Guidelines for CPR and ECC provide the latest treatment recommendations based on current and comprehensive resuscitation literature. Healthcare Provider BLS and ACLS are the typically recommended AHA training courses for adult CR/SP depending on personnel training requirements (guideline 12.4).[13,14]

The concepts of high-quality CPR with minimal interruptions and early defibrillation are of utmost importance to improving resuscitation outcomes in inpatient and outpatient CR/SP programs. Since the advent of the AED, staff members successfully completing BLS and AED training may provide for chest compressions, ventilation, and immediate defibrillation, if indicated, regardless of where the program site is located.[17-19] CR/SP personnel should be authorized, trained, equipped, and directed to operate an AED if their professional responsibilities require them to respond to persons in cardiac arrest when ACLS providers are not immediately available and until a code team arrives. Such may be the case in early-morning or evening maintenance programs staffed by nonmedical personnel (guideline 12.5). Because CR/SP services, whether hospital or freestanding, are medical facilities and under the auspices of a physician medical director, they are not subject to public access defibrillation regulations but rather to the policies and procedures of the supervising physician and parent medical facility.

Professional staff who are qualified, are appropriately licensed, and have successfully completed ACLS may administer medications to cardiovert or defibrillate patients as allowed by state licensure laws, which usually apply to physicians and registered nurses but may include

---

Guideline 12.4 **Professional Staff and Emergency Care in Outpatient Cardiac Rehabilitation: Hospital-Based or Freestanding Center**

- All professional staff will successfully complete the National Cognitive and Skills evaluations in accordance with the AHA curriculum for Healthcare Provider BLS.

- A physician, registered nurse, or other appropriately trained staff member who has successfully completed the National Cognitive and Skills evaluations in accordance with the AHA curriculum for ACLS and has met state and hospital or facility medicolegal requirements for defibrillation and other related practices will provide medical supervision for moderate- to high-risk patients.

- Standing orders or policies and procedures for all emergency situations will be in effect and reviewed

regularly by the staff and the program medical director.

- Regularly scheduled and documented emergency procedure in-services including mock codes (at least four per year) for all staff involved in patient care will be performed and documented (see appendix U).

- Regularly scheduled reviews (monthly is recommended) of emergency cart equipment, emergency medications, and supplies will be performed and appropriately documented.

Guideline 12.5 **Personnel Requirements Related to Emergency Care**

- All staff involved with the patient in exercise and education will successfully complete the National Cognitive and Skills evaluations in accordance with the AHA curriculum for Healthcare Provider BLS (CPR/AED).

- A physician, registered nurse, or other appropriately trained staff member who has successfully completed the National Cognitive and Skills evaluations

in accordance with the AHA curriculum for ACLS and has met state and hospital or facility medicolegal requirements for defibrillation and other related practices will provide medical supervision for moderate- to high-risk patients All professional staff will be aware of the specific emergency procedures required by the agency for inpatients and outpatients and specific patient care units.

other allied health or emergency personnel. Successful completion of either course does not imply licensure or warrant future performance. Tracheal intubation may be performed only by health care providers experienced in this skill and those who obtain regular experience (6-12 times per year). Therefore, most providers employed in CR/SP programs should use alternative, noninvasive techniques for airway management, such as a bag mask device, laryngeal mask airway, esophageal–tracheal Combitube, or pharyngotracheal lumen airway. If tracheal intubation is used, continuous quantitative waveform capnography is recommended during the resuscitation period. It is useful for confirming tracheal tube placement, monitoring CPR quality, and detecting return of spontaneous circulation. ACLS training emphasizes assessments and interventions that improve outcomes. However, vascular access, drug delivery, and advanced airway placement, while recommended, should not cause significant interruptions in the delivery of high-quality chest compressions or delay defibrillation of ventricular fibrillation or pulseless ventricular tachycardia, two critical links in the chain of survival.[19]

Within each facility, the emergency plan must address transportation of patients to a hospital emergency room or other destination (e.g., catheterization lab, coronary care unit). Such a plan must include telephone access to call a code, 911, or the local emergency medical system. For programs not operating within a hospital, staff should be familiar with the emergency transport teams in their geographic area so that access and location of the center are clearly identified. The emergency response team should be met at the appropriate entrance of the facility so that they can be promptly guided to the site of the emergency situation when possible, while the victim remains directly supervised by an appropriate staff member at all times. A number of publications have made recommendations for staff experience and emergency care and are the basis for guidelines regarding professional staff and emergency care.[17,20]

Inpatient programs have a wide range of standing protocols for the treatment of medical emergencies. Because the patient is being seen on an inpatient unit, staff nurses and the code team will be available to respond to an emergency.

Nontraditional Programs

To be able to offer CR/SP to more individuals and to decrease costs, nontraditional programs are offered through Internet-based risk factor reduction and community- or home-based settings. Some existing CR/SP programs have also incorporated home-based CR/SP as a service option.[21-24] The exercise portion of these programs may be managed by remote ECG monitoring, conducted in a supervised setting, or self-managed by patients following recommended exercise prescriptions that they have been given.[25] These options are addressed in the next three subsections.

Remote ECG Monitoring

Remote ECG monitoring is used primarily in patients who require monitored exercise programs but whose geographic location is not within reasonable proximity for travel to an outpatient exercise facility.[26,27] The prime example of such monitoring is its use for at-home programming, but it may be used in more typical types of exercise facilities such as community centers, health clubs, or gymnasiums. The professional staff member supervising the incoming ECG signal is responsible for recognizing impending problems; evaluating a change in patient condition through history, symptoms, and ECG interpretation; and providing direction to the patient and whoever might be with the patient to avert further problems. In cases of patients exercising in a facility where health personnel are providing direct supervision, such staff members should meet personnel requirements as described for outpatient program staff for emergency care. In situations in which patients are exercising without health care staff supervision, however, the plan for the course of action is much different (guideline 12.6).

Home Setting

Secondary prevention services performed in the home may be subject to different personnel requirements inherent in the unique delivery of care. Whereas home health nurses and physical therapists are not typically ACLS prepared and do not carry an ECG monitor or a defibrillator to the patient home, those providing CR/SP should be qualified similarly to those providing the care in a hospital or outpatient setting. Personnel requirements for these staff are listed in guideline 12.7.

Guideline 12.6   Remote Supervision of Exercise in the Absence of On-Site Health Care Providers (in the Home or Nonsupervised Center)

- An open phone line to provide access to the patient will be available not only for routine communication with the patient but also in times of an emergency situation.

- Previous contact with local emergency care providers will have been made, including the development of a plan for and the availability of access to emergency cardiac care to the home or nonsupervised facility.

Guideline 12.7   Home Health Personnel Requirements Related to Emergency Care

- All staff involved with the patient in exercise and education will have successfully completed the National Cognitive and Skills evaluations in accordance with the AHA curriculum for Healthcare Provider BLS.

- All home health nurses who provide CR/SP services will have previous experience in cardiac nursing and will have successfully completed the National

Cognitive and Skills examination in accordance with the AHA curriculum for ACLS.

- All home health nurses and other professional staff providing direct patient care will be familiar with the local EMS access number (911 or other appropriate number).

- Emergency equipment should include BP kit, stethoscope, emergency plan, and possibly an AED.

Other recommendations relative to guideline 12.7 include the following:

- Patient family members will be taught to recognize cardiac arrest, notify emergency medical services (EMS), and perform chest compressions, since early CPR and defibrillation are key to survival.

- The patient's home will be evaluated for ease of emergency access with a stretcher. An emergency plan will be determined and reviewed with the patient and family, including assisting the family in labeling telephones with the local EMS number, such as 911, and home address. This will provide accurate information for anyone needing to place an emergency call.

- Evidence is insufficient to recommend for, or against, the deployment of an AED in homes at this time.[28]

Community-Site Programming

As patients are encouraged to make their exercise program a lifelong commitment, many use a community-site facility. The AHA/ACSM scientific statements "Recommendations for Cardiovascular Screening, Staffing, and Emergency Policies at Health/Fitness Facilities" and "Automated External Defibrillators in Health/Fitness Facilities" offer guidelines for emergencies within these facilities.[17,18] Guideline 12.8 is based on these documents.

Guideline 12.8 Community-Site Personnel Requirements Related to Emergency Care

- All staff will have successfully completed the National Cognitive and Skills evaluations in accordance with the AHA curriculum for BLS and AED training.

- The facility will have a medical liaison, that is, a physician, ACLS-trained registered nurse, or emergency medical technician (EMT), to oversee emergency planning. In medically supervised exercise programs and facilities that serve clinical populations, the liaison should be a licensed physician. The facility will have written emergency policies and procedures.

- Staff will perform and document emergency plan practice drills at least quarterly or more often as staff changes occur.

- Standards for such programming should comply with those for hospital-based centers but should be subject to the particular oversight of the community program medical director.

- Emergency equipment for such programming should comply with guidelines for freestanding centers and include emergency airway supplies, AED, medications, and medication administration supplies as determined by the community program medical director.

- Phones will be available and labeled with the local EMS number and the address of and directions to the building and area.

Summary

It remains the ultimate responsibility of the medical director and the professional staff to provide emergency care to the patient, regardless of the site of the CR/SP service. Regular review of the plan and appropriate modifications to enhance patient outcomes are required. The foundation of emergency care in CR is continued assessment of the patient and recognition of changes in patient condition that may be treated to avert an emergency. The role of manual defibrillation or AED with BLS and ACLS is paramount, as defibrillation may be the first treatment administered to the patient with sudden cardiac arrest. It is important that all CR programs be prepared with an emergency plan of early recognition and activation of the plan, including providing BLS and ACLS as appropriate.

Appendix A

Example of CR/SP Entry Clinical Review

Date:	Diagnosis:
	OR Date: Surgeon/Physician:
	Summary:
	ECG/dysrhythmia/test results:
	Lab values:
	Medications:
	Activity order:
	Plan:

From *Guidelines for Cardiac Rehabilitation and Secondary Prevention Programs, Fifth Edition,* by American Association of Cardiovascular and Pulmonary Rehabilitation, 2013, Human Kinetics, Champaign, IL.

Appendix B

Example of Inpatient Rehabilitation Services Record

Patient information

Date:	Diagnosis:
C.R.	Remarks: (day #)
	Exercise: monitored/unmonitored; O$_2$ Sat:
	Response: HR BP SS Assistance
	Rest:
	Ex period 1:
	Ex period 2:
	Ex period 3:
	Comments:
	Education:
	Instructions:
	Plan:

From *Guidelines for Cardiac Rehabilitation and Secondary Prevention Programs, Fifth Edition,* by American Association of Cardiovascular and Pulmonary Rehabilitation, 2013, Human Kinetics, Champaign, IL.

Appendix C

Sample Informed Consent for Exercise Testing of Patients With Known or Suspected Heart Disease

Name: _____

1. Purpose and Explanation of Test

I hereby consent to voluntarily engage in an exercise test to determine my capacity and state of cardiovascular health. I also consent, if necessary, to the taking of samples of my exhaled air during exercise to properly measure my oxygen uptake. It is my understanding that the information obtained will help me evaluate future physical activities in which I may safely engage and aid my doctor in the determination of an appropriate medical treatment for me.

I understand that my physician has recommended the exercise test and referred me to this particular center for performance of the test. I have provided correct responses to the questions as indicated on the patient medical history form or to those of the interviewer. I understand that based on this information, it will be determined if there are any reasons that would make it undesirable or unsafe for me to take the test. Consequently, I understand that it is important that I provide complete and accurate responses to the interviewer and recognize that my failure to do so could lead to possible unnecessary injury to myself during the test.

The test that I will undergo will be performed on a motor-driven treadmill or bicycle ergometer with the amount of effort gradually increasing. As I understand it, this increase in effort will continue until I feel and verbally report to the operator any symptoms such as fatigue, shortness of breath, or chest discomfort. I have been clearly advised that it is my right to request that a test be stopped at any point and that I should immediately upon experiencing any such symptoms inform the operator.

It is further my understanding that prior to beginning the test, I will be connected by electrodes and cables to an electrocardiographic recorder which will enable personnel to monitor my cardiac (heart) activity. During the test itself, it is my understanding that a physician or trained observer will monitor my responses continuously and take frequent readings of blood pressure, the electrocardiogram, and record my expressed feelings of discomfort or effort.

Once the test has been completed, but before I am released from the test area, I will be given special instructions about showering and the recognition of certain symptoms that may appear within the first 24 hours after the test. I agree to follow these instructions and promptly contact the program personnel or medical providers if such symptoms develop.

2. Risks

It is my understanding, and I have been informed, that there exists the possibility of adverse changes during the actual test. I have been informed that these changes could include abnormal blood pressure, fainting, disorders of heart rhythm, stroke, and very rare instances of heart attack or even death. Every effort, I have been told, will be made to minimize these occurrences by observations taken during the test. I have also been informed that emergency equipment and personnel are readily available to deal with these unusual situations should they occur. I understand that there is a risk of injury, heart attack, or even death as a result of my performance of this test, but knowing those risks, it is my desire to proceed to take the test as herein indicated.

From *Guidelines for Cardiac Rehabilitation and Secondary Prevention Programs, Fifth Edition,* by American Association of Cardiovascular and Pulmonary Rehabilitation, 2013, Human Kinetics, Champaign, IL.

3. Benefits to Be Expected and Alternatives to the Exercise Testing Procedure

I understand that the possible beneficial results of this test depend on my doctor's medical reasons for requesting it. It may be helpful in determining my chances of having heart disease that should be treated medically. If my doctor suspects or knows already that I have heart disease, this test may help to evaluate how this disease affects my ability to safely do certain types of physical work or exercises and how best to treat the disease.

4. Confidentiality and Use of Information

I have been informed that the information obtained from this exercise test will be treated as privileged and confidential and will consequently not be released or revealed to any person without my express written consent. I understand that this information will be used by the cardiac rehabilitation program staff to evaluate my exercise status or needs.

5. Inquiries and Freedom of Consent

I have been given the opportunity to ask questions regarding the procedure.

I further understand that there are remote risks other than those mentioned previously that may be associated with this procedure. Despite the fact that a complete accounting of all remote risks is not entirely possible, I am satisfied with the review of these risks which was provided to me, and it is still my desire to proceed with the test.

I acknowledge that I have read this document in its entirety or that it has been read to me if I have been unable to read same.

I consent to the rendition of all services and procedures as explained herein by all program personnel.

_____

Patient signature   Date

_____

Witness signature   Date

_____

Test supervisor signature   Date

From *Guidelines for Cardiac Rehabilitation and Secondary Prevention Programs, Fifth Edition,* by American Association of Cardiovascular and Pulmonary Rehabilitation, 2013, Human Kinetics, Champaign, IL.

Appendix D

Six-Minute Walk Test Protocol (6MWT)

The 6MWT should be performed indoors, along a long, flat, straight, enclosed corridor with a hard surface that is seldom traveled. The walking course must be 30 m in length. A 100 ft (30.4 m) hallway is, therefore, required. The length of the corridor should be marked every 3 m. The turnaround points should be marked with a cone (such as an orange traffic cone). A starting line, which marks the beginning and end of each 60 m lap, should be marked on the floor using brightly colored tape.

Patient Preparation

1. Comfortable clothing should be worn.
2. Appropriate shoes for walking should be worn.
3. Patients should use their usual walking aids during the test (e.g., cane, walker).
4. The patient's usual medical regimen should be continued.
5. A light meal is acceptable before early morning or early afternoon tests.
6. Patients should not have exercised vigorously within 2 hours of beginning the test.

Measurements

Repeat testing should be performed about the same time of day.

Set the lap counter to zero and the timer to 6 minutes. Assemble all necessary equipment (lap counter, timer, clipboard, worksheet) and move to the starting point.

Instruct the patient as follows:

"The object of this test is to walk as far as possible for 6 minutes. You will walk back and forth in this hallway. Six minutes is a long time to walk, so you will be exerting yourself. You will probably get out of breath or become exhausted. You are permitted to slow down, to stop, and to rest as necessary. You may lean against the wall while resting, but resume walking as soon as you are able. You will be walking back and forth around the cones. You should pivot briskly around the cones and continue back the other way without hesitation. Now I'm going to show you. Please watch the way I turn without hesitation."

Demonstrate by walking one lap yourself. Walk and pivot around a cone briskly.

"Are you ready to do that? I am going to use this counter to keep track of the number of laps you complete. I will click it each time you turn around at this starting line. Remember that the object is to walk AS FAR AS POSSIBLE for 6 minutes, but don't run or jog. Start now or whenever you are ready."

- Position the patient at the starting line. You should also stand near the starting line during the test. Do not walk with the patient. As soon as the patient starts to walk, start the timer. Do not talk to anyone during the walk. Use an even tone of voice when using the standard phrases of encouragement.

- Watch the patient. Do not get distracted and lose count of the laps. Each time the participant returns to the starting line, click the lap counter once (or mark the lap on the worksheet). Let the participant see you do it. Exaggerate the click using body language, like using a stopwatch at a race.

- During the test, after the first minute, tell the patient the following (in even tones*): "You are doing well. You have 5 minutes to go."*

- When the timer shows 4 minutes remaining, tell the patient the following: *"Keep up the good work. You have 4 minutes to go."*

- When the timer shows 3 minutes remaining, tell the patient the following: *"You are doing well. You are halfway done."*

From *Guidelines for Cardiac Rehabilitation and Secondary Prevention Programs, Fifth Edition,* by American Association of Cardiovascular and Pulmonary Rehabilitation, 2013, Human Kinetics, Champaign, IL.

- When the timer shows 2 minutes remaining, tell the patient the following: *"Keep up the good work. You have only 2 minutes left."*

- When the timer shows only 1 minute remaining, tell the patient: *"You are doing well. You have only 1 minute to go."*

- Do not use other words of encouragement (or body language to speed up).

If the patient stops walking during the test and needs a rest, say this: *"You can lean against the wall if you would like; then continue walking whenever you feel able."* Do not stop the timer. If the patient stops before the 6 minutes are up and refuses to continue (or you decide that the patient should not continue), wheel the chair over for the patient to sit on, discontinue the walk, and note on the worksheet the distance, the time stopped, and the reason for stopping prematurely.

When the timer is 15 seconds from completion, say this: *"In a moment I'm going to tell you to stop. When I do, just stop right where you are and I will come to you."*

When the timer rings (or buzzes), say this: *"Stop!"* Walk over to the patient. Consider taking the chair if the patient looks exhausted. Mark the spot where the patient stopped by placing a beanbag or a piece of tape on the floor. Record the number of laps from the counter (or tick marks on the worksheet), that is, the total distance walked in 6 minutes.

Reprinted, by permission, from American Thoracic Society, 2002, "ATS Statement: Guidelines for the six-minute walk test," *American Journal of Respiratory Critical Care Medicine* 166: 111-117.

From *Guidelines for Cardiac Rehabilitation and Secondary Prevention Programs, Fifth Edition,* by American Association of Cardiovascular and Pulmonary Rehabilitation, 2013, Human Kinetics, Champaign, IL.

Appendix E
Example of Quick Look Patient Record

Patient Fact Sheet

Date: _____

Institution Name

Name: _____

Address: _____

City: _____

State: _____ Zip: _____

SS Number (last 4): _____

Patient Phone: _____

Work Phone: _____

Occupation: _____

Race/Ethnicity: _____

Marital Status: _____

Spouse: _____

DOB: _____

Patient Status: _____

Age: _____ Height: _____

Initial Weight: _____

Weight: _____ BMI: _____

Gender: _____

Target HR: _____

Abrev. Dx: _____

Medical History: _____

_____

_____

_____

Detailed Medications: _____

_____

_____

_____

Allergies: _____

_____

_____

_____

Educational Classes: _____

_____

_____

_____

Cardiac Rehabilitation

Referring Physician: _____

Cardiologist: _____

Surgeon: _____

Insurance: _____

Admit to CR Date: _____

Authorization Number: _____

Authorization Dates: _____

Clinic I.D.: _____

System Code: _____

Risk Factors:

☐ Obesity   ☐ Diabetes   ☐ Family Hx

☐ High BP   ☐ Sed. Lifestyle   ☐ Stress

☐ Smoker

Smoking Comments: _____

_____

☐ Hyperlipidemia

Chol: _____

Trig: _____

HDL: _____

LDL: _____

Hgb A1c: _____

Date Drawn: _____

Stress Test Data

Stress Test Date: _____

Stress Test Time: _____

Type: _____

Duration: _____

Stress Test METS: _____

Highest Stage: _____

Peak HR: _____

Peak Ex BP: _____

Resting ECG: _____

Symptoms: _____

ECG Changes: _____

Interpretation: _____

_____

From *Guidelines for Cardiac Rehabilitation and Secondary Prevention Programs, Fifth Edition,* by American Association of Cardiovascular and Pulmonary Rehabilitation, 2013, Human Kinetics, Champaign, IL.

Appendix F

Informed Consent for Exercise Rehabilitation of Patients with Known or Suspected Heart Disease

Name: _____

1. Purpose and Explanation of Procedure

In order to improve my physical capacity and generally aid in my medical treatment for heart disease, I hereby consent to enter a cardiac rehabilitation program that will include cardiovascular monitoring, physical exercise, dietary counseling, smoking cessation, stress reduction, and health education activities. The levels of exercise that I will perform will be based on the condition of my heart and circulation as determined by my physician. I will be given exact instructions regarding the amount and kind of exercise I should do. I agree to participate three times per week in the rehabilitation program. Professionally trained clinical personnel will provide leadership to direct my activities and monitor my electrocardiogram and blood pressure to be certain that I am exercising at the prescribed level. I understand that I am expected to attend every session and to follow physician and staff instructions with regard to any medications that may have been prescribed, exercise, diet, stress management, and smoking cessation. If I am taking prescribed medication, I have already so informed the program staff and further agree to so inform them promptly of any changes my doctor or I have made with regard to use of these.

I have been informed that in the course of my participation in exercise, I will be asked to complete the activities unless such symptoms as fatigue, shortness of breath, chest discomfort, or similar occurrences appear. At that point I have been advised that it is my complete right to stop exercise and that it is my obligation to inform the program personnel of my symptoms. I recognize and hereby state that I have been advised that I should immediately upon experiencing any such symptoms inform the program personnel of my symptoms.

I understand that during the performance of exercise, a trained observer will periodically monitor my performance and perhaps take my electrocardiogram, pulse, blood pressure, or make other observations for the purpose of monitoring my progress and/or condition. I also understand that the observer may reduce or stop my exercise program when findings indicate that this should be done for my safety and benefit.

2. Risks

It is my understanding, and I have been informed, that there exists the possibility during exercise of adverse changes including abnormal blood pressure; fainting; disorders of heart rhythm; and very rare instances of heart attack, stroke, or even death. Every effort, I have been told, will be made to minimize these occurrences by proper staff assessment of my condition before each exercise session, staff supervision during exercise, and my own careful control of exercise effort. I have also been informed that emergency equipment and personnel are readily available to deal with unusual situations should these occur. I understand that there is a risk of injury, heart attack, stroke, or even death as a result of my exercise, but knowing those risks, it is my desire to proceed to participate as herein indicated.

3. Benefits to Be Expected and Alternatives Available

I understand that this medical treatment may or may not benefit my health status or physical fitness. Generally, participation will help determine

From *Guidelines for Cardiac Rehabilitation and Secondary Prevention Programs, Fifth Edition,* by American Association of Cardiovascular and Pulmonary Rehabilitation, 2013, Human Kinetics, Champaign, IL.

what recreational and occupational activities I can safely and comfortably perform. Many individuals in such programs also show improvements in their capacity for physical work. For those who are overweight and able to follow the physician's and dietitian's recommended dietary plan, this program may also aid in achieving appropriate weight education and control.

4. Confidentiality and Use of Information

I have been informed that the information obtained from this rehabilitation program will be treated as privileged and confidential and will consequently not be released or revealed to any person without my express written consent. I do, however, agree to the use of any information for research and statistical purposes as long as same does not identify my person or provide facts that could lead to my identification. Any other information obtained, however, will be used only by the program staff in the course of prescribing exercise for me, planning my rehabilitation program, or advising my personal physician of my progress.

5. Inquiries and Freedom of Consent

I have been given an opportunity to ask certain questions as to the procedures of this program.

I further understand that there are remote risks other than those previously described that may be associated with this program. Despite the fact that a complete accounting of all remote risks is not entirely possible, I am satisfied with the review of these risks that was provided to me, and it is still my desire to participate.

I acknowledge that I have read this document in its entirety or that it has been read to me if I have been unable to read same.

I consent to the rendition of all services and procedures as explained herein by all program personnel.

_____

Patient's Signature   Date

_____

Witness's Signature   Date

_____

Program Staff's Signature   Date

From *Guidelines for Cardiac Rehabilitation and Secondary Prevention Programs, Fifth Edition,* by American Association of Cardiovascular and Pulmonary Rehabilitation, 2013, Human Kinetics, Champaign, IL.

Appendix G

Example of Daily Exercise Session Report

Institution/Program name: _____

Cardiac Rehabilitation: _____

Patient Name: _____

Session #:_____ THR: _____ Session Date: _____

Session Summary				
☐ Meds Taken Comments: _____ _____	Rest HR: _____	Rest BP: _____	Baseline ECG: _____ _____ _____	Class Start Time: _____
Weight: _____	Peak HR: _____	End BP: _____	_____ _____	Class End Time: _____
Pre-BS: _____ Post-BS: _____	End HR: _____	S/S: _____		Session MD: _____
Problems/concerns since last session: _____ _____ Comments: _____ _____				

#	Modality	Ex min	Prescribed work load	Est. MET level	HR	RPE	ECG/symptoms comments	Other data, e.g., BP, SaO$_2$
1	Rest		-	-				
2	Warm-up		-	-				
3	Treadmill		mph/ %grade					
4	Arm ergometer		Watts					
5	Bike ergometer		Watts					
6	Rower		Watts					
7	Resistance training		setting					
8	Treadmill		mph/ %grade					
9	Cool-down		-	-				

Post-Session Comments/Plan: _____

_____

From *Guidelines for Cardiac Rehabilitation and Secondary Prevention Programs, Fifth Edition,* by American Association of Cardiovascular and Pulmonary Rehabilitation, 2013, Human Kinetics, Champaign, IL.

Appendix H

Example of Long-Term Outpatient Program Daily Exercise Record

Name: _____

Target HR: _____

Exercise prescription: _____

Date	Adjustments or comments	Meds	Rest HR	Rest BP	Warm-up	Ex HR 10 min	Ex HR 20 min	Ex HR 30 min	Post-ex BP	Weight

From *Guidelines for Cardiac Rehabilitation and Secondary Prevention Programs, Fifth Edition,* by American Association of Cardiovascular and Pulmonary Rehabilitation, 2013, Human Kinetics, Champaign, IL.

Appendix I

Education Flow Sheet

Patient Identification Information Topics	Teaching needs Please check	Discussed	Reinforced	Verbalized understanding	Teaching materials*	Comments
ORIENTATION TO EARLY OUTPATIENT CARDIAC REHABILITATION						
1. Registration						
2. Medical history—initial evaluation						
3. Risk-factor identification						
4. Orientation to staff and equipment						
5. Explanation of exercise prescription and target HR						
6. Instruction/review pulse check technique						
ANATOMY AND PHYSIOLOGY						
1. MI						
2. CABGS						
3. PTCA						
4. Angina						
5. Other—please list						
RISK FACTORS						
1. Smoking						
2. Hypertension						
3. Hyperlipidemia						
4. Diabetes						
5. Obesity						
6. Stress						
7. Inactivity						
8. Family history						
9. Age/sex						

* H = handout; AV = audiovisual; C = class.

From *Guidelines for Cardiac Rehabilitation and Secondary Prevention Programs, Fifth Edition,* by American Association of Cardiovascular and Pulmonary Rehabilitation, 2013, Human Kinetics, Champaign, IL.

Appendix J

Example of Home Exercise Program

Name: _____

Type of Exercise: _____

_____

_____

Intensity (How Hard to Exercise):

    Warm-up: (heart rate)   _____

    Training or Target Heart Rate: _____

    Cool-down: (heart rate)   _____

    The highest your heart rate should be at any time is: _____

Duration (How Long to Exercise):

    Warm-up: (minutes) _____

    Exercise Training: (minutes) _____

    Cool-down: (minutes) _____

Frequency (How Often to Exercise): _____

This program has been designed specifically for you as of _____. It will need periodic review and revision, especially if there are any changes in your medications or condition. Your program should be re-evaluated:

- Every 6 months
- After any type of exercise stress test
- Changes in medications, especially heart medications
- Changes or new onset of chest discomfort or other symptoms

Program Staff:_____

Phone Extension:_____

Date:_____ **THR:** _____

From *Guidelines for Cardiac Rehabilitation and Secondary Prevention Programs, Fifth Edition,* by American Association of Cardiovascular and Pulmonary Rehabilitation, 2013, Human Kinetics, Champaign, IL.

Date	Type of exercise	Resting pulse	Max pulse	Total time	Comments/symptoms

Appendix K

Smoking History Questionnaire

Name: _____ Date: _____

1. Have you smoked at least one cigarette, cigar, pipe full of tobacco, or cigarillo or had one chew of tobacco in the past month?

    _____ No; do not ask any of the remaining questions on this form.

    _____ Yes; continue.

2. What type of tobacco product do you use predominantly? (Circle one.)

    1 Cigarette   3 Pipe   5 Snuff/chewing tobacco

    2 Cigar   4 Cigarillo

3. On average, in the past 6 months how many cigarettes (or other tobacco products) have you smoked per day?

    _____ # of cigarettes   _____ # pipes full of tobacco   _____ # of chews

    _____ # of cigars   _____ # of cigarillos

4. How old were you when you began to smoke?

    _____ years of age

5. How many years have you smoked on a regular basis?

    _____ # of years

6. How many times have you made a *serious* attempt to quit smoking?

    _____ # of times (if never, go to question 12)

7. What was the longest time you have been off cigarettes?

    _____ # of years   _____ # of months   _____ # of days

8. In what year did this occur?

    _____ (year)

9. When was the last time you made a serious attempt to quit smoking?

    _____ / _____

From *Guidelines for Cardiac Rehabilitation and Secondary Prevention Programs, Fifth Edition,* by American Association of Cardiovascular and Pulmonary Rehabilitation, 2013, Human Kinetics, Champaign, IL.

10. What prompted you to begin smoking after your last attempt to quit? (Choose only one.)

   1 Crisis (death, illness, loss of job, family)

   2 Chronic stress

   3 Social/party situation

   4 Withdrawal symptoms

   5 Boredom

   6 Other; please explain: _____

11. What method of stopping smoking has worked best for you in the past, if any? (Choose only one.)

   1 Quit on own   6 Formal program

   2 Pamphlets   7 Private therapy

   3 Buddy system   8 Other medications

   4 Nicotine gum/patch   9 Other: _____

   5 Hypnosis, acupuncture

12. Have you ever used any prescribed medication(s) like nicotine chewing patch, buproprion, or varenicline to help you stop smoking?

   No

   Yes   Which medication(s)?_____

Questions 13 and 14 relate to addiction. Patients smoking within 30 minutes of waking and always/usually when ill are normally highly addicted to tobacco; pharmacological therapy may be highly beneficial.

13. How soon after you wake up do you smoke your first cigarette? (Circle only one.)

   1. When you first open your eyes

   2. Within the first 15 minutes of waking up

   3. Between 15 and 30 minutes after waking up

   4. Between 30 and 60 minutes after waking up

   5. Between 1 and 2 hours after waking up

   6. More than 2 hours after waking up

14. Do you smoke on the days that you are so ill that you are in bed most of the day? (Circle only one.)

   5 Always

   4 Usually

   3 Sometimes

   2 Rarely

   1 Never

15. Does the person you are closest to (spouse, companion) smoke?

No

Yes   Who is this? _____

16. Do you intend to stay off cigarettes, or other tobacco products, in the next month?

1	2	3	4	5	6	7
Definitely no	Probably	Possibly no	Maybe no	Possibly yes	Probably yes	Definitely yes

17. How often do you drink some kind of alcoholic beverage? (If you choose an answer other than "never," proceed to question 18.)

_____ Daily or almost every day

_____ 3 or 4 times a week

_____ Once or twice a week

_____ Once or twice a month

_____ Less than once a month

_____ Never (go to question 23)

Questions 18 to 21 are the CAGE questions related to alcohol. A score of 2 or greater significantly increases the probability of alcoholism; additional screening is warranted.

18. Have you ever felt you ought to CUT DOWN on your drinking?

No

Yes

19. Have people ever ANNOYED you by criticizing your drinking?

No

Yes

20. Have you ever felt bad or GUILTY about your drinking?

No

Yes

21. Have you ever had a drink first thing in the morning (EYE OPENER) to steady your nerves or get rid of a hangover?

No

Yes

22. How many of these alcoholic beverages do you drink during an average week?

_____ # of 12 oz bottles or cans of beer, ale, etc.

_____ # of 4 oz glasses of wine, sherry, port, etc.

_____ # of shots (a shot = 1.5 ounces) of vodka, rum, Scotch whiskey, bourbon, tequila, or gin (including mixed drinks and cocktails)

_____ # of after-dinner drinks

23. How hard has it been for you not to smoke since you've been in the hospital?

1	2	3	4	5
Very easy	Easy	Moderately easy	Hard	Very hard

24. How severe have withdrawal symptoms been for you?

1	2	3	4	5
Not at all severe	Mildly severe	Moderately severe	Severe	Very severe

Question 25: A response of 5 or greater may indicate moderate problems with depression, suggesting a need for further screening or intervention; pharmacological therapy (buproprion SR) may be highly beneficial.

25. How troubled are you by feeling miserable and depressed?

1	2	3	4	5	6	7	8	9
Hardly		Slightly		Moderately		Markedly		Very severely

26. How confident are you that you will be able to stay off cigarettes once you are discharged from the hospital? (0% = no confidence, 100% = total confidence)

0%   10%   20%   30%   40%   50%   60%   70%   80%   90%   100%

From *Guidelines for Cardiac Rehabilitation and Secondary Prevention Programs, Fifth Edition,* by American Association of Cardiovascular and Pulmonary Rehabilitation, 2013, Human Kinetics, Champaign, IL.

Appendix L

CAGE Questionnaire

_____ No _____ Yes Have you ever felt you ought to CUT DOWN on your drinking?

_____ No _____ Yes Have people ever ANNOYED you by criticizing your drinking?

_____ No _____ Yes Have you ever felt bad or GUILTY about your drinking?

_____ No _____ Yes Have you ever had a drink first thing in the morning (EYE OPENER) to steady your nerves or get rid of a hangover?

_____TOTAL (No = 0; Yes = 1)

A total score of 2 or greater significantly increases the probability of alcoholism—additional screening is warranted.

From _Guidelines for Cardiac Rehabilitation and Secondary Prevention Programs, Fifth Edition,_ by American Association of Cardiovascular and Pulmonary Rehabilitation, 2013, Human Kinetics, Champaign, IL.

Appendix M

Algorithm for Assessment of Patient Willingness to Quit Smoking

Are you willing to quit smoking now?

No	Yes
• Provide strong, unequivocal advice. • Ask about knowledge of negative consequences (risks). • Identify potential benefits. • Ask patient to limit number of cigarettes/tobacco products. • Protect cardiac disease status (i.e., antiplatelet agents, beta-blockers). • Provide resources regarding smoking programs, if applicable. • Ask about capability of follow-up.	• Determine need for cessation or relapse prevention.

	Cessation
	• Set quit date.
	• Determine method for cessation:
	  • Cold turkey
	  • Decreasing number of cigarettes
	  • Switching brands
	• Ask patient to self-monitor.
	• Offer pharmacotherapy as needed before quitting

	Relapse prevention
	• Identify high-risk situations.
	• Offer cognitive and behavioral strategies.
	• Contract to remain nonsmoker.
	• Provide counseling for the following:
	  • Weight gain
	  • Alcohol use
	  • Loss/deprivation
	  • Social support
	  • Exercise
	  • Depression
	• What about slips?
	  • Recommend pharmacologic therapy for all eligible patients.
	  • Provide medication instruction.
	  • Offer instruction sheets.

From *Guidelines for Cardiac Rehabilitation and Secondary Prevention Programs, Fifth Edition,* by American Association of Cardiovascular and Pulmonary Rehabilitation, 2013, Human Kinetics, Champaign, IL.

Appendix N

Example of Standing Orders To Initiate Outpatient Cardiac Rehabilitation

1. Initiate monitored exercise program per outpatient CR/SP policies and procedures.

2. Determine target heart rate (THR) via sign- or symptom-limited graded exercise testing (GXT) or sign- or symptom-limited responses to submaximal exercise.

3. Begin with a training duration of up to 30 minutes to tolerance, one to five times a week.

4. Gradually increase duration of training exercise if patient cardiovascular and physiological responses are within normal limits.

5. Observe participant for signs of exercise intolerance and adapt or terminate exercise as indicated in policies and procedures.

6. Assess lipid profile approximately 6 weeks postevent.

7. Administer nitroglycerin 0.3 or 0.4 mg sublingually every 5 minutes $\times$ 3 as needed for angina discomfort or ischemic symptoms.

8. Provide regular, periodic progress reports to the referring physician. Provide copies of reports to other physicians as needed.

9. Initiate patient education and counseling sessions as patient needs indicate.

10. Consult patient personal physician or CR/SP supervising physician for any necessary orders.

11. Notify the CR/SP dietitian to provide individualized nutrition education for each participant.

12. Enter the patient into a non–ECG-monitored maintenance program upon completion of early outpatient CR program.

Physician's signature

Date

From *Guidelines for Cardiac Rehabilitation and Secondary Prevention Programs, Fifth Edition,* by American Association of Cardiovascular and Pulmonary Rehabilitation, 2013, Human Kinetics, Champaign, IL.

Appendix O

Example of Outpatient Cardiac Rehabilitation Emergency Standing Orders*

Table of Contents

Protocols for Emergencies in the Cardiac Rehabilitation Area

  I. Cardiopulmonary Arrest—Code 99
  II. Chest Pain
  III. Hypoglycemia
  IV. Hyperglycemia
  V. Hypotension
  VI. Hypertension
  VII. Arrhythmias
  VIII. Dyspnea
  IX. Placement of Intravenous Line
  X. Patient Transportation

I. Cardiopulmonary Arrest/Code 99

A. Identify unresponsiveness and determine if breathing is absent or abnormal (gasping).

B. Call out for help/call a code/activate emergency medical system (EMS).

1. Call out for help from coworker. If no one responds and if no other staff member is available to assist, go to the nearest phone and dial code number or EMS. (Emergency numbers with specific scripted instructions are posted at each phone.) Get defibrillator/automated external defibrillator (AED). If no pulse, attach defibrillator/AED and shock if indicated. Begin cardiopulmonary resuscitation (CPR) with compressions.

2. If a second responder is available to assist, that person should go to the nearest phone and dial code number or EMS and then get the defibrillator/AED while the first responder stays with the patient to start compressions until the defibrillator/AED is available.

3. When the call is answered, state "Code 99."

4. Identify the area or room the patient is in. Do not hang up until the operator repeats the information to verify location.

5. The operator will announce "Code 99" and the location over the intercom system.

6. The assigned code team will proceed immediately to that area.

7. The operator will then call 911 to initiate notification of EMS for assistance and transport.

8. Operator will notify EMS which entrance to use.

9. The operator will page the group Code 99 number so that 99 appears on the code team pagers. The code team personnel will call the operator for location information (if the overhead page is not heard).

10. The operator will also call the hospital emergency department and notify the charge nurse of the Code 99 situation and impending transfer of the patient.

11. A runner from the communication center will be dispatched to the appropriate entrance to direct the EMS team to the Code 99 area.

First Responder

1. Determine unresponsiveness and absent or abnormal breathing.

---

*Appendix N should be used only as an example of standing orders that might be considered and adopted for use in freestanding outpatient or community-based programs.

From *Guidelines for Cardiac Rehabilitation and Secondary Prevention Programs, Fifth Edition,* by American Association of Cardiovascular and Pulmonary Rehabilitation, 2013, Human Kinetics, Champaign, IL.

2. Send someone to call a code and get defibrillator/AED.

3. If pulseless, begin chest compressions until defibrillator/AED arrives. Push hard, push fast at a depth of at least 2 inches and a rate of at least 100 per minute, using a compression to ventilation ratio of 30:2. Allow for complete chest recoil, minimize interruptions to <10 seconds, and avoid excessive ventilation.

Second Responder

1. After calling a code, take crash cart with defibrillator/AED to the patient. (See "Emergency on Track" or "Emergency in Locker Room" for these areas.)

2. Place defibrillator pads on patient and assess cardiac rhythm or place on AED.

3. Shock if indicated, resume compressions. Follow appropriate algorithm according to ACLS guidelines.

Third Responder if available

1. Direct remaining patients to another area and dismiss class.

2. Direct and control incoming emergency response team and patients.

3. Obtain extra supplies and equipment as needed.

4. Act as the recorder of events until the code team arrives.

5. Prepare records to be sent with patient to the emergency department (ED) if needed.

6. Notify patient physician/cardiologist and family.

Emergency on Track

1. First responder will remove the backpack, defibrillator, and portable suction from the crash cart and take them to the track.

2. Initiate standard Code 99 procedure.

Emergency in Locker Rooms

1. Remove patient from locker room to a dry area when appropriate.

2. Appropriately dry patient with bath towels or blanket.

3. Initiate standard Code 99 procedure.

II. Chest Pain

A. If a patient develops chest pain while in the exercise area, the patient should immediately discontinue exercise and sit or lie down. Note the exercise workloads and rate–pressure product at which the symptoms occurred.

B. The following protocol should be followed by the cardiac rehabilitation staff:

1. Check pulse, blood pressure, cardiac rhythm (attach telemetry monitor if not already monitored), and oxygen saturation.

2. Rate angina on a scale of 1 to 10.

3. If no relief with 1 to 3 minutes of rest, give 1 nitroglycerine (NTG) 0.4 mg SL or spray.

4. Obtain 12-lead ECG and call supervising physician.

C. If pain is relieved:

1. If this angina is of new onset, the patient should be evaluated by the supervising physician. The patient primary physician should be notified of the results of the evaluation and recommended treatment, if any.

2. If the patient experiences chronic stable angina, he or she will stop exercising until the angina is relieved. Patient may resume the exercise at a lower workload dependent on the clinical judgment of the professional staff. This patient should be observed closely for recurrent angina.

OR

The patient may be sent home and instructed to report any increase in frequency or severity of angina episodes to primary physician.

D. If pain is not relieved:

1. Monitor pulse, blood pressure, cardiac rhythm, and oxygen saturation closely.

2. Place on oxygen at 2 to 4 L per nasal prongs if oxygen saturation ≤94%.

3. Patient to chew aspirin 160 to 325 mg.

4. Repeat NTG 0.4 mg SL or spray every 5 minutes for unrelieved angina symptoms.

---

*Appendix N should be used only as an example of standing orders that might be considered and adopted for use in freestanding outpatient or community-based programs.

From *Guidelines for Cardiac Rehabilitation and Secondary Prevention Programs, Fifth Edition,* by American Association of Cardiovascular and Pulmonary Rehabilitation, 2013, Human Kinetics, Champaign, IL.

5. The supervising physician will evaluate and consult with primary physician to determine the course of action or transfer patient to the ED, cath lab, or coronary care unit (CCU) for evaluation and treatment.

6. Establish IV access.

III. Hypoglycemia

A. Be alert to signs and symptoms of hypoglycemia, which may include:

1. Headache, weakness, diaphoresis, nervousness, and shakiness

2. Faintness, numbness, tingling of tongue and lips, blurred or double vision, and unsteady gait

3. Tachycardia, pallor, or chilling

4. Confusion, aggressive or erratic behavior

5. Convulsions or unconsciousness

B. If patient displays any of these symptoms:

1. Obtain finger-stick blood glucose level.

2. If blood glucose results are below 70 mg/dL, or if patient remains symptomatic, give 15 g carbohydrate (CHO), juice, or three glucose tablets.

3. Retest blood glucose in 15 minutes. If blood glucose is not >90 mg/dL, repeat 15 g CHO and recheck blood glucose in 15 minutes.

4. If patient is uncooperative or unconscious, call supervising physician, give glucose gel, or establish intravenous (IV) access, and give 50 cc (1 amp) 50% dextrose solution IV. Arrange for transport to ED.

IV. Hyperglycemia

A. A participant with a blood sugar greater than 300 mg/dL may not exercise. In situations in which patient's referring physician and rehabilitation medical director have given their permission, this policy may be superseded.

B. Participants who have demonstrated reliable home blood sugar evaluations will have occasional blood sugar evaluations by the professional staff.

C. Participants who are found to be unreliable with home blood sugar evaluations will need their blood sugar levels evaluated more frequently by the rehabilitation staff.

D. The cardiac rehabilitation staff may request a blood sugar evaluation on any patient based on suspected signs and symptoms of hyperglycemia (nausea, flushing, polyuria, polydypsia, fruity breath, tachypnea).

V. Hypotension

A. Remove the patient from the exercise area if possible.

B. Place patient in a supine position. May elevate legs or place in Trendelenberg position.

C. Attach a telemetry monitor if not already monitored.

D. Check blood pressure, pulse, cardiac rhythm, and oxygen saturation.

E. If no response to position change (SBP remains <90 mmHg and/or patient remains symptomatic), call supervising physician. If the patient condition continues to deteriorate or becomes progressively symptomatic, or if BP continues to drop, start an IV of normal saline NS at 100 mL/hour and call the supervising physician. After evaluation and treatment of the patient, the supervising physician should notify the patient's primary physician of the hypotensive episode and discuss any further treatment if necessary.

F. If patient does respond to the supine position, keep supine until BP is greater than 100 systolic, then gradually assist to sitting position. Continue to carefully monitor BP, pulse, and rhythm. Encourage fluids. Notify the patient's primary physician of the episode.

VI. Hypertension

A. Check every patient's blood pressure before exercise and compare with previous recordings.

---

*Appendix N should be used only as an example of standing orders that might be considered and adopted for use in freestanding outpatient or community-based programs.

From *Guidelines for Cardiac Rehabilitation and Secondary Prevention Programs, Fifth Edition,* by American Association of Cardiovascular and Pulmonary Rehabilitation, 2013, Human Kinetics, Champaign, IL.

B. If the systolic reading is greater than 170 mmHg or the diastolic reading is greater than 100 mmHg, have the patient sit and recheck the blood pressure in 5 minutes.

C. If the blood pressure remains elevated, do not have patient exercise. May notify primary care physician or call supervising physician to evaluate and/or refer the patient to his or her physician when appropriate.

D. Investigate whether patient is complying with taking medications, following diet, sodium restriction, and so on.

VII. Dysrhythmias

Premature Ventricular Contractions (PVCs)

A. Observe for the following:

1. Frequency

2. Whether multifocal or unifocal

3. Pairs or runs, sustained, or paroxymal

4. Associated signs or symptoms

5. Palpate pulse to evaluate for peripheral perfusion

B. Document any new arrhythmias or increase in severity with a rhythm strip and make notation on chart. Notify supervising physician or referring physician or both, where appropriate, to discuss treatment.

C. Decrease workloads for frequent single PVCs (>10 minutes) and discontinue exercise if PVCs are a new event, or if they develop into bigeminy or pairs, or if the patient becomes symptomatic. Contact patient referring physician regarding new PVCs or a change in the severity of PVCs.

D. If the patient condition deteriorates and becomes symptomatic, check pulse, BP, oxygen saturation, and notify supervising physician, place oxygen at 2 to 4 L/NP, establish IV access.

E. Chronic asymptomatic PVCs:

1. If patient primary physician has been consulted to evaluate PVCs, and if it is determined that patient is benign, the patient may continue to exercise unless he or she becomes symptomatic.

2. Continue to document arrhythmias and closely observe for any developing signs and symptoms.

Bradycardia

A. If patient develops symptomatic bradycardia, stop exercise.

B. Monitor heart rate and rhythm, BP, and oximetry. Oxygen at 2 to 4 L for oxygen sats <94%. Get 12-lead ECG if available.

C. Assess for symptoms of instability or altered mental status, ischemic chest discomfort, heart failure, or hypotension. If present, notify supervising physician, obtain IV access, and prepare to administer atropine 0.5 mg IV bolus every 3 to 5 minutes to a maximum of 3 mg and transfer of patient to ED. May utilize external pacing if available.

Tachycardia

A. If patient develops a new wide or narrow complex tachycardia, stop exercise.

B. Monitor heart rate and rhythm, BP, and oximetry. Oxygen at 2 to 4 L for oxygen sats <94%. Get 12-lead ECG if available to determine type of tachycardia.

C. Assess for symptoms of instability or altered mental status, ischemic chest discomfort, heart failure, or hypotension. If present, notify supervising physician, obtain IV access, and prepare for synchronized cardioversion. If stable, may utilize vagal maneuvers or antiarrhythmic agents per advanced cardiac life support tachycardia algorithm.

D. Prepare for transfer to ED.

VIII. Dyspnea

A. If patient develops acute dyspnea, stop exercise and have patient sit down.

B. Monitor heart rate and rhythm, BP, respiratory rate, lung sounds, and oximetry. Oxygen at 2 to 4 L for oxygen sats <94%.

C. If patient has a metered dose inhaler, it may be administered as prescribed.

D. If condition deteriorates, notify supervising physician to evaluate for treatment options and possible transfer to ED.

*Appendix N should be used only as an example of standing orders that might be considered and adopted for use in freestanding outpatient or community-based programs.

From *Guidelines for Cardiac Rehabilitation and Secondary Prevention Programs, Fifth Edition,* by American Association of Cardiovascular and Pulmonary Rehabilitation, 2013, Human Kinetics, Champaign, IL.

E. If condition improves, notify primary physician for further recommendations.

IX. Placement of Intravenous Line

Purpose: To provide immediate access to administer emergency medication and intravenous fluids.

A. An attempt will be made to notify the supervising physician.

B. Place a saline lock in participant when one or more of the following apply:

    1. Chest pain protocol has been followed and chest pain persists.

    2. ECG, vital signs, or participant appears to be clinically unstable or symptomatic.

    3. Physician directs the placement of IV line.

X. Patient Transportation

The cardiac rehabilitation program has contracted with ambulance service to provide emergency transportation to the hospital. Their personnel include trained medical technicians. The ambulance service phone number is posted at each phone extension.

A. Ambulance emergency transportation: Notify ambulance service personnel as above and instruct them to use the front entrance at the facility address.

B. Nonemergency transportation: In the event the patient is stable but needs transportation to the hospital for a procedure or nonemergent admission, the program shuttle van will be used. A nurse from the cardiac rehabilitation area will accompany the patient to the hospital to ensure safety.

C. The physician will be called before transfer to see which method of transportation is required. Document physician decision (if it is to transfer in shuttle van). Cardiac rehabilitation nursing personnel will document patient condition before, during, and at the time of transfer to the hospital.

Cardiac Rehabilitation Department Emergency Procedures and Standing Orders Were Reviewed and Approved

_____

Physician's name

_____

Signature

_____

Date of most recent review

*Appendix N should be used only as an example of standing orders that might be considered and adopted for use in freestanding outpatient or community-based programs.

From *Guidelines for Cardiac Rehabilitation and Secondary Prevention Programs, Fifth Edition,* by American Association of Cardiovascular and Pulmonary Rehabilitation, 2013, Human Kinetics, Champaign, IL.

Appendix P

Cardiac Rehabilitation Untoward Event—Physician Notification

Patient name:_____ DOB:_____ Date:_____

To: Physician _____ Date physician notified: _____

Phone: _____ Time physician notified:_____

Fax: _____

Physician orders:

_____ May resume CR at next scheduled visit

_____ May not resume CR until _____

_____ Limit exercise as directed below

_____ Will be evaluated on _____

_____ No follow-up needed

Additional physician orders or comments:

_____

_____

_____

_____

Physician signature: _____ **Date:** _____

Please return this page, completed and signed, to Cardiac Rehabilitation.

Patient name: _____DOB: _____ Diagnosis: _____

Date of event: _____ Time: _____ Rehab week/visit #: _____

Reason for report:

_____ New sign or symptom

_____ Change from previous condition

_____ Findings exceed acceptable parameters

_____ Other:_____

Attach appropriate physiological data such as 12-lead ECG, BP measurement, code form, and so on.

From *Guidelines for Cardiac Rehabilitation and Secondary Prevention Programs, Fifth Edition,* by American Association of Cardiovascular and Pulmonary Rehabilitation, 2013, Human Kinetics, Champaign, IL.

Type of event:

_____ Angina symptoms

_____ Dysrhythmia or ECG changes

_____ BP abnormality

_____ Dyspnea or abnormal O_2 saturation

_____ Heart failure symptoms

_____ Blood glucose abnormality

_____ Other:_____

Description of occurrence: _____

_____

Description of action:

_____ Managed by rehab staff

_____ Seen in rehab by supervising physician

_____ Transferred to emergency room

_____ Sent to clinic or physician office

_____ Appt made with _____ on _____

Treatment:

_____ NTG _____ mg × _____

_____ Oxygen @ _____ L/m

_____ 12-lead ECG

_____ Aspirin _____ mg

Recommendations: _____

_____

Disposition:

_____ ER

_____ Physician's office or clinic

_____ Home

Accompanied by:

_____ Self

_____ Spouse/family

_____ Rehab staff

_____ Other

Status upon departure:

_____ Stable

_____ Unstable

_____ Other

Report completed by: _____

Attach appropriate physiological data such as 12-lead ECG, BP measurement, code form, and so on.

From *Guidelines for Cardiac Rehabilitation and Secondary Prevention Programs, Fifth Edition,* by American Association of Cardiovascular and Pulmonary Rehabilitation, 2013, Human Kinetics, Champaign, IL.

Appendix Q

Guidelines for Completing the Get With the Guidelines-Resuscitation (GWTG-R) Code Sheet

The following is a list of general guidelines for completing the Get With the Guidelines-Resuscitation (GWTG-R) Code Sheet. Individual institutions may choose to require additional information, such as recording the patient's actual spontaneous pulse rate instead of indicating only presence with check mark.

1. The GWTG-R Code Sheet should be completed for any patient, visitor, or employee who requires emergency assisted ventilation (mouth to mask, mouth to barrier, bag valve mask, or invasive airway), defibrillation, or chest compressions.

2. Record the patient's name and medical record number in the upper right corner of the record. The patient's label or the addressograph stamp should also be placed in this section before distribution.

3. **The Top Section of the Code Sheet** may be completed immediately after the event.

    A. **Date/Time Event Recognized:** The date and time that the event was recognized should be recorded in this space.

    B. **Location:** Record the location of the patient at the date and time that the event was recognized.

    C. **Witnessed:** Indicate yes if the patient was directly observed by someone (can be family, lay bystander, employee, or health care professional) at onset of event (differs from monitored).

    D. **Age, Weight, and Height (Length):** Record the patient's data in the appropriate space.

    E. **Was a hospital-wide resuscitation response activated?** Indicate if a hospital-wide resuscitation response was activated.

F. **Condition when need for chest compression/defibrillation was identified?**

    1. **Pulse (Poor Perfusion):** Indicate if the patient had a pulse when the need for chest compressions and/or defibrillation was identified.

    2. **Pulseless:** Indicate if the patient was pulseless when the need for chest compressions and/or defibrillation was identified.

G. **Did the patient with a pulse become pulseless?** Indicate yes if the patient had a pulse at onset of chest compressions and/or defibrillation but became pulseless during the event.

H. **Patient Conscious at Onset:** Indicate yes if the patient was conscious at the beginning of the event.

I. **Indicate all monitors present at onset.**

    1. **ECG:** Cardiac monitoring in the form of telemetry (central and/or bedside) monitoring

    2. **Pulse Ox.:** Pulse oximeter in the form of telemetry (central and/or bedside) monitoring

    3. **Apnea:** Apnea/bradycardia monitor in the form of telemetry (central and/or bedside) monitoring

4. **Airway/Ventilation Section** and subsequent sections should be recorded *during* the event for greatest accuracy.

    A. **At Onset:** Indicate the patient's respiratory status when the need for emergency assisted ventilation, chest compressions, and/or defibrillation was recognized.

From *Guidelines for Cardiac Rehabilitation and Secondary Prevention Programs, Fifth Edition,* by American Association of Cardiovascular and Pulmonary Rehabilitation, 2013, Human Kinetics, Champaign, IL.

1. **Spontaneous:** Breathing without mechanical assistance

2. **Apneic:** Not breathing spontaneously

3. **Agonal:** Gasping (ineffective) respirations

4. **Assisted:** Mechanical ventilation being provided

B. **Time of First Assisted Ventilation:** Enter the time that emergency assisted ventilation (noninvasive or invasive) was first initiated during the event.

C. **Ventilation:** Select each type of ventilation/airway used during the event. There is no limit on the number of types that may be selected.

   1. **Bag valve mask:** Bag-valve-mask ventilation provided *(should not be selected if patient had ETT or tracheotomy in place during the entire event)*.

   2. **Endotracheal Tube:** Endotracheal tube in place or placed during the event.

   3. **Tracheostomy:** Tracheostomy tube in place or placed during the event.

   4. **Other:** If "Other" is selected, provide the name(s) of the other airways used.

D. **Intubation: Time, Size, and by Whom:** If an invasive airway was inserted or reinserted during the event, enter the time of achievement, not when the first attempt was made. Also record the size of the invasive airway and the name of the person who successfully intubated the patient.

E. **Confirmation Method:** Method(s) of confirmation used to ensure correct placement of invasive airway. Indicate all that apply.

   1. **Auscultation:** Indicate if the presence of equal bilateral breath sounds was confirmed.

   2. **Exhaled CO_2:** Indicate if expired CO_2 detector such as capnography or colorimetric was used to confirm placement.

   3. **Other:** If "Other" is selected, provide the name(s) of the other method(s) used to confirm placement.

5. **Circulation Section**

   A. **First Rhythm Requiring Compressions:** Record the rhythm identified via ECG monitor when patient with a pulse first received compressions during the event.

   B. **First PULSELESS Rhythm:** Record the first rhythm identified when the patient became pulseless. For the unmonitored patient, select the rhythm first identified when monitor was applied.

   C. **Compressions:** Describe the method used to provide chest compressions during the event. Indicate all that apply:

      1. **None:** Chest compressions were not required during the event.

      2. **Manual:** Manual chest compressions were delivered during the event.

      3. **Device:** If "Device" is selected, provide the name(s) of the device(s) used to provide chest compressions.

   D. **Time Chest Compressions Were Started:** Record the time that the first chest compressions were started.

   E. **Impedance Threshold Device Used?** Indicate if an impedance threshold device was used at any time during the event.

   F. **AED Applied:** Indicate if an automated external defibrillator (AED) was used.

      1. **Time:** If an AED was applied during the event, enter the time AED was applied.

   G. **Defibrillator Type:** Indicate make and model of all defibrillators used.

   H. **Pacemaker On:** Indicate if a pacemaker (transcutaneous or internal) was functioning during the event. Record the type of device in the "Comments" section.

6. **Outcome**

   A. **Time Resuscitation Event Ended:** Record the time chest compressions stopped and did not resume either because it was the beginning of the sustained (>20 min) return of circulation or because of other reasons indicated below under "Reason Resuscitation Ended."

B. **Reason Resuscitation Ended:** Select the reason that the resuscitation event ended from the list below.

1. **Survived—Return of Circulation (ROC) >20 min:** Return of spontaneous pulse, including with pacemaker or extracorporeal membrane oxygenation (ECMO), with good perfusion that was sustained for >20 min.

2. **Died: Efforts Terminated, No Sustained ROC:** Patient did not respond to advanced life support (ALS), unable to achieve a sustained ROC.

3. **Died: Medical Futility:** Advanced life support (ALS) was terminated because of medical futility, such as end-stage disease or organ failure.

4. **Died: Advanced Directives:** Patient had an advanced directive in place that limited the extent of advanced life support procedures.

5. **Died: Restrictions by Family:** There were restrictions placed by the family of the patient, that is, family requested that the event be terminated.

7. **Documentation of the Event**

A. **Time:** Record the time of each intervention/procedure.

B. **Breathing:** Indicate with a check mark in the top half of the box if the patient is breathing spontaneously. Indicate with a check mark in the bottom half of the box if the patient is receiving assisted ventilation (invasive or noninvasive).

C. **Pulse:** Indicate with a check mark in the top half of the box if the patient has a spontaneous pulse. Indicate with a check mark in the bottom half of the box if the patient is receiving chest compression (manual or mechanical). *NOTE: If the patient with a pulse is receiving chest compressions, there should be a check mark in both parts of the box.*

D. **BP:** Indicate the patient's blood pressure (BP) if present. Leave the box blank if BP is not obtainable.

E. **Rhythm:** Identify the rhythm displayed on the monitor after 5 cycles of CPR prior to each intervention.

F. **Defibrillator Type:** Document electrical cardioversion with a "D" representing defibrillation (unsynchronized) and "C" representing synchronized cardioversion. Indicate the type of defibrillator used—AED or manual (conventional)—to deliver each shock.

G. **Joules:** Record the number of joules used for each shock.

H. **Boluses:** Circle the route of the medication at the top of the column and document all drugs administered as a bolus with the dose. Any drug not listed but administered should be recorded in the available blank slots with the dose and route documented as stated above. If route other than IV or OI is used to administer any medication, record the alternate route in the appropriate line in the "Comments" section.

I. **Infusions:** Document all continuous infusions, recording the time started and the rate in mL per hour. The concentration of the infusion and the route (IV or IO) should be recorded under the drug name at the top of the column. Any infusion not listed but administered should be recorded in the available blank slots with the rate (mL) per hour and the concentration and route documented as stated above.

J. **Comments:** The "Comments" section should be used to document any procedures, interventions, lab results, as well as the patient's response to procedures or interventions.

8. **Signatures:** The Recorder, ICU/Code Team Nurse, and Physician must thoroughly review and sign the record in the appropriate places. The physician's name must also be printed in the slot above the physician's signature.

9. **Page _____ of _____:** Record the page number and the total number of pages utilized for the event in the bottom left of the record.

10. **Distribution:** The original record should be placed in the patient's medical record. Other copies should be distributed as indicated on the bottom right of the record.

From *Guidelines for Cardiac Rehabilitation and Secondary Prevention Programs, Fifth Edition*, by American Association of Cardiovascular and Pulmonary Rehabilitation, 2013, Human Kinetics, Champaign, IL.

Appendix R
Daily Emergency Cart Checklist

Month_____/Year_____

1. Defibrillator discharges appropriate test joules (unplugged)

1	2	3	4	5	6	7	8	9	10	11	12	13	14	15	16	17	18	19	20	21	22	23	24	25	26	27	28	29	30	31

2. Defibrillator plugged in

1	2	3	4	5	6	7	8	9	10	11	12	13	14	15	16	17	18	19	20	21	22	23	24	25	26	27	28	29	30	31

3. Defibrillator battery registers full capacity

1	2	3	4	5	6	7	8	9	10	11	12	13	14	15	16	17	18	19	20	21	22	23	24	25	26	27	28	29	30	31

4. Monitor display records ECG accurately (extra roll of paper available)

1	2	3	4	5	6	7	8	9	10	11	12	13	14	15	16	17	18	19	20	21	22	23	24	25	26	27	28	29	30	31

5. Electrode patches and fast patches available

1	2	3	4	5	6	7	8	9	10	11	12	13	14	15	16	17	18	19	20	21	22	23	24	25	26	27	28	29	30	31

6. O₂ tank registers full capacity

1	2	3	4	5	6	7	8	9	10	11	12	13	14	15	16	17	18	19	20	21	22	23	24	25	26	27	28	29	30	31

7. Ambu bag, oral airway, O₂ mask/cannula available

1	2	3	4	5	6	7	8	9	10	11	12	13	14	15	16	17	18	19	20	21	22	23	24	25	26	27	28	29	30	31

From *Guidelines for Cardiac Rehabilitation and Secondary Prevention Programs, Fifth Edition*, by American Association of Cardiovascular and Pulmonary Rehabilitation, 2013, Human Kinetics, Champaign, IL

8. Suction machine functions with appropriate suction capacity

1	2	3	4	5	6	7	8	9	10	11	12	13	14	15	16	17	18	19	20	21	22	23	24	25	26	27	28	29	30	31

9. Suction canister, tubing, Yankauer suction tip available

1	2	3	4	5	6	7	8	9	10	11	12	13	14	15	16	17	18	19	20	21	22	23	24	25	26	27	28	29	30	31

10. Emergency code documentation sheets available

1	2	3	4	5	6	7	8	9	10	11	12	13	14	15	16	17	18	19	20	21	22	23	24	25	26	27	28	29	30	31

11. Sharps container present

1	2	3	4	5	6	7	8	9	10	11	12	13	14	15	16	17	18	19	20	21	22	23	24	25	26	27	28	29	30	31

12. Personal protective equipment available (gloves, eye/face shield)

1	2	3	4	5	6	7	8	9	10	11	12	13	14	15	16	17	18	19	20	21	22	23	24	25	26	27	28	29	30	31

13. Signature of reviewer (Name):

1	2	3	4	5	6	7	8	9	10	11	12	13	14	15	16	17	18	19	20	21	22	23	24	25	26	27	28	29	30	31

From *Guidelines for Cardiac Rehabilitation and Secondary Prevention Programs, Fifth Edition*, by American Association of Cardiovascular and Pulmonary Rehabilitation, 2013, Human Kinetics, Champaign, IL

Appendix S

Monthly Emergency Cart Checklist

1. The entire emergency cart is to be checked monthly and following any cardiac arrest.
2. The defibrillator, monitoring equipment, and oxygen equipment are to be checked by an RN before the first exercise session of the day. (See daily emergency cart checklist.)
3. If there is any problem with the equipment, the RN checking it is responsible for calling the appropriate office and seeing that the equipment is restored to full function as soon as possible.

	Quantity	Jan	Feb	Mar	Apr	May	Jun	Jul	Aug	Sep	Oct	Nov	Dec
Date checklist completed													
TOP OF CART													
Defibrillator	1												
Extra rolls ECG paper	2												
ECG cable and fast patch cable	1												
Electrode sets and fast patches	2												
Adult oral airways (small/medium/large)	3												
ACLS algorithms	1												
Clipboard, pen, resuscitation documentation form	1												
Ambu bag valve mask	1												
Pocket face mask	1												
O_2 nasal prongs	2												
Oxygen mask/tubing	1												
Oxygen extension tubing	1												
Box of gloves	1												
Face shields/masks	2												
Sharps/contaminated box	1												
DRAWER #1 PHARMACY DRUGS													
Adenosine 6 mg/2 mL	2												
Amiodarone 150 mg/3 mL	2												
Atropine sulfate 1 mg/10 mL	3												
Aspirin chewable	2												
Dextrose 50%, 25 g/50 mL	1												
Glucose gel	1												
Epinephrine HCl (1:10,000) 1 mg/10 mL	4												
Lidocaine HCl 100 mg/5 mL	3												
Magnesium sulfate 5 g	1												
Metoprolol 5 mg/5 mL	3												

From *Guidelines for Cardiac Rehabilitation and Secondary Prevention Programs, Fifth Edition,* by American Association of Cardiovascular and Pulmonary Rehabilitation, 2013, Human Kinetics, Champaign, IL.

	Quantity	Jan	Feb	Mar	Apr	May	Jun	Jul	Aug	Sep	Oct	Nov	Dec
Nitroglycerin 0.4 mg SL tablets or spray	1												
Sodium bicarbonate 50 mEq/50 mL	4												
Vasopressin 20 u/1 mL	2												
DRAWER #2 GENERAL SUPPLIES													
Latex-free tourniquets	2												
IV start kits	4												
#18 g. IV catheter	4												
#20 g. IV catheter	4												
#22 g. IV catheter	4												
10 cc syringes	5												
5 cc syringes	5												
3 cc syringes	5												
50 cc syringes	2												
50 cc Toomey Syringe	1												
#18 needles	5												
#19 needles	5												
#22 needles	5												
Plastic anti-stick needle/connectors	10												
Normal saline 20 mL vials or prefilled saline syringes	4												
Silk suture 3-0	2												
Scissors (pair)	1												
Alcohol wipes	30												
1 in. tape (roll)	1												
2 in. tape (roll)	1												
2 × 2s (packages)	2												
4 × 4s (packages)	2												
Sterile gloves: sizes 6, 6 1/2, 7, 7 1/2, 8 (2 of each size)	10												
Suture set	1												
Disposable razor	1												
Saline lock	4												
DRAWER #3 IV SUPPLIES													
Macrodrip IV tubing	3												
Minidrip IV tubing	3												
Infusion pump tubing	2												
Normal saline 1000 cc	2												
D5W 1000 cc	1												
Lactated ringers 1000 cc	1												
D5W 100 cc	2												
D5W 250 cc/400 mg dopamine	1												
IV extension tubing	2												
Three-way stop cocks	2												

(continued)

(continued)

	Quantity	Jan	Feb	Mar	Apr	May	Jun	Jul	Aug	Sep	Oct	Nov	Dec
Cut-down tray	1												
Arrow introducers	2												
Triple lumen catheters	2												
RESPIRATORY DRAWER													
Goggles/shield	1												
ABG kits	2												
1 in. tape	1												
Laryngoscope handle	1												
#2 Miller laryngoscope blade	1												
#3 Miller laryngoscope blade	1												
#2 McIntosh blade	1												
#4 McIntosh blade	1												
Oral airways, 80, 90, and 100 mm (1 each size)	3												
7.0 cm nasal airway	1												
#14F suction catheter	2												
Extra bulbs	2												
Stylette	1												
Flow meter	1												
Endotracheal tubes 6.5, 7.0, 7.5, 8.0, 8.5 cm (1 each size)	5												
12 mL syringe	1												
Water-soluble lubricant	1												
Americaine spray	1												
Extra batteries	2												
Magill forceps	1												
CO_2 detector	1												
BOTTOM DRAWER													
Sterile water or normal saline 1000 cc	1												
Blood pressure cuff	1												
Stethoscope	1												
Flashlight	1												
Blanket	1												
SIDE OF CART													
Oxygen tank	1												
Portable suction machine	1												
Disposable suction canister	1												
Suction tubing	1												
Yankauer suction tip	1												
Back board	1												
Electrical extension cord	1												
Signature of reviewer:													

From *Guidelines for Cardiac Rehabilitation and Secondary Prevention Programs, Fifth Edition,* by American Association of Cardiovascular and Pulmonary Rehabilitation, 2013, Human Kinetics, Champaign, IL.

Appendix T

Emergency Equipment Maintenance Log

Date of most recent maintenance check:_____

Date due for next maintenance check:_____

1. Defibrillator
   - Batteries replaced: _____   _____

2. Electrocardiographic monitor: _____

3. Oxygen tank: _____

4. Suction apparatus: _____

Maintenance problems noted: Date corrected: _____

   1. _____

   2. _____

   3. _____

Other: _____

Program director notified   (yes/no)   Date corrected: _____

   1. _____

   2. _____

   3. _____

Other: _____

From *Guidelines for Cardiac Rehabilitation and Secondary Prevention Programs, Fifth Edition,* by American Association of Cardiovascular and Pulmonary Rehabilitation, 2013, Human Kinetics, Champaign, IL.

Appendix U

Mock Code and Emergency In-Service Log

Date: _____

Location: _____

Brief description of activity: _____

_____

_____

_____

_____

_____

Who attended the in-service?	Understood the required knowledge:	Needs further training and review:
_____	_____	_____
_____	_____	_____
_____	_____	_____
_____	_____	_____
_____	_____	_____
_____	_____	_____
_____	_____	_____
_____	_____	_____
_____	_____	_____
_____	_____	_____
_____	_____	_____
_____	_____	_____
_____	_____	_____

From *Guidelines for Cardiac Rehabilitation and Secondary Prevention Programs, Fifth Edition,* by American Association of Cardiovascular and Pulmonary Rehabilitation, 2013, Human Kinetics, Champaign, IL.

References

Chapter 1

1. Leon RS, Franklin BA, Costa F, et al. Cardiac rehabilitation and secondary prevention of coronary heart disease: an American Heart Association scientific statement, in collaboration with the American Association of Cardiovascular and Pulmonary Rehabilitation. *Circulation.* 2005;111:369-376.

2. Bittner V, Sanderson B. Cardiac rehabilitation as a secondary prevention center. *Coron Artery Dis.* 2006;17:211-218.

3. Ades PA, Balady G, Berra K. Transforming exercise based cardiac rehabilitation programs into secondary prevention centers: a national imperative. *J Cardiopulm Rehabil.* 2001;21:263-272.

4. Brown TM, Hernandez AF, Bittner V. Predictors of cardiac rehabilitation referral in coronary artery disease patients: findings from the American Heart Association's Get With the Guidelines program. *J Am Coll Cardiol.* 2009;54:515-521.

5. Smith SC Jr, Allen J, Blair SN, et al.; AHA/ACC; National Heart, Lung, and Blood Institute. AHA/ACC guidelines for secondary prevention for patients with coronary and other atherosclerotic vascular disease: 2006 update: endorsed by the National Heart, Lung, and Blood Institute. *Circulation.* 2006;113:2363-2372.

6. Epstein AJ, Polsky D, Yang F, Yang L, Groeneveld PW. Coronary revascularization trends in the United States, 2001-2008. *JAMA.* 2011;305:1769-1776.

7. Shah ND, Dunlay SM, Ting HH, et al. Long-term medication adherence after myocardial infarction: experience of a community. *Am J Med.* 2009;122:961.e7-13.

8. Choudhry NK, Avorn J, Glynn RJ, et al. Full coverage for preventive medications after myocardial infarction. *NEJM.* 2011;365:2088-2097.

9. Haskell WL, Alderman EL, Fair JM, et al. Effects of intensive multiple risk factor reduction on coronary atherosclerosis and clinical cardiac events in men and women with coronary artery disease. The Stanford Coronary Risk Intervention Project (SCRIP). *Circulation.* 1994;89:975-990.

10. Bowden WE, O'Rourke RA, Koon KT, et al. Impact of optimal medical therapy with or without percutaneous coronary intervention on long-term cardiovascular end points in patients with stable coronary artery disease (from the COURAGE Trial) on behalf of the COURAGE Trial Investigators. *Am J Cardiol.* 2009;104:1-4.

11. Wood DA, Kotseva K, Connolly S, et al. Nurse-coordinated multidisciplinary, family-based cardiovascular disease prevention programme (EUROACTION) for patients with coronary heart disease and asymptomatic individuals at high risk of cardiovascular disease: a paired, cluster-randomised controlled trial. *Lancet.* 2008;371(9629):1999-2012.

12. Ma J, Berra K, Haskell WL, et al. Case management to reduce risk of cardiovascular disease in a county health care system. *Arch Intern Med.* 2009;169:1988-1995.

13. Balady GJ, Ades PA, Bittner VA, et al. Referral, enrollment, and delivery of cardiac rehabilitation/secondary prevention programs at clinical centers and beyond: a presidential advisory from the American Heart Association. *Circulation.* 2011;124:2951-2960.

14. Rittenhouse DR, Shortell S, Fisher ES. Primary care and accountable care—two essential elements of delivery-system reform. *NEJM.* 2009;361:2301-2303.

15. Ades PA, Balady GJ, Berra K. Transforming exercise-based cardiac rehabilitation programs into secondary prevention centers: a national imperative. *J Cardiopulm Rehabil.* 2001;21:263-272.

16. Clark AM, Catto S, Bowman G, Macintyre PD. Design matters in secondary prevention: individualization and supervised exercise improved the effectiveness of cardiac rehabilitation. *Eur J Cardiovasc Prev Rehabil.* 2011;18:761-769.

17. O'Connor GT, Buring JE, Yusuf S, et al. An overview of randomized trials of rehabilitation after myocardial infarction. *Circulation.* 1989;80:234-244.

18. Oldridge NB, Guyatt GH, Fischer ME, Rimm AA. Cardiac rehabilitation after myocardial infarction: combined experience of randomized clinical trials. *JAMA.* 1988;260:945-950.

19. Pavy B, Iliou MC, Meurin P, Tabet JY, Corone S. Safety of exercise training for cardiac patients. Results of the French Registry of Complications During Cardiac Rehabilitation. *Arch Intern Med.* 2006;166:2329-2334.

20. Hamm LF, Kavanagh T, Campbell MS, et al. Timeline for peak improvements during 52 weeks of outpatient cardiac rehabilitation. *J Cardiopulm Rehabil.* 2004;24:374-382.

21. Smith SC, Benjamin EJ, Bonow RO, et al. AHA/ACCF secondary prevention and risk reduction therapy for patients with coronary and other atherosclerotic vascular disease: 2011 update. *Circulation.* 2011;58:2432-2446.

22. Ellrodt G, Glasener R, Cadorette B, et al. Multidisciplinary rounds (MDR): an implementation system for sustained improvement in the American Heart Association's Get With The Guidelines program. *Crit Pathw Cardiol.* 2007;6:106-116.

23. Maron DJ, Boden WE, O'Rourke RA, et al. Intensive multifactorial intervention for stable coronary artery disease: optimal medical therapy in the COURAGE (Clinical Outcomes Utilizing Revascularization and Aggressive Drug Evaluation) trial. *J Am Coll Cardiol.* 2010;55:1348-1358.

24. Schwalm J-D R, Yusuf S. Commentary: "The end of clinical freedom": relevance in the era of evidence-based medicine. *Int J Epidemiol.* 2011;40:855-858.

25. Savage PD, Sanderson BK, Brown TM, Berra K, Ades PA. Clinical research in cardiac rehabilitation and secondary prevention: looking back and moving forward. *J Cardiopulm Rehabil Prev.* 2011;31:333-341.

26. Berra K. Does nurse case management improve implementation of guidelines for cardiovascular disease reduction? *J Cardiovasc Nurs.* 2011;26:145-167.

Chapter 2

1. Brant-Zawadzki M, Perazzo C, Afable RF. Community hospital to community health system: a blueprint for continuum of care. *Physician Exec.* 2011;37:16-21.

2. Evashwick CJ. Creating a continuum. The goal is to provide an integrated system of care. *Health Prog.* 1989;70:36-39, 56.

3. Oelke ND, Cunning L, Andrews K, et al. Organizing care across the continuum: primary care, specialty services, acute and long-term care. *Healthc Q.* 2009;13:75-79.

4. Aston G. Creating a cardiac care continuum. Hospitals & health networks. *Am Hospital Assoc.* 2010;84:32, 34, 36.

5. Kay D, Blue A, Pye P, Lacy A, Gray C, Moore S. Heart failure: improving the continuum of care. *Care Manag J.* 2006;7:58-63.

6. Miranda MB, Gorski LA, LeFevre JG, Levac KA, Niederstadt JA, Toy AL. An evidence-based approach to improving care of patients with heart failure across the continuum. *J Nurs Care Qual.* 2002;17:1-14.

7. Rockson SG, deGoma EM, Fonarow CG. Reinforcing a continuum of care: in-hospital initiation of long-term secondary prevention following acute coronary syndromes. *Cardiovasc Drugs Ther.* 2007;21:375-388.

8. Blackburn H. Population strategies of cardiovascular disease prevention: scientific base, rationale and public health implications. *Ann Med.* 1989;21:157-162.

9. Capewell S, Lloyd-Jones DM. Optimal cardiovascular prevention strategies for the 21st century. *JAMA.* 2010;304:2057-2058.

10. McNamara RL, Wang Y, Herrin J, et al. Effect of door-to-balloon time on mortality in patients with ST-segment elevation myocardial infarction. *J Am Coll Cardiol.* 2006;47:2180-2186.

11. Fonarow GC, Gawlinski A, Moughrabi S, Tillisch JH. Improved treatment of coronary heart disease by implementation of a Cardiac Hospitalization Atherosclerosis Management Program (CHAMP). *Am J Cardiol.* 2001;87:819-822.

12. Choudhry NK, Winkelmayer WC. Medication adherence after myocardial infarction: a long way left to go. *J Gen Intern Med.* 2008;23:216-218.

13. Shah ND, Dunlay SM, Ting HH, et al. Long-term medication adherence after myocardial infarction: experience of a community. *Am J Med.* 2009;122:961.e7-13.

14. Dunlay SM, Witt BJ, Allison TG, et al. Barriers to participation in cardiac rehabilitation. *Am Heart J.* 2009;158:852-859.

15. Grace SL, Gravely-Witte S, Brual J, et al. Contribution of patient and physician factors to cardiac rehabilitation enrollment: a prospective multilevel study. *Euro J Cardiovasc Prev Rehabil.* 2008;15:548-556.

16. Grace SL, Gravely-Witte S, Brual J, et al. Contribution of patient and physician factors to cardiac rehabilitation referral: a prospective

multilevel study. *Nat Clin Pract Cardiovasc Med.* 2008;5:653-662.

17. Grace SL, Russell KL, Reid RD, et al. Effect of cardiac rehabilitation referral strategies on utilization rates: a prospective, controlled study. *Arch Intern Med.* 2011;171:235-241.

18. Witt BJ, Thomas RJ, Roger VL. Cardiac rehabilitation after myocardial infarction: a review to understand barriers to participation and potential solutions. *Eura Medicophys.* 2005;41:27-34.

19. Thomas RJ. Cardiac rehabilitation/secondary prevention programs: a raft for the rapids: why have we missed the boat? *Circulation.* 2007;116:1644-1646.

20. Grace SL, Krepostman S, Brooks D, et al. Referral to and discharge from cardiac rehabilitation: key informant views on continuity of care. *J Eval Clin Pract.* 2006;12:155-163.

21. Riley DL, Stewart DE, Grace SL. Continuity of cardiac care: cardiac rehabilitation participation and other correlates. *Int J Cardiol.* 2007;119:326-333.

22. Giannuzzi P, Temporelli PL, Marchioli R, et al. Global secondary prevention strategies to limit event recurrence after myocardial infarction: results of the GOSPEL study, a multicenter, randomized controlled trial from the Italian Cardiac Rehabilitation Network. *Arch Intern Med.* 2008;168:2194-2204.

23. Hammill BG, Curtis LH, Schulman KA, Whellan DJ. Relationship between cardiac rehabilitation and long-term risks of death and myocardial infarction among elderly Medicare beneficiaries. *Circulation.* 2010;121:63-70.

24. Oldridge NB, Guyatt GH, Fischer ME, Rimm AA. Cardiac rehabilitation after myocardial infarction. Combined experience of randomized clinical trials. *JAMA.* 1988;260:945-950.

25. Squires RW, Montero-Gomez A, Allison TG, Thomas RJ. Long-term disease management of patients with coronary disease by cardiac rehabilitation program staff. *J Cardiopulm Rehabil Prev.* 2008;28:180-186.

26. Suaya JA, Stason WB, Ades PA, Normand SL, Shepard DS. Cardiac rehabilitation and survival in older coronary patients. *J Am Coll Cardiol.* 2009;54:25-33.

27. Taylor RS, Unal B, Critchley JA, Capewell S. Mortality reductions in patients receiving exercise-based cardiac rehabilitation: how much can be attributed to cardiovascular risk factor improvements? *Euro J Cardiovasc Prev Rehabil.* 2006;13:369-374.

28. Williams MA, Ades PA, Hamm LF, et al. Clinical evidence for a health benefit from cardiac rehabilitation: an update. *Am Heart J.* 2006;152:835-841.

29. Witt BJ, Jacobsen SJ, Weston SA, et al. Cardiac rehabilitation after myocardial infarction in the community. *J Am Coll Cardiol.* 2004;44:988-996.

30. Gupta R, Sanderson BK, Bittner V. Outcomes at one-year follow-up of women and men with coronary artery disease discharged from cardiac rehabilitation: what benefits are maintained? *J Cardiopulm Rehabil Prev.* 2007;27:11-18.

31. Balady GJ, Williams MA, Ades PA, et al. Core components of cardiac rehabilitation/secondary prevention programs: 2007 update: a scientific statement from the American Heart Association and the American Association of Cardiovascular and Pulmonary Rehabilitation. *J Cardiopulm Rehabil Prev.* 2007;27:121-129.

32. Riggio JM, Sorokin R, Moxey ED, Mather P, Gould S, Kane GC. Effectiveness of a clinical-decision-support system in improving compliance with cardiac-care quality measures and supporting resident training. *Acad Med.* 2009;84:1719-1726.

33. Gravely-Witte S, Leung YW, Nariani R, et al. Effects of cardiac rehabilitation referral strategies on referral and enrollment rates. *Nat Rev Cardiol.* 2010;7:87-96.

34. Mueller E, Savage PD, Schneider DJ, Howland LL, Ades PA. Effect of a computerized referral at hospital discharge on cardiac rehabilitation participation rates. *J Cardiopulm Rehabil Prev.* 2009;29:365-369.

35. Suaya JA, Shepard DS, Normand SL, Ades PA, Prottas J, Stason WB. Use of cardiac rehabilitation by Medicare beneficiaries after myocardial infarction or coronary bypass surgery. *Circulation.* 2007;116:1653-1662.

36. Thomas RJ, Miller NH, Lamendola C, et al. National survey on gender differences in cardiac rehabilitation programs. Patient characteristics and enrollment patterns. *J Cardiopulm Rehabil.* 1996;16:402-412.

37. Tricoci P, Peterson ED, Roe MT. Patterns of guideline adherence and care delivery for patients with unstable angina and non-ST-segment elevation myocardial infarction (from the CRUSADE Quality Improvement Initiative). *Am J Cardiol.* 2006;98:30Q-35Q.

38. Jacobson PD. Legal and policy considerations in using clinical practice guidelines. *Am J Cardiol.* 1997;80:74H-79H.

39. Spertus JA, Eagle KA, Krumholz HM, Mitchell KR, Normand SL. American College of Cardiology and American Heart Association methodology for the selection and creation of performance measures for quantifying the quality of cardiovascular care. *J Am Coll Cardiol.* 2005;45:1147-1156.

40. Fonarow GC, Abraham WT, Albert NM, et al. Association between performance measures and clinical outcomes for patients hospitalized with heart failure. *JAMA.* 2007;297:61-70.

41. Fonarow GC, Peterson ED. Heart failure performance measures and outcomes: real or illusory gains. *JAMA.* 2009;302:792-794.

42. Spertus JA, Bonow RO, Chan P, et al. ACCF/AHA new insights into the methodology of performance measurement. *Circulation.* 2010;122:2091-2106.

43. Thomas RJ, King M, Lui K, et al. AACVPR/ACC/AHA 2007 performance measures on cardiac rehabilitation for referral to and delivery of cardiac rehabilitation/secondary prevention services. *J Cardiopulm Rehabil Prev.* 2007;27:260-290.

44. Thomas RJ. King M, Lui K, et al. AACVPR/ACCF/AHA 2010 update: performance measures on cardiac rehabilitation for referral to cardiac rehabilitation/secondary prevention services. *J Cardiopulm Rehabil Prev.* 2010;30:279-288.

45. Krumholz HM, Anderson JL, Bachelder BL, et al. ACC/AHA 2008 performance measures for adults with ST-elevation and non-ST-elevation myocardial infarction. *Circulation.* 2008;118:2596-2648.

46. Artham SM, Lavie CJ, Milani RV. Cardiac rehabilitation programs markedly improve high-risk profiles in coronary patients with high psychological distress. *South Med J.* 2008;101:262-267.

47. Milani RV, Lavie CJ. Impact of cardiac rehabilitation on depression and its associated mortality. *Am J Med.* 2007;120:799-806.

48. Oldridge N, Guyatt G, Jones N, et al. Effects on quality of life with comprehensive rehabilitation after acute myocardial infarction. *Am J Cardiol.* 1991;67:1084-1089.

49. Ades PA, Pashkow FJ, Fletcher G, Pina IL, Zohman LR, Nestor JR. A controlled trial of cardiac rehabilitation in the home setting using electrocardiographic and voice transtelephonic monitoring. *Am Heart J.* 2000;139:543-548.

50. DeBusk RF, Miller NH, Superko HR, et al. A case-management system for coronary risk factor modification after acute myocardial infarction. *Ann Intern Med.* 1994;120:721-729.

51. Gordon NF. New methods of delivering secondary preventive services: the promise of the Internet. *J Cardiopulm Rehabil.* 2003;23:349-351.

52. Vandelanotte C, Dwyer T, Van Itallie A, Hanley C, Mummery WK. The development of an internet-based outpatient cardiac rehabilitation intervention: a Delphi study. *BMC Cardiovasc Disord.* 2010;10:27.

53. Varnfield M, Karunanithi MK, Särelä A, et al. Uptake of a technology-assisted home-care cardiac rehabilitation program. *Med J Aust.* 2011;194:S15-19.

54. Bradley EH, Holmboe ES, Mattera JA, Roumanis SA, Radford MJ, Krumholz HM. A qualitative study of increasing beta-blocker use after myocardial infarction: why do some hospitals succeed? *JAMA.* 2001;285:2604-2611.

55. Curry LA, Spatz E, Cherlin E, et al. What distinguishes top-performing hospitals in acute myocardial infarction mortality rates? A qualitative study. *Ann Intern Med.* 2011;154:384-390.

Chapter 3

1. Glanz K, Rimer BK, Viswanath K, eds. *Health Behavior and Health Education: Theory, Research, and Practice.* 4th ed. San Francisco: Jossey-Bass, 2008.

2. Anderson NB, ed. *Encyclopedia of Health & Behavior, Vols. 1 and 2.* Thousand Oaks, CA: Sage, 2004.

3. Bandura A. *Self-efficacy: The Exercise of Control.* New York: Freeman, 1997.

4. Bandura A. *Social Foundations of Thought and Action: A Social-Cognitive Theory.* Englewood Cliffs, NJ: Prentice-Hall, 1986.

5. Prochaska J. Why do we behave the way we do? *Can J Cardiol.* 1995;11:20A-25A.

6. Prochaska J, DiClemente C. Stages and processes of self-change of smoking: toward an integrative model of change. *J Consult Clin Psychol.* 1983;51:390-395.

7. Rogers R. A protection motivation theory of fear appeals and attitude change. *J Psychol.* 1975;91:93-114.

8. Becker MH, ed. The Health Belief Model and personal health behavior. *Health Education Monographs*. 1974;2:324-473.

9. Fishbein M, Ajzen I. *Belief, Attitude, Intention, and Behavior: An Introduction to Theory and Research*. Boston: Addison-Wesley, 1975.

10. Hausenblas H, Carron A, Mack D. Application of the Theories of Reasoned Action and Planned Behavior to exercise behavior: a meta-analysis. *J Sport Exerc Psychol*. 1997;19:36-51.

11. Caulin-Glaser T, Maciejewski PK, Snow R, et al. Depressive symptoms and sex affect completion rates and clinical outcomes in cardiac rehabilitation. *Prev Cardiol*. 2007;10:15-21.

12. Chaiken S, Liberman A, Eagly A. Heuristic and systematic processing within and beyond the persuasion context. In: J Uleman, J Bargh, eds. *Unintended Thought*. New York: Guilford Press, 1989:212-252.

13. Petty R, Cacioppo J. *Communication and Persuasion: Central and Peripheral Routes to Attitude Change*. New York: Springer-Verlag, 1986.

14. Bandura A. Self-efficacy. In: NB Anderson, ed. *Encyclopedia of Health & Behavior, Vol. 2*. Thousand Oaks, CA: Sage, 2004:708-714.

15. Falvo DR. *Effective Patient Education: A Guide to Increased Compliance*. 3rd ed. Sudbury, MA: Jones and Bartlett, 2004.

16. U.S. Department of Education, National Center for Education Statistics. 1992 National Adult Literacy Survey (NALS) and 2003 National Assessment of Adult Literacy (NAAL). A first look at the literacy of America's adults in the 21st century. Washington, DC: U.S. Department of Education, 2005. http://nces.ed.gov/pubsearch/pubsinfo.asp?pubid=2006470. Accessed August 8, 2011.

17. U.S. Department of Education, National Center for Education Statistics. The health literacy of America's adults: results from the 2003 National Assessment of Adult Literacy. Washington, DC: U.S. Department of Education, 2006. http://nces.ed.gov/pubsearch/pubsinfo.asp?pubid=2006483. Accessed August 8, 2011.

18. Cornett S. Assessing and addressing health literacy. *OJIN*. 2009;14(3), Manuscript 2. www.nursingworld.org/MainMenuCategories/ANA-Marketplace/ANAPeriodicals/OJIN/TableofContents/Vol142009/No3Sept09/Assessing-Health-Literacy-.html#Estey. Accessed January 23, 2012.

19. National Cancer Institute, Office of Cancer Communications. *Making Health Communication Programs Work*. Bethesda, MD: National Cancer Institute, 2001. www.cancer.gov/cancertopics/cancerlibrary/pinkbook/page1. Accessed August 8, 2011.

20. Liberman A, Chaiken S. Defensive processing of personally relevant health messages. *Pers Soc Psychol Bull*. 1992;18:669-679.

21. Weinstein N. Unrealistic optimism about illness susceptibility: conclusions from a community-wide sample. *J Behav Med*. 1987;10:481-500.

22. Weinstein N. Unrealistic optimism about susceptibility to health problems. *J Behav Med*. 1982;5:441-460.

23. Weinstein N. Why it won't happen to me: perceptions of risk factors and susceptibility. *Health Psychol*. 1984;3:431-457.

24. Rothman A, Schwarz N. Constructing perceptions of vulnerability: personal relevance and the use of experiential information in health judgments. *Pers Soc Psychol Bull*. 1998;24:1053-1064.

25. Rossi JS. Transtheoretical model of behavior change. In: NB Anderson, ed. *Encyclopedia of Health & Behavior. Vol. 2*. Thousand Oaks, CA: Sage, 2004:803-806.

26. University of Rhode Island, Cancer Prevention Research Center. Exercise: Stages of Change (Short Form). www.uri.edu/research/cprc/measures/ex_stages_change_shrt.html. Accessed August 8, 2011.

27. Marcus BH, Selby VC, Niaura RS, Rossi, JS. Self-efficacy and the stages of exercise behavior change. *Res Q Exerc Sport*. 1992;63:60-66.

28. Doran GT. There's a S.M.A.R.T. way to write management's goals and objectives. *Manag Rev*. 1981;70:35-36.

29. DeBusk RF, Miller NH, Superko HR, et al. A case management system for coronary risk factor modification. *Ann Intern Med*. 1994;120:721-729.

30. Curnier DY, Savage PD, Ades PA. Geographic distribution of cardiac rehabilitation programs in the United States. *J Cardiopulm Rehabil*. 2005;25:80-84.

31. Rollnick S, Miller W, Butler CC. *Motivational Interviewing in Health Care. Helping Patients Change Behavior*. New York: Guilford Press, 2008.

32. Madson MB, Loignon AC, Lane C. Training in motivational interviewing: a systematic review. *J Subst Abuse Treat*. 2009;36:101-109.

33. Moyers TB, Miller WR, Hendrickson SML. How does Motivational Interviewing work? Therapist interpersonal skill predicts client involvement within Motivational Interviewing sessions. *J Consult Clin Psychol*. 2005;73:590-598.

34. Ayala C, Orenstein D, Greenlund KJ, et al. Division of Adult and Community Health, National Center for Chronic Disease Prevention and Health Promotion, Centers for Disease Control and Prevention. Receipt of cardiac rehabilitation services among heart attack survivors – 19 states and the District of Columbia, 2001. *MMWR*. 2003;52:1072-1075.

35. Caulin-Glaser T, Blum M, Schmeizl R, et al. Gender differences in referral to cardiac rehabilitation programs after revascularization. *J Cardiopulm Rehabil*. 2001;21:24-30.

36. Barber K, Stommel M, Kroll J, et al. Cardiac rehabilitation for community-based patients with myocardial infarction: factors predicting discharge recommendation and participation. *J Clin Epidemiol*. 2001;54:1025-1030.

37. Benz Scott LA, Ben-Or K, Allen JK. Why are women missing from outpatient cardiac rehabilitation programs? A review of multilevel factors affecting referral, enrollment, and completion. *J Women's Health*. 2002;11:773-791.

38. Missik E. Women and cardiac rehabilitation: accessibility issues and policy recommendations. *Rehabil Nurs*. 2001;26:141-147.

39. Sanderson BK, Phillips MM, Gerald L, et al. Factors associated with the failure of patients to complete cardiac rehabilitation for medical and nonmedical reasons. *J Cardiopulm Rehabil*. 2003;23:281-289.

40. Thomas RJ, Miller NH, Lamendola C, et al. National survey on gender differences in cardiac rehabilitation programs. *J Cardiolpulm Rehabil*. 1996;16:402-412.

41. Allen JK, Benz Scott LA, Stewart K, Young D. Disparities in women's referral to and enrollment in outpatient cardiac rehabilitation. *J Gen Intern Med*. 2004;19:747-753.

42. Yohannes AM, Yalfani A, Doherty P, Bundy C. Predictors of drop-out from an outpatient cardiac rehabilitation programme. *Clin Rehabil*. 2007;21:222-229.

Chapter 5

1. Begs VAL, Willis SB, Mails EL, et al. Patient education for discharge after coronary bypass surgery in the 1990s: are patients adequately prepared? *J Cardiovasc Nurs*. 1998;12:72-86.

2. Brezynskie H, Pendon E, Lindsay P, Adam M. Identification of the perceived learning needs of balloon angioplasty patients. *J Cardiovasc Nurs*. 1998;9:8-14.

3. AACVPR. Resources for Patients. www.aacvpr.org/Resources/ResourcesforPatients/tabid/500/Default.aspx. Accessed May 11, 2012 (link may require login to view material).

4. Seconds Count. www.scai.org/secondscount/Default.aspx. Accessed May 11, 2012.

5. American College of Cardiology. Cardiosmart. www.cardiosmart.org/. Accessed May 11, 2012.

6. Drozda J Jr, Messer JV, Spertus J, et al. ACCF/AHA/AMA-PCPI 2011 performance measures for adults with coronary artery disease and hypertension: a report of the American College of Cardiology Foundation/American Heart Association and the American Medical Association–Physician Consortium for Performance Improvement. *J Am Coll Cardiol*. 2011;58:316-336.

7. AACVPR/ACCF/AHA 2010 update: performance measures on cardiac rehabilitation for referral to cardiac rehabilitation/secondary prevention services. *J Cardiopulm Rehabil Prev*. 2010;30:279-288.

8. Thomas RJ, King M, Lui K, et al. AACVPR/ACC/AHA 2007 performance measures on cardiac rehabilitation for referral to and delivery of cardiac rehabilitation/secondary prevention services. *J Cardiopulm Rehabil Prev*. 2007;27:260-290.

9. Mueller E, Savage PD, Schneider DJ, Howland LL, Ades PA. Effect of a computerized referral at hospital discharge on cardiac rehabilitation participation rates. *J Cardiopulm Rehabil Prev*. 2009;29:365-369.

10. Arena R, Williams M, Forman DE, et al. Increasing referral and participation rates to outpatient cardiac rehabilitation: the valuable role of healthcare professionals in the inpatient and home health settings: a science advisory from the American Heart Association. *Circulation*. 2012;125:1321-1329.

11. Titler MG, Pettit DM. Discharge readiness assessment. *J Cardiovasc Nurs*. 1995;9:64-74.

12. Meyer JW, Feingold MG. Using standard treatment protocols to manage costs and quality of hospital services. *Hospital Technology Special Report*. 1993;12:1-23.

13. Edwardson SR. The consequences and opportunities of shortened lengths of stay for cardiovascular patients. *J Cardiovasc Nurs*. 1999;14:1-11.

14. Hamm LF, Sanderson BK, Ades PA, et al. Core competencies for cardiac rehabilitation/secondary prevention professionals: 2010 update: position statement of the American Association of Cardiovascular and Pulmonary Rehabilitation. *J Cardiopulm Rehabil Prev*. 2011;31:2-10.

15. Joint Commission on Accreditation of Healthcare Organizations. www.jointcommission.org. Accessed January 23, 2012.

16. Anderson JA, Petersen NJ, Kistner C, Soltero ER, Willson P. Determining predictors of delayed recovery and the need for transitional cardiac rehabilitation after cardiac surgery. *J Am Acad Nurs Pract*. 2006;18:386-392.

17. Sansone GR, Alba A, Frengley JD. Analysis of FIM instrument scores for patients admitted to an inpatient cardiac rehabilitation program. *Arch Phys Med Rehabil*. 2002;83:506-512.

18. Kong KH, Kevorkian CG, Rossi CD. Functional outcomes of patients on a rehabilitation unit after open heart surgery. *J Cardiopulm Rehabil*. 1996;16:413-418.

19. Keith RA, Granger CV, Hamilton BB, Sherwin FS. The Functional Independence Measure: a new tool for rehabilitation. *Adv Clin Rehabil*. 1987;1:6-18.

20. Fiedler RC, Granger CV, Ottenbacher KJ. The uniform data system for medical rehabilitation: report of first admissions for 1994. *Am J Phys Med Rehabil*. 1996;75:125-129.

21. Doran K, Sampson B, Status R, et al. Clinical pathways across tertiary and community care after an interventional cardiology procedure. *J Cardiovasc Nurs*. 1997;11:2:1-14.

Chapter 6

1. Smith SC Jr, Benjamin EJ, Bonow R, et al. AHA/ACCF secondary prevention and risk reduction therapy for patients with coronary and other atherosclerotic vascular disease: 2011 update. *Circulation*. 2011;124:2458-2473.

2. Sargent LA, Seyfer AE, Hollinger J, et al. The healing sternum: a comparison of osseous healing with wire versus rigid fixation. *Ann Thorac Surg*. 1991;52:490-494.

3. Losanoff JE, Jones JW, Richman BW. Primary closure of median sternotomy: techniques and principles. *Cardiovasc Surg*. 2002;10:102-110.

4. Gibbons RJ, Balady GJ, Bricker JT, et al. ACC/AHA 2002 guideline update for exercise testing: summary article. *J Am Coll Cardiol*. 2002;40:1531-1540.

5. Myers J, Arena R, Franklin B, et al. Recommendations for clinical exercise laboratories: a scientific statement from the American Heart Association. *Circulation*. 2009;119:3144-3161.

6. American College of Sports Medicine. *ACSM Guidelines for Exercise Testing and Prescription*. 9th ed. Philadelphia: Lippincott Williams & Wilkins, 2014.

7. Fletcher GF, Balady GJ, Amsterdam EA, et al. Exercise standards for testing and training: a statement for healthcare professionals from the American Heart Association. *Circulation*. 2001;104:1694-1740.

8. Wilke NA, Sheldahl LM, Dougherty SM, et al. Baltimore Therapeutic Equipment work simulator: energy expenditure of work activities in cardiac patients. *Arch Phys Med Rehabil*. 1993;74:419-424.

9. Fletcher GF, Ades PA, Kligfield P, et al. Exercise standards for testing and training. A scientific statement from the American Heart Association. *Circulation*. In Press 2013.

10. Balady GJ, Arena R, Sietsema K, et al. Clinician's guide to cardiopulmonary exercise testing in adults. *Circulation*. 2010;122:191-225.

11. Keteyian SJ, Isaac D, Thadani U, et al. Safety of symptom-limited cardiopulmonary exercise testing in patients with chronic heart failure due to severe left ventricular systolic dysfunction. *Am Heart J*. 2009;158:S72-S77.

12. Physical Activity Readiness Questionnaire. www.csep.ca/CMFiles/publications/parq/par-q.pdf. Accessed February 28, 2012.

13. Myers J, Arena R, Franklin B, et al. Recommendations for clinical exercise laboratories: a scientific statement from the American Heart Association. *Circulation*. 2009;119:3144-3161.

14. Rodgers GP, Ayanian JZ, Balady G, et al. American College of Cardiology/American Heart Association Clinical Competence statement on stress testing. *Circulation*. 2000;102:1726-1738.

15. Cardiovascular Credentialing International. www.cci-online.org. Accessed February 28, 2012.

16. Gibbons RJ, Balady GJ, Bricker JT, et al. ACC/AHA 2002 guideline update for exercise testing: summary article. *Circulation*. 2002;106:1883-1892.

17. Myers J, Bader D, Madhavan R, Froelicher V. Validation of a specific activity questionnaire to estimate exercise tolerance in patients referred for exercise testing. *Am Heart J.* 2001;142:1041-1046.

18. Maeder M, Wolber T, Atefy R, et al. A nomogram to select the optimal treadmill ramp protocol in subjects with high exercise capacity: validation and comparison with the Bruce protocol. *J Cardiopulm Rehabil.* 2006;26:16-23.

19. Arena R, Myers J, Williams MA, et al. Assessment of functional capacity in clinical and research settings: a scientific statement from the American Heart Association. *Circulation.* 2007;116:329-343.

20. Myers J, Buchanan N, Walsh D, et al. Comparison of the ramp versus standard exercise protocols. *J Am Coll Cardiol.* 1991;17:1334-1342.

21. Wasserman K, Hansen J, Sue D, et al. *Principles of Exercise Testing and Interpretation.* 4th ed. Philadelphia: Lippincott Williams & Wilkins, 2004.

22. Jones N. *Clinical Exercise Testing.* Philadelphia: Saunders, 1997.

23. Hansen JE, Sue DY, Wasserman K. Predicted values for clinical exercise testing. *Am Rev Respir Dis.* 1984;129:S49-S55.

24. Morris CK, Myers J, Froelicher VF, et al. Nomogram based on metabolic equivalents and age for assessing aerobic exercise capacity in men. *J Am Coll Cardiol.* 1993;22:175-182.

25. Cole CR, Blackstone EH, Pashkow FJ, et al. Heart-rate recovery immediately after exercise as a predictor of mortality. *NEJM.* 1999;341:1351-1357.

26. Gauri AJ, Raxwal VK, Roux L, et al. Effects of chronotropic incompetence and beta-blocker use on the exercise treadmill test in men. *Am Heart J.* 2001;142:136-141.

27. Frolkis JP, Pothier CE, Blackstone EH, et al. Frequent ventricular ectopy after exercise as a predictor of death. *NEJM.* 2003;348:781-790.

28. Pinkstaff S, Peberdy MA, Kontos MC, Finucane S, Arena R. Quantifying exertion level during exercise stress testing using percentage of age-predicted maximal heart rate, rate pressure product, and perceived exertion. *Mayo Clin Proc.* 2010;85:1095-1100.

29. Fletcher GF, Balady GJ, Amsterdam EA, et al. Exercise Standards for Testing and Training. A Statement for Healthcare Professionals From the American Heart Association. http://circ.ahajournals.org/content/104/14/1694.Accessed 4/9/13.

30. Cheitlin MD, Armstrong WF, Aurigemma GP, et al. ACC/AHA/ASE 2003 guideline update for the clinical application of echocardiography. *Circulation.* 2003;108:1146-1162.

31. Kohli P, Gulati M. Exercise stress testing in women: going back to the basics. *Circulation.* 2010;122:2570-2580.

32. Klocke FJ, Baird MG, Lorell BH, et al. ACC/AHA/ASNC guidelines for the clinical use of cardiac radionuclide imaging. *Circulation.* 2003;108:1404-1418.

33. American Thoracic Society statement: guidelines for the six-minute walk test. *Am J Respir Crit Care Med.* 2002;166:111-117.

34. Ainsworth B, Haskell W, Leon AS. Compendium of physical activities: classification of energy costs of human physical activities. In: J Roitman, ed. *ACSM's Resource Manual for Guidelines for Exercise Testing and Prescription.* Philadelphia: Lippincott Williams & Wilkins, 2001:673-686.

35. Myers J, Do D, Herbert W, et al. A nomogram to predict exercise capacity from a specific activity questionnaire and clinical data. *Am J Cardiol.* 1994;73:591-596.

36. Pereira MA, FitzerGerald SJ, Gregg EW, et al. A collection of Physical Activity Questionnaires for health-related research. *Med Sci Sports Exerc.* 1997;29:S1-205.

37. Goldman L, Hashimoto B, Cook EF, et al. Comparative reproducibility and validity of systems for assessing cardiovascular functional class: advantages of a new specific activity scale. *Circulation.* 1981;64:1227-1234.

38. Hlatky MA, Boineau RE, Higginbotham MB, et al. A brief self-administered questionnaire to determine functional capacity (the Duke Activity Status Index). *Am J Cardiol.* 1989;64:651-654.

39. Borg GA. Psychophysical bases of perceived exertion. *Med Sci Sports Exerc.* 1982;14:377-381.

Chapter 7

1. Smith SC Jr, Benjamin EJ, Bonow RO, et al. AHA/ACC secondary prevention and risk reduction therapy for patients with coronary and other atherosclerotic vascular disease: 2011 update. *Circulation.* 2011;124:2458-2473.

2. DeBusk RF, Miller NH, Superko HR, et al. A case-management system for coronary risk factor modification after acute myocardial infarction. *Ann Intern Med.* 1994;120:721-729.

3. Gordon NF, English CD, Contractor AS, et al. Effectiveness of three models for comprehensive cardiovascular risk reduction. *Am J Cardiol.* 2002;89:1263-1268.

4. Haskell WL, Aldernam EL, Fair JM, et al. Effects of intensive multiple risk factor reduction on coronary atherosclerosis and clinical cardiac events in men and women with coronary artery disease. The Stanford Coronary Risk Intervention Project (SCRIP). *Circulation.* 1994;89:975-990.

5. King DE, Mainous AG, Carnemolla M, Everett CJ. Adherence to healthy lifestyle habits in U.S. adults, 1988-2006. *Am J Med.* 2009;122:528-534.

6. Taylor R, Brown A, Ebrahim S, et al. Exercise-based rehabilitation for patients with coronary heart disease: systematic review and meta-analysis of randomized controlled trials. *Am J Med.* 2004;116:682-692.

7. Clark A, Hartling L, Vandermeer B, McAlister F. Meta-analysis: secondary prevention programs for patients with coronary artery disease. *Ann Intern Med.* 2005;143:659-672.

8. Suaya JA, Stason WB, Ades PA, Normand S-LT, Shepard DS. Cardiac rehabilitation and survival in older coronary patients. *J Am Coll Cardiol.* 2009;54:25-33.

9. Gravely-Witte S, Leung YW, Nariani R, et al. Effects of cardiac rehabilitation referral strategies on referral and enrollment rates. *Nat Rev Cardiol.* 2010;7:87-96.

10. Grace SL, Russell KL, Reid RD, et al. for the Cardiac Rehabilitation Care Continuity Through Automatic Referral Evaluation (CRCARE) investigators. Effect of cardiac rehabilitation referral strategies on utilization rates: a prospective, controlled study. *Arch Intern Med.* 2011;171:235-241.

11. Thomas RJ, King M, Lui K, Oldridge N, Piña Il. AACVPR/ACCF/AHA 2010 update: performance measures on cardiac rehabilitation for referral to cardiac rehabilitation/secondary prevention services. *J Cardiopulm Rehabil Prev.* 2010;30:279-288.

12. Balady GJ, Williams MA, Ades PA, et al. Core components of cardiac rehabilitation/secondary prevention programs: 2007 update. *J Cardiopulm Rehabil Prev.* 2007;27:121-129.

13. Graham I, Atar D, Borch-Johnsen K, et al. European guidelines on cardiovascular disease prevention in clinical practice. Fourth Joint Task Force of the European Society of Cardiology and Societies on Cardiovascular Disease Prevention in Clinical Practice. *Eur J Cardiovasc Prev Rehabil.* 2007;14(suppl 2):S1-S113.

14. Ornish D, Scherwitz LW, Billings JH, et al. Intensive lifestyle changes for reversal of coronary heart disease. *JAMA.* 1998;280:2001-2007.

15. Vogel RA, Corretti MC, Plotnik GD. The postprandial effect of components of the Mediterranean diet on endothelial function. *J Am Coll Cardiol.* 2000;36:1455-1460.

16. Gould KL, Ornish D, Scherwitz L, et al. Changes in myocardial perfusion abnormalities by positron emission tomography after long-term, intense risk factor modification. *JAMA.* 1995;274:894-899.

17. Qureshi AL, Suri FK, Guterman LR, et al. Ineffective secondary prevention in survivors of cardiovascular events in the US population. *Arch Intern Med.* 2001;161:1621-1628.

18. Hamm LF, Sanderson BK, Ades PA, et al. Core competencies for cardiac rehabilitation/secondary prevention professionals: 2010 update: position statement of the American Association of Cardiovascular and Pulmonary Rehabilitation. *J Cardiopulm Rehabil Prev.* 2011;31:2-10.

19. Moore M, Boothroyd L. White paper: The obesity epidemic: a confidence crisis calling for professional coaches. Wellcoaches, Inc. www.wellcoaches.com/images/whitepaper.pdf. Accessed May 23, 2011.

20. Libby P, Ridker P, Hansson GK. Inflammation in atherosclerosis: from pathophysiology to practice. *J Am Coll Cardiol.* 2009;54:2129-2139.

21. Libby P. Atherosclerosis: the new view. *Scientific American.* 2002;286:47-53.

22. Framingham Heart Study. www.framinghamheartstudy.org/.

23. Grundy SM. Metabolic syndrome: a multiplex cardiovascular risk factor. *J Clin Endocrinol Metab.* 2007;92:399-404.

24. Okun MA, Karoly P. Perceived goal ownership, regulatory goal cognition and health behavior change. *Am J Health Behav.* 2007;31:98-109.

25. Bovend'Eerdt TJH, Botell RE, Wade DT. Writing SMART rehabilitation goals and achieving goal attainment scaling: a practical guide. *Clin Rehabil.* 2009;23:352-361.

26. Anderson JV, Mavis BE, Robinson JI, Stoffelmayr BE. A work-site weight management

program to reinforce behavior. *J Occup Med.* 1993;35:800-804.

27. O'Keefe JH, Carter MD, Lavie CJ. Primary and secondary prevention of cardiovascular diseases: a practical evidence-based approach. *Mayo Clin Proc.* 2009;84:741-757.

28. Verani MS, Mahmarian JJ. Nonexercise stress testing. In: AS Iskandrian, ed. *American Journal of Cardiology, Continuing Education Series, Myocardial Perfusion Imaging.* 1993;4:10.

29. Foster C, Porcari JP. The risks of exercise training. *J Cardiopulm Rehabil.* 2001;21:347-352.

30. Franklin B. Cardiovascular events associated with exercise: the risk-protection paradox. *J Cardiopulm Rehabil.* 2005;25:189-195.

31. Lavie CJ, Thomas RJ, Squires RW, Allison TG, Milani RV. Exercise training and cardiac rehabilitation in primary and secondary prevention of coronary heart disease. *Mayo Clin Proc.* 2009;84:373-383.

32. O'Connor CM, Whelan DJ, Lee KL, et al. Efficacy and safety of exercise training in patients with chronic heart failure: HF-ACTION randomized controlled trial. *JAMA.* 2009;301:1439-1450.

33. McKelvie RS. Exercise training in patients with heart failure: clinical outcomes, safety, and indications. *Heart Fail Rev.* 2008;13:3-11.

34. Mittleman MA, Maclure M, Tofler GH, Sherwood JB, Goldberg RJ, Muller JE, for the Determinants of Myocardial Infarction Onset Study investigators. Triggering of acute myocardial infarction by heavy physical exertion. *Heart.* 1996;75:323-325.

35. Dahabreh IJ, Paulus JK. Association of episodic physical and sexual activity with triggering of acute cardiac events: systematic review and meta-analysis. *JAMA.* 2011;305:1225-1233.

36. Scheinowitz M, Harpaz D, Safety of cardiac rehabilitation in a medically supervised, community-based program. *Cardiology.* 2005;103:113-117.

37. Pavy B, Iliou MC, Meurin P, Tabet JY, Corone S, for the Functional Evaluation and Cardiac Rehabilitation Working Group of the French Society of Cardiology. Safety of exercise training for cardiac patients results of the French Registry of Complications During Cardiac Rehabilitation. *Arch Intern Med.* 2006;166:2329-2334.

38. Hossack KF, Hartwig R. Cardiac arrest associated with supervised cardiac rehabilitation. *J Card Rehabil.* 1982;2:405-408.

39. Centers for Medicare and Medicaid Services. Title 42 Code of Federal Regulations, Section 410.49: Cardiac rehabilitation program and intensive cardiac rehabilitation program. Conditions of coverage. http://edocket.access.gpo.gov/cfr_2010/octqtr/pdf/42cfr410.49.pdf. Accessed March 12, 2011.

40. Verrill D, Ashley R, Witt K, Forkner T. Recommended guidelines for monitoring and supervision of North Carolina Phase II/III cardiac rehabilitation programs: a position paper by the North Carolina Cardiopulmonary Rehabilitation Association. *J Cardiopulm Rehabil.* 1996;2:9-24.

41. Ades PA, Savage PD, Toth MJ, Harvey-Berino J, David J. High-calorie-expenditure exercise: a new approach to cardiac rehabilitation for overweight coronary patients. *Circulation.* 2009;119;2671-2678.

42. Seki E, Watanabe Y, Shimada K, et al. Effects of a phase III cardiac rehabilitation program on physical status and lipid profiles in elderly patients with coronary artery disease: J-CARP. *Circ J.* 2008;72:1230-1234.

43. Seki E, Watanabe Y, Sunayama S, et al. Effects of phase III cardiac rehabilitation programs on health-related quality of life in elderly patients with coronary artery disease: J-CARP. *Circ J.* 2003;67:73-77.

44. Tkatch R, Artinan NT, Abrams J, et al. Social network and health outcomes among African American cardiac rehabilitation patients. *Heart Lung.* 2011;40:193-200.

45. Shen BJ, Wachowiak PS, Brooks LG. Psychosocial factors and assessment in cardiac rehabilitation. *Eur Medicophys.* 2005;41:75-91.

46. Hancock K, Davidson P, Daly J, Webber D, Chang E. An exploration of the usefulness of motivational interviewing in facilitating secondary prevention gains in cardiac rehabilitation. *J Cardiopulm Rehabil.* 2005;25:200-206.

47. Hardcastle S, Taylor A, Baily M, Castle R. A randomized controlled trial on the effectiveness of a primary health care based counseling intervention on physical activity, diet and CHD risk factors. *Patient Educ Couns.* 2008;70:31-39.

48. Bennett JA, Lyons KS, Winters-Stone K, Nail LM, Scherer J. Motivational interviewing to increase physical activity in long-term cancer survivors. *Nurs Res.* 2007;56:18-27.

49. Carels RA, Darby L, Cacciapaglia HM, et al. Using motivational interviewing as a supplement to obesity treatment: a stepped-care approach. *Health Psychol.* 2007;26:369-374.

50. Harland J, White M, Drinkwater C, Chinn D, Farr L, Howel D. The Newcastle exercise project: a randomised controlled trial of methods to promote physical activity in primary care. *BMJ*. 1999;319:828-832.

51. Duncan KA, Pozehl B. Staying on course: the effects of an adherence facilitation intervention on home exercise prescription. *Prog Cardiovasc Nurs*. 2002;17:59-65, 71.

52. Papadakis S, Reid RD, Coyle D, et al. Cost-effectiveness of cardiac rehabilitation program delivery models in patients at varying cardiac risk, reason for referral, and sex. *Eur J Cardiovasc Prev Rehabil*. 2008;15:347-353.

53. Papadakis S, Oldridge NB, Coyle D, et al. Economic evaluation of cardiac rehabilitation: a systematic review. *Eur J Cardiovasc Prev Rehabil*. 2005;12:513-520.

54. Oldridge N, Furlong W, Perkins A, et al. Community or patient preferences for cost-effectiveness of cardiac rehabilitation: does it matter? *Eur J Cardiovasc Prev Rehabil*. 2008;15:608-615.

55. Thomas RJ. Cardiac rehabilitation/secondary prevention programs: a raft for the rapids: why have we missed the boat? *Circulation*. 2007;116:1644-1646.

Chapter 8

Introduction

1. Smith SC, Benjamin EJ, Bonow RO, et al. AHA/ACCF secondary prevention and risk reduction therapy for patients with coronary and other atherosclerotic vascular disease: 2011 update. *Circulation*. 2011;124:2458-2473.

2. Hamm LF, Sanderson BK, Ades PA, et al. Core competencies for cardiac rehabilitation/secondary prevention professionals: 2010 Update. Position Statement of the American Association of Cardiovascular and Pulmonary Rehabilitation. *J Cardiopulm Rehabil*. 2011;31:2-10.

3. Lavie CJ, Thomas RJ, Squires RW, Allison TG, Milani RV. Exercise training and cardiac rehabilitation in primary and secondary prevention of coronary heart disease. Mayo Clin Proc. 2009;84:373-383.

Tobacco Use section

1. American Heart Association. *Heart and Stroke Statistical Update*. Dallas: American Heart Association, 2010.

2. Critchley JA, Capwell S. Mortality risk reduction associated with smoking cessation in patients with coronary heart disease: a systematic review. *JAMA*. 2003;290:86-97.

3. Fiore MC, Jaen MC, Baker TB, et al. *Treating Tobacco Use and Dependence: 2008 Update. Clinical Practice Guideline*. Rockville, MD: U.S. Department of Health and Human Services, Public Health Service, 2008.

4. Benowitz NL. Nicotine addiction. *NEJM*. 2010;362:2295-2303.

5. Pipe AL, Papadakis S, Reid RD. The role of smoking cessation in the prevention of coronary artery disease. *Curr Atheroscler Rep*. 2010;12:145-150.

6. Taylor CB, Miller NH, Smith PM, DeBusk RF. The effect of a home-based, case-managed, multifactorial risk-reduction program on reducing psychological distress in patients with cardiovascular disease. *J Cardiopulm Rehabil*. 1997;17:157-162.

7. Ewing JA. Detecting alcoholism: the CAGE Questionnaire. *JAMA*. 1984;252:1905-1907.

8. Kalman D, Kim S, DiGirolamo G, Smelson D, Ziedonis D. Addressing tobacco use disorder in smokers in early remission from alcohol dependence: the case for integrating smoking cessation services in substance use disorder treatment programs. *Clin Psychol Rev*. 2010;30:12-24.

9. Reid RD, Mullen KA, Pipe AL. Systematic approaches to smoking cessation in the cardiac setting. *Curr Opin Cardiol*. 2011;26:443-448.

10. Taylor CB, Miller NH, Killen JD, et al. Smoking cessation after myocardial infarction: effects of a nurse-managed intervention. *Ann Intern Med*. 1990;113:118-123.

11. Abrams DB, et al. Boosting population quits through evidence-based cessation treatment and policy. *Am J Prev Med*. 2010;38:S351-S363.

12. Prochaska JO, DiClemente CC, Norcross JC. In search of how people change: applications to addictive behaviors. *Am Psychologist*. 1992;47:1102-1114.

13. Miller NH, Smith PM. Smoking cessation. In: J Roitman et al., eds. *ACSM's Resource Manual for Guidelines for Exercise Testing and Prescription*. 3rd ed. Baltimore: Williams & Wilkins, 1998.

14. Benowitz NL, Gourlay SG. Cardiovascular toxicity of nicotine: implications for nicotine replacement therapy. *J Am Coll Cardiol*. 1997;29:1422-1431.

15. Joseph AM, Norman SM, Ferry LH, et al. The safety of transdermal nicotine as an aid to smoking cessation in patients with cardiac disease. *NEJM*. 1996;335:1792-1798.

16. Mahmarian JJ, Moye LA, Nasser GA, et al. Nicotine patch therapy in smoking cessation reduces the extent of exercise-induced myocardial ischemia. *J Am Coll Cardiol*. 1997;30:125-130.

17. U.S. Food and Drug Administration. FDA Drug Safety Communication: Chantix (varenicline) drug label now contains updated efficacy and safety information. www.fda.gov/Drugs/DrugSafety/ucm264436.htm. Accessed January 23, 2012.

18. Miller NH, Smith PM, DeBusk RF, et al. Smoking cessation and hospitalized patients: results of a randomized trial. *Arch Intern Med*. 1997;157:409-415.

Abnormal Lipids section

1. Grundy SM, Cleemanm JI, Mertz C, et al. Implications of recent clinical trials for the National Cholesterol Education Program Adult Treatment Panel III guidelines. *Circulation*. 2004;110:227-239.

2. Heart Protection Study Collaborative Group. MRC/BHF Heart Protection Study of cholesterol lowering with simvastatin in 20,536 high-risk individuals: a randomised placebo-controlled trial. *Lancet*. 2002;360(9326):7-22.

3. Cholesterol Treatment Trialists' (CTT) collaborators. Efficacy and safety of cholesterol-lowering treatment: prospective meta-analysis of data from 90,056 participants in 14 randomised trials of statins. *Lancet*. 2005;306:1267-1278.

4. Cholesterol Treatment Trialists' (CTT) collaboration. Efficacy and safety of more intensive lowering of LDL: a meta-analysis of data from 170,000 participants in 26 randomised trials. *Lancet*. 2010;376:1670-1681.

5. Gotto AM. Lipid lowering, regression, and coronary events. *Circulation*. 1995;92:646-656.

6. Simvastatin Survival Study Group. Randomised trial of cholesterol lowering in 4444 patients with coronary heart disease: the Scandinavian Simvastatin Survival Study (4S). *Lancet*. 1994;344:1383-1389.

7. Shepherd J, Blauw GJ, Murphy MB, et al, for Prosper study group. Pravastatin in elderly individuals at risk of vascular disease (PROSPER): a randomized controlled trial. *Lancet*. 2002;360(9346):1623-1630.

8. Mosca L, Benjamin EJ, Berra K, et al. Effectiveness-based guidelines for the prevention of cardiovascular disease in women—2011 update: a guideline from the American Heart Association. *Circulation*. 2011;123:1243-1262.

9. Sacks FM, Pfeffer MA, Moye LA, et al. The effect of pravastatin on coronary events after myocardial infarction with average cholesterol levels. Cholesterol and Recurrent Events Trial investigators. *NEJM*. 1996;335:1001-1009.

10. Schedlbauer A, Davies P, Fahey T. Interventions to improve adherence to lipid lowering medication. *Cochrane Database Syst Rev*. 2010;3:CD004371.

11. Allen JK, Blumenthal RS. Coronary risk factors in women six months after coronary artery bypass grafting. *Am J Cardiol*. 1995;75:1092-1095.

12. Cannistra L, O'Malley CJ, Balady GJ. Comparison of outcome of cardiac rehabilitation in black women and white women. *Am J Cardiol*. 1995;75:890-893.

13. Lavie C, Milani R. Effects of cardiac rehabilitation, exercise training, and weight reduction on exercise capacity, coronary risk factors, behavior characteristics, and quality of life in obese coronary patients. *Am J Cardiol*. 1997;79:397-401.

14. National Cholesterol Education Program (NCEP). Executive summary of the third report of the Expert Panel on Detection, Evaluation and Treatment of High Blood Cholesterol in Adults (Adult Treatment Panel III). *JAMA*. 2001;285:2486-2497.

15. Gardner C, Fortmann S, Krauss R. Association of small low density lipoprotein particles with the incidence of coronary artery disease in men and women. *JAMA*. 1996;276:875-881.

16. Schwartz GG, Olsson AG, Ezekowitz MD, et al. Effects of atorvastatin on early recurrent ischemic events in acute coronary syndromes (the MIRACL study): a randomized controlled trial. *JAMA*. 2001;285:1711-1718.

17. Smith SC Jr, Blair SN, Bonow RO, et al. Guidelines for preventing heart attack and death in patients with atherosclerotic cardiovascular disease: 2001 update: a statement for healthcare professionals from the AHA/ACC. *Circulation*. 2001;104:1577-1579.

18. Greenland P, Alpert JS, Beller GA, et al. 2010 ACCF/AHA guideline for assessment of cardiovascular risk in asymptomatic adults. *J Am Coll Cardiol*. 2010;56:e50-103.

19. Krauss RM, Eckel RH, Howard B, et al. AHA Dietary Guidelines: revision 2000. *Circulation.* 2000;102:2284-2299.

20. Pyörälä M, Miettinen H, Laakso M, Pyörälä K. Hyperinsulinemia predicts coronary heart disease risks in healthy middle-aged men: the 22-year follow-up results of the Helsinki policeman study. *Circulation.* 1998;98:398-404.

21. Reaven G. Pathophysiology of insulin resistance in human disease. *Physiol Rev.* 1995;75:473-486.

22. Reinhart SL. Uncomplicated acute myocardial infarction: a critical path. *J Cardiovasc Nurs.* 1995;31:1-7.

23. Zavaroni I, Bonini L, Gasparini P, et al. Hyperinsulinemia in a normal population as a predictor of non-insulin dependent diabetes mellitus, hypertension, and coronary heart disease: the Barilla factory revisited. *Metabolism.* 1999;48:989-994.

24. Mayer-Davis E, D'Agostino R, Karter A, et al. Intensity and amount of physical activity in relation to insulin sensitivity. *JAMA.* 1998;279:669-674.

25. Stefanick M, Mackey S, Sheehan M, et al. Effects of diet and exercise in men and postmenopausal women with low levels of HDL-cholesterol and high levels of LDL-cholesterol. *NEJM.* 1998;339:12-20.

26. Reaven GM. Role of insulin resistance in human disease. *Diabetes.* 1998;37:1595-1607.

27. Austin M, Hokanson J, Edwards K. Hypertriglyceridemia as a cardiovascular risk factor. *Am J Cardiol.* 1998;81(4A):7B-12B.

28. Stampfer M, Krauss R, Ma J, et al. A prospective study of triglyceride level, low-density lipoprotein particles diameter, and risk of myocardial infarction. *JAMA.* 1996;276:882-888.

29. Frost P, Havel R. Rationale for use of non-high-density lipoprotein cholesterol rather than low-density lipoprotein cholesterol as a tool for lipoprotein cholesterol screening and assessment of risk and therapy. *Am J Cardiol.* 1998;81(4A):26B-31B.

30. Campbell NC, Grimshaw JM, Ritchie LD, Rawles JM. Outpatient cardiac rehabilitation: are the potential benefits being realized? *J R Coll Physicians Lond.* 1996;30:514-519.

31. Chan AW, Bhatt DL, Chew DP, et al. Early and sustained survival benefit associated with statin therapy at the time of percutaneous coronary intervention. *Circulation.* 2002;105:691-696.

32. Heeschen C, Hamm CW, Laufs U, et al. Withdrawal of statins increases event rates in patients with acute coronary syndromes. *Circulation.* 2002;15:1446-1452.

33. Lefer DJ. Statins as potent anti-inflammatory drugs. *Circulation.* 2002;106:2041-2042.

34. Pruefer D, Makowski J, Schnell M, et al. Simvastatin inhibits inflammatory properties of staphylococcus aureus alphatoxin. *Circulation.* 2002;106:2104-2110.

35. Ridker PM, Rifai N, Pfeffer M, et al. Long term effects of pravastatin on plasma concentration of C-reactive protein. *Circulation.* 1999;100:230-235.

36. Ross R. Atherosclerosis: an inflammatory disease. *NEJM.* 1999;340:115-126.

Hypertension section

1. Roger VL, Go AS, Lloyd-Jones DM. Heart disease and stroke statistics—2011 update. A report from the American Heart Association. *Circulation.* 2011;123:e18-e209.

2. Audelin MC, Savage PD, Ades PA. Changing clinical profile of patients entering cardiac rehabilitation/secondary prevention programs: 1996 to 2006. *J Cardiopulm Rehabil Prev.* 2008;28:299-306.

3. Chobodian AV, Bakris GL, Black HR, et al, and the National High Blood Pressure Education Program Coordinating Committee. Seventh report of Joint National Committee on Prevention, Detection, Evaluation, and Treatment of High Blood Pressure. *Hypertension.* 2003;42:1206-1252.

4. Smith SC, Benjamin EJ, Bonow RO, et al. AHA/ACCF secondary prevention and risk reduction therapy for patients with coronary and other atherosclerotic vascular disease: 2011 update. *Circulation.* 2011;124:2458-2473.

5. Lichtenstein AH, Appel LJ, Brands M, et al. AHA 2006 diet and lifestyle recommendations. *Circulation.* 2006;114:82-96.

6. Appel LJ, Frohlich ED, Hall JE, et al. The importance of population-wide sodium reduction as a means to prevent cardiovascular disease and stroke: a call to action from the American Heart Association. *Circulation.* 2011;123:1138-1143.

7. U.S. Department of Agriculture and U.S. Department of Health and Human Services. *Dietary Guidelines for Americans, 2010.* 7th ed. Washington, DC: U.S. Government Printing Office, 2010.

8. Appel LJ, Moore TJ, Obarzanek E, et al. A clinical trial of the effects of dietary patterns on blood pressure. DASH Collaborative Research Group. *NEJM*. 1997;336:1117-1124.

9. Svetkey LP, Simons-Morton D, Vollmer WM, et al. Effects of dietary patterns on blood pressure: subgroup analysis of the Dietary Approaches to Stop Hypertension (DASH) randomized clinical trial. *Arch Intern Med*. 1999;159:285-293.

10. Bray GA, Vollmer WM, Sacks FM, Obarzanek E, Svetkey LP, Appel LJ, DASH Collaborative Research Group. A further subgroup analysis of the effects of the DASH diet and three dietary sodium levels on blood pressure: results of the DASH-Sodium Trial. *Am J Cardiol*. 2004;94:222-227.

11. Adrogue HJ, Madias NE. Sodium and potassium in the pathogenesis of hypertension. *NEJM*. 2007;356:1966-1978.

12. Yusuf S, Hawken S, Ounpuu S, et al. Effect of potentially modifiable risk factors associated with myocardial infarction in 52 countries (the INTERHEART study): case-control study. *Lancet*. 2004;364:937.

Physical Inactivity section

1. Haskell W, Lee I-M, Pate R, et al. Physical activity and public health: updated recommendation for adults from the American College of Sports Medicine and the American Heart Association. *Circulation*. 2007;116:1081-1093.

2. U.S. Department of Health and Human Services. *2008 Physical Activity Guidelines for Americans*. www.health.gov/paguidelines/pdf/paguide.pdf

3. Thompson PD, Buchner D, Pina IL, et al. AHA scientific statement: exercise and physical activity in the prevention and treatment of atherosclerotic cardiovascular disease. *Circulation*. 2003;107:3109-3116.

4. Pate RR, Pratt M, Blair SN, et al. Physical activity and public health: a recommendation from the Centers for Disease Control and Prevention and the American College of Sports Medicine. *JAMA*. 1995;273:402-407.

5. U.S. Department of Health and Human Services. *Clinical Practice Guidelines: Cardiac Rehabilitation*. U.S. Department of Health and Human Services; Public Health Service, Agency for Health Care Policy and Research, National Heart, Lung and Blood Institute, 1995.

6. U.S. Department of Health and Human Services. *Physical Activity and Health: A Report of the Surgeon General*. Atlanta: U.S. Department of Health and Human Services, Centers for Disease Control and Prevention, National Center for Chronic Disease Prevention and Health Promotion, 1996.

7. Myers J, Prakash M, Froelicher V, et al. Exercise capacity and mortality among men referred for exercise testing. *NEJM*. 2002;346:793-801.

8. Blair SN, Kohl HW 3rd, Paffenbarger RS Jr, et al. Physical fitness and all-cause mortality. A prospective study of healthy men and women. *JAMA*. 1989;262:2395-2401.

9. Katzmarzyk P, Church T, Craig C, et al. Sitting time and mortality from all causes, cardiovascular disease, and cancer. *Med Sci Sports Exerc*. 2009;41:998-1005.

10. Stamatakis E, Hamer M, Dunstan D. Screen-based entertainment time, all-cause mortality, and cardiovascular events: population-based study with ongoing mortality and hospital events follow-up. *J Am Coll Cardiol*. 2011;57:292-299.

11. Paffenbarger RS, Kampert JB, Lee IM, et al. Changes in physical activity and other lifeway patterns influencing longevity. *Med Sci Sports Exerc*. 1994;26:857-865.

12. Oldridge NB, Guyatt GH, Fischer ME, et al. Cardiac rehabilitation after myocardial infarction: combined experience of randomized clinical trials. *JAMA*. 1988;260:945-950.

13. Caspersen CJ, Powell KE, Christenson GM. Physical activity, exercise, and physical fitness: definitions and distinctions for health-related research. *Public Health Rep*. 1985;100:126-131.

14. Lloyd-Jones D, Hong Y, Labarthe D, et al. Defining and setting national goals for cardiovascular health promotion and disease reduction: the American Heart Association's Strategic Impact Goal through 2020 and beyond. *Circulation*. 2010;121:586-613.

15. Blair SN, Kohl HW 3rd, Barlow CE, et al. Changes in physical fitness and all-cause mortality. A prospective study of healthy and unhealthy men. *JAMA*. 1995;273:1093-1098.

16. Warren JM, Ekelund U, Besson H, et al. Assessment of physical activity—a review of methodologies with reference to epidemiological research: a report of the exercise physiology section of the European Association of Cardiovascular Preven-

tion and Rehabilitation. *Eur J Cardiovasc Prev Rehabil.* 2010;17:127-139.

17. Balady GJ, Arena R, Sietsema K, et al. Clinician's guide to cardiopulmonary exercise testing in adults: a scientific statement from the American Heart Association. *Circulation.* 2010;122:191-225.

18. Lauer M, Froelicher ES, Williams M, Kligfield P. Exercise testing in asymptomatic adults: a statement for professionals from the American Heart Association. *Circulation.* 2005;112:771-776.

19. Fletcher GF, Balady GJ, Amsterdam EA, et al. Exercise standards for testing and training: a statement for healthcare professionals from the American Heart Association. *Circulation.* 2001;104:1694-1740.

20. American College of Sports Medicine. *ACSM's Guidelines for Exercise Testing and Prescription.* 9th ed. Philadelphia: Lippincott Williams & Wilkins, 2014.

21. Williams M. Exercise testing in cardiac rehabilitation: exercise prescription and beyond. *Cardiol Clin.* 2001;19:415-431.

22. Williams M, Haskell W, Ades P, et al. Resistance training in individuals with and without cardiovascular disease: 2007 update: a scientific statement from the American Heart Association. *Circulation.* 2007;116:572-584.

23. Saris W, Blair SN, van Baak M, et al. How much physical activity is enough to prevent unhealthy weight gain? Outcome of the IASO 1st Stock Conference and consensus statement. *Obesity Rev.* 2003;4:101-114.

24. Hambrecht R, Niebauer J, Marburger C, et al. Various intensities of leisure time physical activity in patients with coronary artery disease: effects on cardiorespiratory fitness and progression of coronary atherosclerotic lesions. *J Am Coll Cardiol.* 1993;22:468-477.

25. Ayabe M, Brubaker PH, Dobrosielski D, et al. The physical activity patterns of cardiac rehabilitation program participants. *J Cardiopulm Rehabil.* 2004;24:80-86.

26. McConnell TR, Palm RJ, Shearn WM, et al. Body fat distribution's impact on physiologic outcomes during cardiac rehabilitation. *J Cardiopulm Rehabil.* 1999;19:162-169.

27. Savage PD, Brochu M, Scott P, et al. Low caloric expenditure in cardiac rehabilitation. *Am Heart J.* 2000;140:527-533.

28. Schairer JR, Keteyian SJ, Ehrman JK, et al. Leisure time physical activity of patients in maintenance cardiac rehabilitation. *J Cardiopulm Rehabil.* 2003;23:260-265.

29. Schairer JR, Kostelnik T, Proffitt SM, et al. Caloric expenditure during cardiac rehabilitation. *J Cardiopulm Rehabil.* 1998;18:290-294.

30. McConnell TR, Klinger TA, Gardner JK, et al. Cardiac rehabilitation without exercise tests for post-myocardial infarction and post-bypass surgery patients. *J Cardiopulm Rehabil.* 1998;18:458-463.

31. Ades PA, Savage PD, Harvey-Berino J. The treatment of obesity in cardiac rehabilitation. *J Cardiopulm Rehabil Prev.* 2010;30:289-298.

32. Ayabe M, Brubaker PH, Dobrosielski D, et al. Target step count for the secondary prevention of cardiovascular disease. *Circ J.* 2008;72:299-303.

33. Stevenson TG, Riggin K, Nagelkirk PR, et al. Physical activity habits of cardiac patients participating in an early outpatient rehabilitation program. *J Cardiopulm Rehabil Prev.* 2009;29:299-303.

34. Jones NL, Schneider PL, Kaminsky LA, et al. An assessment of the total amount of physical activity of patients participating in a phase III cardiac rehabilitation program. *J Cardiopulm Rehabil Prev.* 2007;27:81-85.

35. Ayabe M, Brubaker PH, Kumahara H, Kiyonaga A, Tanaka H, Aoki J. Self-monitoring moderate-vigorous physical activity versus steps/day is more effective in chronic disease exercise programs. *J Cardiopulm Rehabil Prev.* 2010;30:111-115.

36. Bravata DM, Smith-Spangler C, Sundaram V, et al. Using pedometers to increase physical activity and improve health: a systematic review. *JAMA.* 2007;298:2296-2304.

37. Healy GN, Matthews CE, Dunstan DW, et al. Sedentary time and cardio-metabolic biomarkers in US adults: NHANES 2003-06. *Eur Heart J.* 2011;32:590-597.

38. Stewart KJ, Ratchford EV, Williams MA. Exercise for restoring health and preventing vascular disease. In: RS Blumenthal. JM Foody, ND Wong, eds. *Preventive Cardiology.* Philadelphia: Elsevier, 2011:541-551.

Diabetes section

1. Centers for Disease Control and Prevention. 2011 national diabetes fact sheet. www.cdc.gov/diabetes/pubs/estimates11.htm#1.

2. Sacks FM. Lipid-lowering therapy in acute coronary syndromes. *JAMA*. 2001;285:1758-1760.

3. Colberg SR, Albright AL, Blissmer BJ, et al. American College of Sports Medicine and the American Diabetes Association joint position statement. Exercise and type 2 diabetes. *Med Sci Sports Exerc*. 2010;42:2282-2303.

4. Knowler WC, Barrett-Connor E, Fowler SE, et al. Reduction in the incidence of type 2 diabetes with lifestyle intervention or metformin. *NEJM*. 2002;346:393-403.

5. Kokkinos P, Myers J, Nylen E, et al. Exercise capacity and all-cause mortality in African American and Caucasian men with type 2 diabetes. *Diabetes Care*. 2009;32:623-628.

6. Gill JM. Physical activity, cardiorespiratory fitness and insulin resistance: a short update. *Curr Opin Lipidol*. 2007;18:47-52.

7. Horowitz JF. Exercise-induced alterations in muscle lipid metabolism improve insulin sensitivity. *Exerc Sport Sci Rev*. 2007;35:192-196.

8. American Diabetes Association. Physical activity/exercise and diabetes. Diabetes Care. 2004;27:s58-s62.

9. Sigal RJ, Kenny GP, Wasserman DH, et al. Physical activity/exercise and type 2 diabetes: a consensus statement from the American Diabetes Association. *Diabetes Care*. 2006;29:1433-1438.

10. Hornsby WG, Albright AL. Diabetes. In: *ACSM's Exercise Management for Persons with Chronic Diseases and Disabilities*. Champaign, IL: Human Kinetics, 2009:182-191.

11. American College of Sports Medicine. *ACSM's Guidelines for Exercise Testing and Prescription*. 9th ed. Baltimore: Lippincott Williams & Wilkins, 2010:281.

12. Pinzur MS, Slovenkai MP, Trepman E, et al. Guidelines for diabetic foot care. *Foot Ankle Int*. 2005;26:113-119.

13. Lopez-Jimenez F, Kramer VC, Masters B, et al. Recommendations for managing patients with diabetes mellitus in cardiopulmonary rehabilitation. An American Association of Cardiovascular and Pulmonary Rehabilitation statement. *J Cardiopulm Rehabil Prev*. 2012;32:101-112.

14. American Diabetes Association. Standards of Medical Care In Diabetes–2013. Exercise in the presence of nonoptimal glycemic control-hypoglycemia. http://care.diabetesjournals.org/content/36/supplement_S11.full (accessed 6/24/2013).

Psychosocial Considerations section

1. Kolman L, Shin N, Krishnan SM, et al. Psychological distress in cardiac rehabilitation participants. *J Cardiopulm Rehabil Prev*. 2011;31:81-86.

2. Barth J, Schneider S, von Känel R. Lack of social support in the etiology and prognosis of coronary heart disease: a systematic review and meta-analysis. *Psychosom Med*. 2010;72:229-238.

3. Hughes JW, Bon-Wilson A, Eichenauer K, Feltz G. Behavioral medicine for patients with heart disease-the case of depression and cardiac rehabilitation. *US Cardiol*. 2010;7:55-60.

4. Oldridge NB, Pashkow FJ. Compliance and motivation in cardiac rehabilitation. In: FJ Pashkow, WA Dafoe, eds. *Clinical Rehabilitation: A Cardiologist's Guide*. Baltimore: Williams & Wilkins, 1993:335-348.

5. Hamm LF, Sanderson BK, Ades PA, et al. Core competencies for cardiac rehabilitation/secondary prevention professionals: 2010 update: position statement of the American Association of Cardiovascular and Pulmonary Rehabilitation. *J Cardiopulm Rehabil Prev*. 2010;31:2-10.

6. Livneh H. Denial of chronic illness and disability: part 1. Theoretical, functional and dynamic perspectives. *Rehabil Couns Bull*. 2009;52:225-236.

7. Perkins-Porras L, Whitehead DL, Strike PC, Steptoe A. Causal beliefs, cardiac denial and pre-hospital delays following the onset of acute coronary syndromes. *J Behav Med*. 2008;31:498-505.

8. Frasure-Smith N. Recent evidence linking coronary heart disease and depression. *Can J Psychiatry*. 2006;51:730-737.

9. Chida Y, Steptoe A. The association of anger and hostility with future coronary heart disease: a meta-analytic review of prospective evidence. *J Am Coll Cardiol*. 2009;53:936-946.

10. Pederson SS, Denollet J. Type D personality, cardiac events, and impaired quality of life: a review. *Eur J Cardiovasc Prev Rehab*. 2003;10:241-248.

11. O'Dell KR, Masters KS, Spielmans G, Maisto SA. Does type-D personality predict outcomes among patients with cardiovascular disease? A meta-analytic review. *J Psychosom Res*. 2011;71:199-206.

12. Rose MI, Robbins B. Psychosocial recovery issues and strategies in cardiac rehabilitation. In: FJ Pashkow, WA Dafoe, eds. *Clinical Rehabilitation: A Cardiologist's Guide*. Baltimore: Williams & Wilkins, 1993:248-262.

13. Beck AT, Steer RA, Brown GK. *BDI-II Manual.* San Antonio: Psychological Corporation, 1996.

14. Derogatis LR. *SCL-90-R: Administration, Scoring and Procedure Manual.* Baltimore: Clinical Psychometric Research, 1983.

15. McNair D, Lorr M, Dropplemann L. *Profile of Mood States.* San Diego: Educational and Industrial Testing Service, 1971.

16. Radloff L. The C.E.S.-D Scale: a self-report depression scale for research in the general population. *Appl Psychol Meas.* 1977;1:385-401.

17. Spielberger C, Gorsuch R, Luschene R. *Manual for the State Trait Anxiety Inventory.* Palo Alto, CA: Consulting Psychologists Press, 1970.

18. Pizzi C, Rutjes AW, Costa GM, Fontana F, Mezzetti A, Manzoli L. Meta-analysis of selective serotonin reuptake inhibitors in patients with depression and coronary heart disease. *Am J Cardiol.* 2011;107:972-979.

19. Taylor CB, Miller NH, Herman S, et al. Smoking cessation after myocardial infarction: effects of a nurse-managed intervention. *Ann Intern Med.* 1990;113:118-123.

20. Allen JP, Eckardt MJ, Wallen J. Screening for alcoholism: techniques and issues. *Public Health Rep.* 1988;10:586-592.

21. Dracup K, Bryan-Brown CW. An open door policy in ICU. *Am J Crit Care.* 1992;2:16-18.

22. Sotile WM, Sotile MO, Ewen GS, Sotile LJ. Marriage and family factors relevant to effective cardiac rehabilitation: a review of risk factor literature. *Sports Med Training Rehabil.* 1993;4:115-128.

23. Sotile WM, Sotile MO, Sotile LJ, Ewan GS. Martial and family factors relevant to cardiac rehabilitation: a integrative review of the psychosocial literature. *Sports Med Training Rehabil.* 1993;4:217-236.

24. Swenson JR, Abbey SE. Management of depression and anxiety disorders in the cardiac patient. In: FJ Pashkow, WA Dafoe, eds. *Clinical Rehabilitation: A Cardiologist's Guide.* Baltimore: Williams & Wilkins, 1993;263-286.

25. Cahill K, Stead LF, Lancaster T. Nicotine receptor partial agonists for smoking cessation. *Cochrane Database Syst Rev.*; April 2012. CD006103.pub6.

26. Sotile WM. The intimacy factor in cardiopulmonary rehabilitation: a practical model for structuring interventions. *J Cardiopulm Rehabil.* 1993;13:237-242.

27. Sotile WM. *Heart Illness and Intimacy: How Caring Relationships Aid Recovery.* Baltimore: Johns Hopkins University Press, 1992.

28. Sotile WM. *Psychosocial Interventions for Cardiopulmonary Patients: A Guide for Health Professionals.* Champaign, IL: Human Kinetics, 1996.

29. Walbroehl GS. Sexual concerns of the patient with pulmonary disease. *Postgrad Med.* 1992;91:455-460.

30. Allan R, Scheidt S. *Heart and Mind: The Practice of Cardiac Psychology.* Washington, DC: American Psychological Association, 1996.

31. Matano RA, Bronstone AB. Assessment, intervention, and referral of patients suffering from alcoholism. *J Cardiopulum Rehabil.* 1994;14:27-29.

32. Williams RB, Williams V. *Anger Kills: Seventeen Strategies for Controlling the Hostility That Can Harm Your Health.* New York: Times Books, 1993.

Overweight/Obesity section

1. Klein S, Burke LE, Bray GA, et al.; American Heart Association Council on Nutrition, Physical Activity, and Metabolism. Clinical implications of obesity with specific focus on cardiovascular disease. *Circulation.* 2004;110:2952-2967.

2. Poirier P, Giles TD, Bray GA, et al. American Heart Association. Obesity and cardiovascular disease: pathophysiology, evaluation, and effect of weight loss: an update. *Circulation.* 2006;113:898-918.

3. Bader DS, Maguire TE, Spahn CM, O'Malley CJ, Balady GJ. Clinical profile and outcomes of obese patients in cardiac rehabilitation stratified according to National Heart, Lung, and Blood Institute criteria. *J Cardiopulm Rehabil.* 2001;21:210-217.

4. Lavie CJ, Milani RV. Effects of cardiac rehabilitation, exercise training, and weight reduction on exercise capacity, coronary risk factors, behavioral characteristics, and quality of life in obese coronary patients. *Am J Cardiol.* 1997;79:397-401.

5. Brochu M, Poehlman ET, Ades PA. Obesity, body fat distribution, and coronary artery disease. *J Cardiopulm Rehabil.* 2000;20:96-108.

6. Audelin MC, Savage PD, Ades PA. Changing clinical profile of patients entering cardiac rehabilitation/secondary prevention programs: 1996 to 2006. *J Cardiopulm Rehabil Prev.* 2008;28:299-306.

7. Zullo M, Dolansky MA, Jackson LW. Incorporation of core guidelines into cardiac rehabilitation practice. *J Cardiopulm Rehabil Prev.* 2010;30:267.

8. Brochu M, Poehlman ET, Savage P, Fragnoli-Munn K, Ross S, Ades PA. Modest effects of exercise training alone on coronary risk factors and body composition in coronary patients. *J Cardiopulm Rehabil.* 2000;20:180-188.

9. Milani RV, Lavie CJ. Prevalence and profile of metabolic syndrome in patients following acute coronary events and effects of therapeutic lifestyle change with cardiac rehabilitation. *Am J Cardiol.* 2003;92:50-54.

10. Eilat-Adat S, Eldar M, Goldbourt U. Association of intentional changes in body weight with coronary heart disease event rates in overweight subjects who have an additional coronary risk factor. *Am J Epidemiol.* 2005;161:352-358.

11. Sierra-Johnson J, Romero-Corral A, Somers VK, et al. Prognostic importance of weight loss in patients with coronary heart disease regardless of initial body mass index. *Eur J Cardiovasc Prev Rehabil.* 2008;15:336-340.

12. Ades PA, Savage PD, Toth MJ, et al. High-caloric expenditure exercise: a new approach to cardiac rehabilitation for overweight coronary patients. *Circulation.* 2009;119:2671-2678.

13. Savage PD, Ludlow M, Toth MJ, et al. Exercise and weight loss improves endothelial dependent vasodilatory capacity in overweight individuals with coronary heart disease. *J Cardiopulm Rehabil Prev.* 2009;29:264.

14. Keating FK, Schneider DJ, Savage PD, Bunn JY, Toth MJ, Ades PA. Platelet reactivity decreases after exercise training and weight loss in overweight patients with coronary artery disease. *Circulation.* 2009;120:S512.

15. Pope L, Harvey-Berino J, Savage P, et al. The impact of high-calorie-expenditure exercise on quality of life in older adults with coronary heart disease. *J Aging Phys Act.* 2011;19:99-116.

16. Seidell JC, Flegal KM. Assessing obesity: classification and epidemiology. *Br Med Bull.* 1997;53:238-252.

17. Expert Panel on Detection, Evaluation, and Treatment of High Blood Cholesterol in Adults. Executive summary of the Third Report of the National Cholesterol Education Program (NCEP) Expert Panel on Detection, Evaluation, and Treatment of High Blood Cholesterol in Adults (Adult Treatment Panel III). *JAMA.* 2001;285:2486-2497.

18. Savage PD, Banzer JA, Balady GJ, Ades PA. Prevalence of metabolic syndrome in cardiac rehabilitation/secondary prevention programs. *Am Heart J.* 2005;149:627-631.

19. Ford ES, Giles WH, Dietz WH. Prevalence of the metabolic syndrome among US adults: findings from the Third National Health and Nutrition Survey. *JAMA.* 2002;287:356-359.

20. Rana JS, Mukamal KJ, Morgan JP, Muller JE, Mittleman MA. Obesity and the risk of death after acute myocardial infarction. *Am Heart J.* 2004;147:841-846.

21. Wolk R, Berger P, Lennon RJ, Brilakis ES, Somers VK. Body mass index: a risk factor for unstable angina and myocardial infarction in patients with angiographically confirmed coronary artery disease. *Circulation.* 2003;108:2206-2211.

22. Wilson PW, D'Agostino RB, Sullivan L, Parise H, Kannel WB. Overweight and obesity as determinants of cardiovascular risk: the Framingham experience. *Arch Intern Med.* 2002;162:1867-1872.

23. Schwartz GG, Olsson AG, Szarek M, Sasiela WJ. Relation of characteristics of metabolic syndrome to short-term prognosis and effects of intensive statin therapy after acute coronary syndrome: an analysis of the Myocardial Ischemia Reduction with Aggressive Cholesterol Lowering (MIRACL) trial. *Diabetes Care.* 2005;28:2508-2513.

24. Levantesi G, Macchia A, Marfisi R, et al. Metabolic syndrome and risk of cardiovascular events after myocardial infarction. *J Am Coll Cardiol.* 2005;46:277-283.

25. Daly CA, Hildebrandt P, Bertrand M, et al. Adverse prognosis associated with the metabolic syndrome in established coronary artery disease: data from the EUROPA trial. *Heart.* 2007;93:1406-1411.

26. Lamonte MJ, Ainsworth BE. Quantifying energy expenditure and physical activity in the context of dose response. *Med Sci Sports Exerc.* 2001;33(6 suppl):S370-378; discussion S419-420.

27. Brownell K. *The LEARN Program for Weight Control.* Dallas: American Health, 2000.

28. Prochaska J, DiClemente C. Stages and processes of self-change of smoking: toward an integrative model of change. *J Consult Clin Psychol.* 1983;51:390-395.

29. Ades PA, Savage PD, Harvey-Berino J. The treatment of obesity in cardiac rehabilitation. *J Cardiopulm Rehabil Prev.* 2010;30:289-298.

30. Harvey-Berino J. Weight loss in the clinical setting: applications for cardiac rehabilitation. *Coron Artery Dis.* 1998;9:795-798.

31. Savage PD, Lee M, Harvey-Berino J, Brochu M, Ades PA. Weight reduction in the cardiac rehabilitation setting. *J Cardiopulm Rehabil.* 2002;22:154-160.

32. Wadden TA, Butryn ML, Wilson C. Lifestyle modification for the management of obesity. *Gastroenterology.* 2007;132:2226-2238.

33. Lichtenstein AH, Appel LJ, Brands M, et al. Summary of American Heart Association diet and lifestyle recommendations revision. *Arterioscler Thromb Vasc Biol.* 2006;26:2186-2191.

34. Larsen TM, Dalskov SM, van Baak M, et al. Diets with high or low protein content and glycemic index for weight-loss maintenance. Diet, Obesity, and Genes (Diogenes) Project. *NEJM.* 2010;363:2102-2113.

35. Noakes M, Keogh JB, Foster PR, Clifton PM. Effect of an energy-restricted, high-protein, low-fat diet relative to a conventional high-carbohydrate, low-fat diet on weight loss, body composition, nutritional status, and markers of cardiovascular health in obese women. *Am J Clin Nutr.* 2005;81:1298-1306.

36. Claessens M, van Baak MA, Monsheimer S, Saris WH. The effect of a low-fat, high-protein or high-carbohydrate ad libitum diet on weight loss maintenance and metabolic risk factors. *Int J Obes (Lond).* 2009;33:296-304.

37. Gardner CD, Kiazand A, Alhassan S, et al. Comparison of the Atkins, Zone, Ornish, and LEARN diets for change in weight and related risk factors among overweight premenopausal women: the A TO Z Weight Loss Study: a randomized trial. *JAMA.* 2007;297:969-977. Erratum in: *JAMA.* 2007;298:178.

38. Mertens DJ, Kavanagh T, Campbell RB, Shephard RJ. Exercise without dietary restriction as a means to long-term fat loss in the obese cardiac patient. *J Sports Med Phys Fitness.* 1998;38:310-316.

39. Savage PD, Brochu M, Poehlman ET, Ades PA. Reduction in obesity and coronary risk factors after high caloric exercise training in overweight coronary patients. *Am Heart J.* 2003;146:317-323.

40. Donnelly JE, Blair SN, Jakicic JM, Manore MM, Rankin JW, Smith BK. American College of Sports Medicine position stand. Appropriate physical activity intervention strategies for weight loss and prevention of weight regain for adults. *Med Sci Sports Exerc.* 2009;41:459-471. Erratum in: *Med Sci Sports Exerc.* 2009;41:1532.

41. Swain DP, Franklin BA. Is there a threshold intensity for aerobic training in cardiac patients? *Med Sci Sports Exerc.* 2002;34:1071-1075.

42. Hamm LF, Kavanagh T, Campbell RB, et al. Timeline for peak improvements during 52 weeks of outpatient cardiac rehabilitation. *J Cardiopulm Rehabil.* 2004;24:374-380.

43. Zeni AI, Hoffman MD, Clifford PS. Energy expenditure with indoor exercise machines. *JAMA.* 1996;275:1424-1427.

44. Levine JA. Nonexercise activity thermogenesis—liberating the life-force. *J Intern Med.* 2007;262:273-287.

45. U.S. Department of Health and Human Services. 2008. *Physical Activity Guidelines for Americans.* Washington, DC: USDHHS. www.health.gov/paguidelines.

46. American College of Sports Medicine. *ACSM's Guidelines for Exercise Testing and Prescription.* 9th ed. Baltimore: Lippincott Williams & Wilkins, 2014:320.

47. Healy GN, Dunstan DW, Salmon J, et al. Breaks in sedentary time: beneficial associations with metabolic risk. *Diabetes Care.* 2008;31:661-666.

Emerging Risk Factors section

1. Khot UN, Khot MB, Bajer CT, et al. Prevalence of conventional risk factors in patients with coronary heart disease. *JAMA.* 2003;290:898-904.

2. Greenland P, Knoll MD, Stamler J, et al. Major risk factors as antecedents of fatal and non-fatal coronary heart disease events. *JAMA.* 2003;290:891-897.

3. Iqbal R, Anand S, Ounpuu S, et al. Dietary patterns and risk of myocardial infarction in 52 countries: results of the INTERHEART study. *Circulation.* 2008;118:1929-1937.

4. Anand S, Islam S, Rosengren A, et al. Risk factors for myocardial infarction in women and men: insights from the INTERHEART study. *Eur Heart J.* 2008;29:932-940.

5. van Dam RM, Willett WC. Unmet potential for cardiovascular disease prevention in the United States. *Circulation.* 2009;120:1171-1173.

6. Clarke R, Halsey J, Lewington S, et al. Effects of lowering homocysteine levels with B vitamins

on cardiovascular disease, cancer, and cause-specific mortality: meta-analysis of 8 randomized trials involving 37,485 individuals. *Arch Intern Med.* 2010;170:1622-1631.

7. Ebbing M, Bonaa KH, Arnesen E, et al. Combined analyses and extended follow-up of two randomized controlled homocysteine-lowering B-vitamin trials. *J Intern Med.* 2010;268:367-382.

8. Miller ER, Juraschek S, Pastor-Barriuso R, et al. Meta-analysis of folic acid supplementation trials on risk of cardiovascular disease and risk interaction with baseline homocysteine levels. *Am J Cardiol.* 2010;106:517-527.

9. Armitage JM, Bowman L, Clarke RJ, et al. Effects of homocysteine-lowering with folic acid plus vitamin B12 vs placebo on mortality and major morbidity in myocardial infarction survivors: a randomized trial. *JAMA.* 2010;303:2486-2494.

10. Gudnason V. Lipoprotein(a): a causal independent risk factor for coronary heart disease? *Curr Opin Cardiol.* 2009;24:490-495.

11. Kamstrup PR. Lipoprotein(a) and ischemic heart disease-a causal association? A review. *Atherosclerosis.* 2010;211:15-23.

12. Erqou S, Kaptoge S, Perry PL, et al. Lipoprotein(a) concentration and the risk of coronary heart disease, stroke, and nonvascular mortality. *JAMA.* 2009;302:412-433.

13. Bermudez V, Arraiz N, Aparicio D, et al. Lipoprotein(a): from molecules to therapeutics. *Am J Ther.* 2010;17:263-273.

14. Tziomalos K, Athyros G, Wierzbicki AS, Mikhailidis DP. Lipoprotein(a): where are we now? *Curr Opin Cardiol.* 2009;24:351-357.

15. Nordestgaard BG, Chapman MJ, Ray K, et al. Lipoprotein(a) as a cardiovascular risk factor: current status. *Eur Heart J.* 2010;23:2844-2853.

16. Myers GL, Christenson RHM, Cushman M, et al. National Academy of Clinical Biochemistry Laboratory Medicine practice guidelines: emerging biomarkers for primary prevention of cardiovascular disease. *Clin Chem.* 2009;55:378-384.

17. He LP, Tang XY, Ling WH, Chen WQ, Chen YM. Early C-reactive protein in the prediction of long-term outcomes after acute coronary syndromes: a meta-analysis of longitudinal studies. *Heart.* 2010;96:339-346.

18. Li JJ, Ren Y, Chen KJ, et al. Impact of C-reactive protein on in-stent restenosis: a meta-analysis. *Tex Heart Inst J.* 2010;37:49-57.

19. Ridker PM, MacFayden J, Libby P, Glynn RJ. Relation of baseline high-sensitivity C-reactive protein level to cardiovascular outcomes with rosuvastatin in Justification for Use of statins in Prevention: an Intervention Trial Evaluating Rosuvastatin (JUPITER). *Am J Cardiol.* 2010;106:204-209.

Chapter 9

Cardiac Rehabilitation and Secondary Prevention in Older and Younger Adults section

1. Audelin MC, Savage PD, Ades PA. Changing clinical profile of patients entering cardiac rehabilitation/secondary prevention programs: 1996 to 2006. *J Cardiopulm Rehabil Prev.* 2008;28:299-306.

2. Pinsky JL, Jette AM, Branch LG, Kannel WB, Feinleib M. The Framingham Disability Study: relationship of various coronary heart disease manifestations to disability in older persons living in the community. *Am J Public Health.* 1990;80:1363-1367.

3. Alexander KP, Newby LK, Cannon CP, et al. Acute coronary care in the elderly, part I: non-ST-segment-elevation acute coronary syndromes: a scientific statement for healthcare professionals from the American Heart Association in collaboration with the Society of Geriatric Cardiology. *Circulation.* 2007;115:2549-2569.

4. Tresch DD, Alla HR. Diagnosis and management of myocardial ischemia (angina) in the elderly patient. *Am J Geriatr Cardiol.* 2001;10:337-344.

5. Madala MC, Franklin BA, Chen AY, et al. Obesity and age of first non-ST-segment elevation myocardial infarction. *Am J Coll Cardiol.* 2008;52:979-985.

6. De S, Searles G, Haddad H. The prevalence of cardiac risk factors in women 45 years of age or younger undergoing angiography for evaluation of undiagnosed chest pain. *Can J Cardiol.* 2002;18:945-948.

7. Audelin MC, Savage PD, Ades PA. Exercise-based cardiac rehabilitation for very old patients (≥75 years): focus on physical function. *J Cardiopulm Rehabil Prev.* 2008;28:163-173.

8. Suaya JA, Stason WB, Ades PA, Normand, SLT, Shepard DS. Cardiac rehabilitation and survival

in older coronary patients. *J Am Coll Cardiol.* 2009;54:25-33.

9. Ades PA, Pashkow F, Nestor J. Cost-effectiveness of cardiac rehabilitation after myocardial infarction. *J Cardiopulm Rehabil.* 1997;17:222-231.

10. Lee AJ, Shepard DS. Costs of cardiac rehabilitation and enhanced lifestyle modification programs. *J Cardiopulm Rehabil Prev.* 2009;29:348-357.

11. Suaya JA, Shepard DS, Normand SLT, Ades PA, Prottas J, Stason WB. Use of cardiac rehabilitation by Medicare beneficiaries after myocardial infarction or coronary bypass surgery. *Circulation.* 2007;116:1653-1662.

12. Ades PA, Waldmann ML, McCann W, Weaver SO. Predictors of cardiac rehabilitation participation in older coronary patients. *Arch Intern Med.* 1992;152:1033-1035.

13. Curnier D, Savage PD, Ades PA. Geographic distribution of cardiac rehabilitation programs in the U.S. *J Cardiopulm Rehabil.* 2005;25:80-84.

14. Gurewich D, Prottas J, Bhalotra S, Suaya JA, Shepard DS. System-level factors and use of cardiac rehabilitation. *J Cardiopulm Rehabil Prev.* 2008;28:380-385.

15. Ades PA, Savage PD, Brawner CA, et al. Aerobic capacity in patients entering cardiac rehabilitation. *Circulation.* 2006;113:2706-2712.

16. Ades PA, Savage PD, Tischler MD, Poehlman ET, Dee J, Niggel J. Determinants of disability in older coronary patients. *Am Heart J.* 2002;143:151-156.

17. Sanderson B, Bittner V. Practical interpretation of 6-minute walk data using healthy adult reference equations. *J Cardiopulm Rehabil.* 2006;26:167-171.

18. Ades PA, Savage PD, Cress ME, Brochu M, Lee NM, Poehlman ET. Resistance training improves performance of daily activities in disabled older women with coronary heart disease. *Med Sci Sports Exerc.* 2003;35:1265-1270.

19. Brochu M, Savage P, Lee M, et al. Effects of resistance training on physical function in older disabled women with coronary heart disease. *J Appl Physiol.* 2002;92:672-678.

20. Ades PA, Ballor DL, Ashikage T, Utton JL, Nair KS. Weight training improves walking endurance in the healthy elderly. *Ann Intern Med.* 1996;124:568-572.

21. Williams MA, Fleg JL, Ades PA, et al. Secondary prevention of coronary heart disease in the elderly (with emphasis on patients ≥75 years of age): an American Heart Association scientific statement. *Circulation.* 2002;105:1735-1743.

22. Wannamethee SG, Shaper AG, Walker M. Physical activity and mortality in older men with diagnosed coronary heart disease. *Circulation.* 2000;102:1358-1363.

23. Williams MA, Haskell WL, Ades PA, et al. Resistance exercise in individuals with and without cardiovascular disease: 2007 update: a scientific statement from the American Heart Association. *Circulation.* 2007;116:572-584.

24. American College of Sports Medicine. *ACSM's Guidelines for Exercise Testing and Prescription.* 8th ed. Philadelphia: Lippincott Williams & Wilkins, 2009.

25. Ades PA, Maloney AE, Savage P, Carhart RL Jr. Determinants of physical function in coronary patients: response to cardiac rehabilitation. *Arch Intern Med.* 1999;159:2357-2360.

26. Miettinen TA, Pyorala K, Olsson AG, et al. Cholesterol-lowering therapy in women and elderly patients with myocardial infarction or angina pectoris: findings from the Scandinavian Simvastatin Survival Study (4S). *Circulation.* 1997;96:4211-4218.

27. Fleg JL, Aronow WS, Frishman WH. Cardiovascular drug therapy in the elderly: benefits and challenges. *Nat Rev Cardiol.* 2011;8:13-28.

28. Grundy SM, Cleeman JI, Merz CN, et al. Implications of recent clinical trials for the National Cholesterol Education Program Adult Treatment Panel III guidelines. *J Am Coll Cardiol.* 2004;44:720-732.

29. Ades PA, Savage PD, Poehlman ET, Brochu M, Fragnoli-Munn K, Carhart RL Jr. Lipid lowering in the cardiac rehabilitation setting. *J Cardiopulm Rehabil.* 1999;19:255-260.

30. Siebenhofer A, Jeitler K, Berghold A, et al. Long-term effects of weight-reducing diets in hypertensive patients. *Cochrane Database Syst Rev.* 2011;9:CD008274.

31. Pescatello LS, Franklin BA, Fagard R, et al. American College of Sports Medicine position stand. Exercise and hypertension. *Med Sci Sports Exerc.* 2004;36:533-553.

32. Appel LJ, Moore TJ, Obarzanek E, et al.; DASH Collaborative Research Group. A clinical trial of the effects of dietary patterns on blood pressure. *NEJM.* 1997;336:1117-1124.

33. Savage PD, Banzer JA, Balady GJ, Ades PA. Prevalence of metabolic syndrome in cardiac rehabilitation/secondary prevention programs. *Am Heart J.* 2005;149:627-631.

34. Grundy SM, Cleeman JI, Daniels SR, et al. Diagnosis and management of the metabolic syndrome: an American Heart Association/National Heart, Lung, and Blood Institute scientific statement. *Circulation.* 2005;112:2735-2752.

35. Milani RV, Lavie CJ. Prevalence and profile of metabolic syndrome in patients following acute coronary events and effects of therapeutic lifestyle change with cardiac rehabilitation. Am J Cardiol. 2003;92:50-54.

36. Ades PA, Savage PD, Toth MJ, et al. High-caloric expenditure exercise: a new approach to cardiac rehabilitation for overweight coronary patients. *Circulation.* 2009;119:2671-2678.

37. Brownell K. *The LEARN Program for Weight Control.* 10th ed. Dallas: American Health, 2004.

38. Harvey-Berino J. Weight loss in the clinical setting: applications for cardiac rehabilitation. *Coron Artery Dis.* 1998;9:795-798.

39. Savage PD, Ades PA. Pedometer step counts predict cardiac risk factors at entry to cardiac rehabilitation. *J Cardiopulm Rehabil Prev.* 2008;28:370-377.

40. Romanelli J, Fauerbach JA, Bush DE, Ziegelstein RC. The significance of depression in older patients after myocardial infarction. *J Am Geriatr Soc.* 2002;50:817-882.

41. Somberg TC, Arora RR. Depression and heart disease: therapeutic implications. *Cardiology.* 2008;11:75-81.

42. Whalley B, Rees K, Davies P, et al. Psychological interventions for coronary heart disease. *Cochrane Database Syst Rev.* 2011;8:CD002902.

43. Blumenthal JA, Babyak MA, Carney RM, et al. Exercise, depression, and mortality after myocardial infarction in the ENRICHD trial. *Med Sci Sports Exerc.* 2004;3:746-755.

44. Yesavage JA, Brink TL, Rose TL, et al. Development and validation of a geriatric depression screening scale: a preliminary report. *J Psychiatr Res.* 1982-1983;17:37-49.

45. Kroenke K, Spitzer RL, Williams JB. The PHQ-9: validity of a brief depression severity measure. *J Gen Intern Med.* 2001;1:606-613.

46. Heffner JE, Barbieri C. Involvement of cardiovascular rehabilitation programs in advance directive education. *Arch Intern Med.* 1996;156:1746-1751.

47. Iso H, Date C, Yamamoto A, et al. Smoking cessation and mortality from cardiovascular disease among Japanese men and women: the JACC Study. *Am J Epidemiol.* 2005;161: 170-179.

48. Hermanson B, Omenn GS, Kronmal RA, Gersh BJ. Beneficial six-year outcome of smoking cessation in older men and women with coronary artery disease. Results from the CASS registry. *NEJM.* 1988;319:1365-1369.

49. Reid RD, Mullen KA, Pipe AL. Systematic approaches to smoking cessation in the cardiac setting. *Curr Opin Cardiol.* 2011;5:443-448.

50. Lavie CJ, Milani RV. Adverse psychological and coronary risk profiles in young patients with coronary artery disease and benefits of formal cardiac rehabilitation. *Arch Intern Med.* 2006;166:1878-1883.

Women section

1. Roger VL, Go AS, Lloyd-Jones DM, et al. Heart disease and stroke statistics—2011 update: a report from the American Heart Association. *Circulation.* 2011;123:e18-e209.

2. Ruff CT, Braunwald E. The evolving epidemiology of acute coronary syndromes. *Nat Rev Cardiol.* 2011;8:140-147.

3. Hemingway H, Langenberg C, Damant J, Frost C, Pyorala K, Barrett-Connor E. Prevalence of angina in women versus men: a systematic review and meta-analysis of international variations across 31 countries. *Circulation.* 2008;117:1526-1536.

4. Canto JG, Rogers WJ, Goldberg RJ, et al. Association of age and sex with myocardial infarction symptom presentation and in-hospital mortality. *JAMA.* 2012;307:813-822.

5. Mosca L, Barrett-Connor E, Wenger NK. Sex/gender differences in cardiovascular disease prevention: what a difference a decade makes. *Circulation.* 2011;124:2145-2154.

6. Anand SS, Islam S, Rosengren A, et al. Risk factors for myocardial infarction in women and men: insights from the INTERHEART study. *Eur Heart J.* 2008;29:932-940.

7. Jacobs AK. Coronary intervention in 2009: are women no different than men? *Circ Cardiovasc Interv.* 2009;2:69-78.

8. Vaccarino V, Parsons L, Peterson ED, Rogers WJ, Kiefe CI, Canto J. Sex differences in mortality after acute myocardial infarction: changes from 1994 to 2006. *Arch Intern Med.* 2009;169:1767-1774.

9. Kramer MC, Rittersma SZ, de Winter RJ, et al. Relationship of thrombus healing to underlying plaque morphology in sudden coronary death. *J Am Coll Cardiol.* 2010;55:122-132.

10. Poon S, Goodman SG, Yan RT, et al. Bridging the gender gap: insights from a contemporary analysis of sex-related differences in the treatment and outcomes of patients with acute coronary syndromes. *Am Heart J.* 2012;163:66-73.

11. Ford ES, Ajani UA, Croft JB, et al. Explaining the decrease in U.S. deaths from coronary disease, 1980-2000. *NEJM.* 2007;356:2388-2398.

12. Nguyen HL, Saczynski JS, Gore JM, et al. Long-term trends in short-term outcomes in acute myocardial infarction. *Am J Med.* 2011;124:939-946.

13. Humphries SE, Drenos F, Ken-Dror G, Talmud PJ. Coronary heart disease risk prediction in the era of genome-wide association studies: current status and what the future holds. *Circulation.* 2010;121:2235-2248.

14. Levit RD, Reynolds HR, Hochman JS. Cardiovascular disease in young women: a population at risk. *Cardiol Rev.* 2011;19:60-65.

15. Beckie TM, Groer MW, Beckstead JW. The relationship between polymorphisms on chromosome 9p21 and age of onset of coronary heart disease in black and white women. *Genet Test Mol Biomarkers.* 2011;15:435-442.

16. Beckie TM, Beckstead JW, Groer MW. The association between variants on chromosome 9p21 and inflammatory biomarkers in ethnically diverse women with coronary heart disease: a pilot study. *Biol Res Nurs.* 2011;13:306-319.

17. Preis SR, Hwang SJ, Coady S, et al. Trends in all-cause and cardiovascular disease mortality among women and men with and without diabetes mellitus in the Framingham Heart Study, 1950 to 2005. *Circulation.* 2009;119:1728-1735.

18. Mente A, Yusuf S, Islam S, et al. Metabolic syndrome and risk of acute myocardial infarction: a case-control study of 26,903 subjects from 52 countries. *J Am Coll Cardiol.* 2010;55:2390-2398.

19. Freund KM, Jacobs AK, Pechacek JA, White HF, Ash AS. Disparities by race, ethnicity, and sex in treating acute coronary syndromes. *J Womens Health.* 2012;21:126-132.

20. Mosca L, Mochari-Greenberger H, Dolor RJ, Newby LK, Robb KJ. Twelve-year follow-up of American women's awareness of cardiovascular disease risk and barriers to heart health. *Circ Cardiovasc Qual Outcomes.* 2010;3:120-127.

21. Mochari-Greenberger H, Mills T, Simpson SL, Mosca L. Knowledge, preventive action, and barriers to cardiovascular disease prevention by race and ethnicity in women: an American Heart Association national survey. *J Womens Health.* 2010;19:1243-1249.

22. Arslanian-Engoren C, Patel A, Fang J, et al. Symptoms of men and women presenting with acute coronary syndromes. *Am J Cardiol.* 2006;98:1177-1181.

23. McSweeney JC, Cleves MA, Zhao W, Lefler LL, Yang S. Cluster analysis of women's prodromal and acute myocardial infarction symptoms by race and other characteristics. *J Cardiovasc Nurs.* 2010;25:311-322.

24. McSweeney JC, O'Sullivan P, Cleves MA, et al. Racial differences in women's prodromal and acute symptoms of myocardial infarction. *Am J Crit Care.* 2010;19:63-73.

25. Berger JS, Elliott L, Gallup D, et al. Sex differences in mortality following acute coronary syndromes. *JAMA.* 2009;302:874-882.

26. Vaccarino V, Lin ZQ, Kasl SV, et al. Sex differences in health status after coronary artery bypass surgery. *Circulation.* 2003;108:2642-2647.

27. Ware JE, Kosinski M, Dewey JE. *How to Score Version 2 of the SF-36 Health Survey.* Lincoln, RI: QualityMetric Inc., 2000.

28. Balady GJ, Williams MA, Ades PA, et al. Core components of cardiac rehabilitation/secondary prevention programs: 2007 update: a scientific statement from the American Heart Association and the American Association of Cardiovascular and Pulmonary Rehabilitation. *J Cardiopulm Rehabil Prev.* 2007;27:121-129.

29. Pischke CR, Weidner G, Elliott-Eller M, et al. Comparison of coronary risk factors and quality of life in coronary artery disease patients with versus without diabetes mellitus. *Am J Cardiol.* 2006;97:1267-1273.

30. Lau-Walker M. Importance of illness beliefs and self-efficacy for patients with coronary heart disease. *J Adv Nurs.* 2007;60:187-198.

31. Husak L, Krumholz HM, Lin ZQ, et al. Social support as a predictor of participation in cardiac

rehabilitation after coronary artery bypass graft surgery. *J Cardiopulm Rehabil.* 2004;24:19-26.

32. Moore SM. Women's views of cardiac rehabilitation programs. *J Cardiopulm Rehabil.* 1996;16:123-129.

33. Beckie TM, Fletcher GF, Beckstead JW, Schocken DD, Evans ME. Adverse baseline physiological and psychosocial profiles of women enrolled in a cardiac rehabilitation clinical trial. *J Cardiopulm Rehabil Prev.* 2008;28:52-60.

34. Mead H, Andres E, Katch H, Siegel B, Regenstein M. Gender differences in psychosocial issues affecting low-income, underserved patients' ability to manage cardiovascular disease. *Womens Health Issues.* 2010;20:308-315.

35. Pilote L, Dasgupta K, Guru V, et al. A comprehensive view of sex-specific issues related to cardiovascular disease. *Can Med Assoc J.* 2007;176:S1-44.

36. Frasure-Smith N, Lesperance F, Habra M, et al. Elevated depression symptoms predict long-term cardiovascular mortality in patients with atrial fibrillation and heart failure. *Circulation.* 2009;120:134-140.

37. Todaro JF, Shen BJ, Niaura R, Tilkemeier PL. Prevalence of depressive disorders in men and women enrolled in cardiac rehabilitation. *J Cardiopulm Rehabil.* 2005;25:71-75.

38. Mallik S, Spertus JA, Reid KJ, et al. Depressive symptoms after acute myocardial infarction: evidence for highest rates in younger women. *Arch Intern Med.* 2006;166:876-883.

39. Whooley MA, de Jonge P, Vittinghoff E, et al. Depressive symptoms, health behaviors, and risk of cardiovascular events in patients with coronary heart disease. *JAMA.* 2008;300:2379-2388.

40. Mallik S, Krumholz HM, Lin ZQ, et al. Patients with depressive symptoms have lower health status benefits after coronary artery bypass surgery. *Circulation.* 2005;111:271-277.

41. Swardfager W, Herrmann N, Dowlati Y, Oh P, Kiss A, Lanctot KL. Relationship between cardiopulmonary fitness and depressive symptoms in cardiac rehabilitation patients with coronary artery disease. *J Rehabil Med.* 2008;40:213-218.

42. Rutledge T, Linke SE, Krantz DS, et al. Comorbid depression and anxiety symptoms as predictors of cardiovascular events: results from the NHLBI-sponsored Women's Ischemia Syndrome Evaluation (WISE) study. *Psychosom Med.* 2009;71:958-964.

43. Frasure-Smith N, Lesperance F, Juneau M, Talajic M, Bourassa MG. Gender, depression, and one-year prognosis after myocardial infarction. *Psychosom Med.* 1999;61:26-37.

44. Frasure-Smith N, Lesperance F, Talajic M. Depression following myocardial infarction. Impact on 6-month survival. *JAMA.* 1993;270:1819-1825.

45. Williams SA, Kasl SV, Heiat A, Abramson JL, Krumholz HM, Vaccarino V. Depression and risk of heart failure among the elderly: a prospective community-based study. *Psychosom Med.* 2002;64:6-12.

46. Mendes de Leon CF, Krumholz HM, Seeman TS, et al. Depression and risk of coronary heart disease in elderly men and women: New Haven EPESE, 1982-1991. Established Populations for the Epidemiologic Studies of the Elderly. *Arch Intern Med.* 1998;158:2341-2348.

47. Wenger NK. Current status of cardiac rehabilitation. *J Am Coll Cardiol.* 2008;51:1619-1631.

48. Caulin-Glaser T, Maciejewski PK, Snow R, LaLonde M, Mazure C. Depressive symptoms and sex affect completion rates and clinical outcomes in cardiac rehabilitation. *Prev Cardiol.* 2007;10:15-21.

49. Komorovsky R, Desideri A, Rozbowsky P, Sabbadin D, Celegon L, Gregori D. Quality of life and behavioral compliance in cardiac rehabilitation patients: a longitudinal survey. *Int J Nurs Stud.* 2008;45:979-985.

50. Casey E, Hughes JW, Waechter D, Josephson R, Rosneck J. Depression predicts failure to complete phase-II cardiac rehabilitation. *J Behav Med.* 2008;31:421-431.

51. Kronish IM, Rieckmann N, Halm EA, et al. Persistent depression affects adherence to secondary prevention behaviors after acute coronary syndromes. *J Gen Intern Med.* 2006;21:1178-1183.

52. Gehi A, Haas D, Pipkin S, Whooley MA. Depression and medication adherence in outpatients with coronary heart disease: findings from the Heart and Soul Study. *Arch Intern Med.* 2005;165:2508-2513.

53. Hammill BG, Curtis LH, Schulman KA, Whellan DJ. Relationship between cardiac rehabilitation and long-term risks of death and myocardial infarction among elderly Medicare beneficiaries. *Circulation.* 2010;121:63-70.

54. Lichtman JH, Bigger JT Jr, Blumenthal JA, et al. Depression and coronary heart disease: recom-

mendations for screening, referral, and treatment: a science advisory from the American Heart Association. *Circulation.* 2008;118:1768-1775.

55. Kroenke K, Spitzer RL, Williams JB. The Patient Health Questionnaire-2: validity of a two-item depression screener. *Med Care.* 2003;41:1284-1292.

56. Kroenke K, Spitzer RL, Williams JB. The PHQ-9: validity of a brief depression severity measure. *J Gen Intern Med.* 2001;16:606-613.

57. Hamm LF, Sanderson BK, Ades PA, et al. Core competencies for cardiac rehabilitation/secondary prevention professionals: 2010 update: position statement of the American Association of Cardiovascular and Pulmonary Rehabilitation. *J Cardiopulm Rehabil Prev.* 2011;31:2-10.

58. Mosca L, Benjamin EJ, Berra K, et al. Effectiveness-based guidelines for the prevention of cardiovascular disease in women—2011 update: a guideline from the American Heart Association. *Circulation.* 2011;123:1243-1262.

59. Piepoli MF, Corra U, Benzer W, et al. Secondary prevention through cardiac rehabilitation: from knowledge to implementation. A position paper from the Cardiac Rehabilitation Section of the European Association of Cardiovascular Prevention and Rehabilitation. *Eur J Cardiovasc Prev Rehabil.* 2010;17:1-17.

60. Balady GJ, Ades PA, Bittner VA, et al. Referral, enrollment, and delivery of cardiac rehabilitation/secondary prevention programs at clinical centers and beyond: a presidential advisory from the American Heart Association. *Circulation.* 2011;124:2951-2960.

61. Suaya JA, Stason WB, Ades PA, Normand SL, Shepard DS. Cardiac rehabilitation and survival in older coronary patients. *J Am Coll Cardiol.* 2009;54:25-33.

62. Smith SC Jr, Benjamin EJ, Bonow RO, et al. AHA/ACCF secondary prevention and risk reduction therapy for patients with coronary and other atherosclerotic vascular disease: 2011 update: a guideline from the American Heart Association and American College of Cardiology Foundation. *Circulation.* 2011;124:2458-2473.

63. Allen JK, Scott LB, Stewart KJ, Young DR. Disparities in women's referral to and enrollment in outpatient cardiac rehabilitation. *J Gen Intern Med.* 2004;19:747-753.

64. Suaya JA, Shepard DS, Normand SL, Ades PA, Prottas J, Stason WB. Use of cardiac rehabilitation by Medicare beneficiaries after myocardial infarction or coronary bypass surgery. *Circulation.* 2007;116:1653-1662.

65. Scott LA, Ben-Or K, Allen JK. Why are women missing from outpatient cardiac rehabilitation programs? A review of multilevel factors affecting referral, enrollment, and completion. *J Womens Health.* 2002;11:773-791.

66. Bethell H, Lewin R, Dalal H. Cardiac rehabilitation in the United Kingdom. *Heart.* 2009;95:271-275.

67. Beckie TM, Mendonca MA, Fletcher GF, Schocken DD, Evans ME, Banks SM. Examining the challenges of recruiting women into a cardiac rehabilitation clinical trial. *J Cardiopulm Rehabil Prev.* 2009;29:13-21.

68. Ades PA, Waldmann ML, Polk DM, Coflesky JT. Referral patterns and exercise response in the rehabilitation of female coronary patients aged greater than or equal to 62 years. *Am J Cardiol.* 1992;69:1422-1425.

69. Grace SL, Gravely-Witte S, Kayaniyil S, Brual J, Suskin N, Stewart DE. A multisite examination of sex differences in cardiac rehabilitation barriers by participation status. *J Womens Health.* 2009;18:209-216.

70. Rolfe DE, Sutton EJ, Landry M, Sternberg L, Price JA. Women's experiences accessing a women-centered cardiac rehabilitation program: a qualitative study. *J Cardiovasc Nurs.* 2010;25:332-341.

71. Witt BJ, Jacobsen SJ, Weston SA, et al. Cardiac rehabilitation after myocardial infarction in the community. *J Am Coll Cardiol.* 2004;44:988-996.

72. Sanderson BK, Bittner V. Women in cardiac rehabilitation: outcomes and identifying risk for dropout. *Am Heart J.* 2005;150:1052-1058.

73. Audelin MC, Savage PD, Ades PA. Changing clinical profile of patients entering cardiac rehabilitation/secondary prevention programs: 1996 to 2006. *J Cardiopulm Rehabil Prev.* 2008;28:299-306.

74. Worcester MU, Murphy BM, Mee VK, Roberts SB, Goble AJ. Cardiac rehabilitation programmes: predictors of non-attendance and drop-out. *Eur J Cardiovasc Prev Rehabil.* 2004;11:328-335.

75. Marzolini S, Brooks D, Oh PI. Sex differences in completion of a 12-month cardiac rehabilitation programme: an analysis of 5922 women and men. *Eur J Cardiovasc Prev Rehabil.* 2008;15:698-703.

76. Brual J, Gravely-Witte S, Suskin N, Stewart DE, Macpherson A, Grace SL. Drive time to cardiac rehabilitation: at what point does it affect utilization? *Int J Health Geogr.* 2010;9:27.

77. Emslie C. Women, men and coronary heart disease: a review of the qualitative literature. *J Adv Nurs.* 2005;51:382-395.

78. Beckie TM, Beckstead JW. Predicting cardiac rehabilitation attendance in a gender-tailored randomized clinical trial. *J Cardiopulm Rehabil Prev.* 2010;30:147-156.

79. Glazer KM, Emery CF, Frid DJ, Banyasz RE. Psychological predictors of adherence and outcomes among patients in cardiac rehabilitation. *J Cardiopulm Rehabil.* 2002;22:40-46.

80. Parkosewich JA. Cardiac rehabilitation barriers and opportunities among women with cardiovascular disease. *Cardiol Rev.* 2008;16:36-52.

81. Beckie TM, Beckstead JW, Schocken DD, Evans ME, Fletcher GF. The effects of a tailored cardiac rehabilitation program on depressive symptoms in women: a randomized clinical trial. *Int J Nurs Stud.* 2011;48:3-12.

82. Clark AM, Barbour RS, White M, MacIntyre PD. Promoting participation in cardiac rehabilitation: patient choices and experiences. *J Adv Nurs.* 2004;47:5-14.

83. Jackson L, Leclerc J, Erskine Y, Linden W. Getting the most out of cardiac rehabilitation: a review of referral and adherence predictors. *Heart.* 2005;91:10-14.

84. Reid RD, Morrin LI, Pipe AL, et al. Determinants of physical activity after hospitalization for coronary artery disease: the Tracking Exercise After Cardiac Hospitalization (TEACH) Study. *Eur J Cardiovasc Prev Rehabil.* 2006;13:529-537.

85. Davidson PM, Daly J, Hancock K, Moser D, Chang E, Cockburn J. Perceptions and experiences of heart disease: a literature review and identification of a research agenda in older women. *Eur J Cardiovasc Nurs.* 2003;2:255-264.

86. Beckie TM. A behavior change intervention for women in cardiac rehabilitation. *J Cardiovasc Nurs.* 2006;21:146-153.

87. Lloyd GW. Preventive cardiology and cardiac rehabilitation programmes in women. *Maturitas.* 2009;63:28-33.

88. Daly J, Sindone AP, Thompson DR, Hancock K, Chang E, Davidson P. Barriers to participation in and adherence to cardiac rehabilitation programs: a critical literature review. *Prog Cardiovasc Nurs.* 2002;17:8-17.

89. Davidson P, Digiacomo M, Zecchin R, et al. A cardiac rehabilitation program to improve psychosocial outcomes of women with heart disease. *J Womens Health.* 2008;17:123-134.

90. Beckie TM, Beckstead JW. The effects of a cardiac rehabilitation program tailored for women on their perceptions of health: a randomized clinical trial. *J Cardiopulm Rehabil Prev.* 2011;31:25-34.

91. Beckie TM, Beckstead JW. The effects of a cardiac rehabilitation program tailored for women on global quality of life: a randomized clinical trial. *J Womens Health.* 2010;19:1977-1985.

92. Miller WR, Rollnick S. Ten things that motivational interviewing is not. *Behav Cogn Psychother.* 2009;37:129-140.

93. Prochaska JO, Norcross JC, DiClemente CC. *Changing for Good.* New York: HarperCollins, 1994.

94. Rollnick S, Miller W, Butler C. *Motivational Interviewing in Health Care: Helping Patients Change Behavior.* New York: Guilford Press, 2008.

95. Jolly K, Taylor RS, Lip GY, Stevens A. Home-based cardiac rehabilitation compared with centre-based rehabilitation and usual care: a systematic review and meta-analysis. *Int J Cardiol.* 2006;111:343-351.

96. Oerkild B, Frederiksen M, Hansen JF, Simonsen L, Skovgaard LT, Prescott E. Home-based cardiac rehabilitation is as effective as centre-based cardiac rehabilitation among elderly with coronary heart disease: results from a randomised clinical trial. *Age Ageing.* 2011;40:78-85.

97. Walters DL, Sarela A, Fairfull A, et al. A mobile phone-based care model for outpatient cardiac rehabilitation: the care assessment platform (CAP). *BMC Cardiovasc Disord.* 2010;10:5.

98. Maddison R, Whittaker R, Stewart R, et al. HEART: heart exercise and remote technologies: a randomized controlled trial study protocol. *BMC Cardiovasc Disord.* 2011;11:26.

99. Artinian NT, Fletcher GF, Mozaffarian D, et al. Interventions to promote physical activity and dietary lifestyle changes for cardiovascular risk factor reduction in adults: a scientific statement from the American Heart Association. *Circulation.* 2010;122:406-441.

100. Riegel B, Moser DK, Anker SD, et al. State of the science: promoting self-care in persons with heart failure: a scientific statement from the American Heart Association. *Circulation.* 2009;120:1141-1163.

101. Thomas D, Vydelingum V, Lawrence J. E-mail contact as an effective strategy in the maintenance of weight loss in adults. *J Hum Nutr Diet.* 2011;24:32-38.

102. Brown TM, Hernandez AF, Bittner V, et al. Predictors of cardiac rehabilitation referral in coronary artery disease patients: findings from the American Heart Association's Get With the Guidelines program. *J Am Coll Cardiol.* 2009;54:515-521.

103. Sanderson BK, Shewchuk RM, Bittner V. Cardiac rehabilitation and women: what keeps them away? *J Cardiopulm Rehabil Prev.* 2010;30:12-21.

104. Arena R, Williams M, Forman DE, et al. Increasing referral and participation rates to outpatient cardiac rehabilitation: the valuable role of healthcare professionals in the inpatient and home health settings: a science advisory from the American Heart Association. *Circulation.* 2012;125:1321-1329.

105. Stuart-Shor EM, Berra KA, Kamau MW, Kumanyika SK. Behavioral strategies for cardiovascular risk reduction in diverse and underserved racial/ethnic groups. *Circulation.* 2012;125:171-184.

Racial and Cultural Diversity section

1. National Partnership for Action. *National Stakeholder Strategy for Achieving Health Equity.* Rockville, MD: Department of Health and Human Services. http://minorityhealth.hhs.gov/npa/templates/content.aspx?lvl=1&lvlid=39&ID=288. Accessed March 28th, 2013.

2. Benz J, Espinosa O, Welsh V, Fontes A. Awareness of racial and ethnic health disparities has improved only modestly over a decade. *Health Aff.* 2011;30:1860-1867.

3. Engebretson J, Mahoney J, Carlson E. Cultural competence in the era of evidence-based practice. *J Prof Nurs.* 2008;24:172-178.

4. Maier-Lorentz M. Transcultural nursing: its importance in nursing practice. *J Cult Divers.* 2008;15:37-43.

5. Humes K, Jones N, Rameriz R. *Overview of Race and Hispanic Origin: 2010 Census Briefs.* Washington, DC: U.S. Department of Commerce and Economics and Statistics Administration, U.S. Census Bureau, 2011:1-24.

6. United States Bureau of the Census. http://www.census.gov/newsroom/releases/archives/population/cb08-123.html. Accessed March 29th, 2013.

7. Smedley BD, Stith AY, Nelson AR; Institute of Medicine Committee on Understanding and Eliminating Racial and Ethnic Disparities in Health Care. *Unequal Treatment: Confronting Racial and Ethnic Disparities in Health Care.* Washington, DC: National Academy Press, 2003.

8. Betancourt JR, Maina AW. The Institute of Medicine report "Unequal Treatment": implications for academic health centers. *Mt Sinai J Med.* 2004;71:314-321.

9. Centers for Disease Control and Prevention. Healthy People 2020. http://www.healthypeople.gov/2020/default.aspx. Accessed July 26, 2012.

10. Blanton M, Maddox T, Rushing O, Mensah G. Disparities in cardiac care: rising to the challenge of Healthy People 2010. *J Am Coll Cardiol.* 2004;44:503-508.

11. Sullivan L.W. *Missing Persons: Minorities in the Health Professions.* Washington, DC: Sullivan Commission, 2004. http://www.aacn.nche.edu/media-relations/SullivanReport.pdf.

12. American Association of Cardiovascular and Pulmonary Rehabilitation. *AACVPR Membership Survey.* Chicago: AACVPR, 2010.

13. U.S. Department of Health and Human Services, AHRQ Publication No. 11-0005. Rockville, MD: Agency for Healthcare Research and Quality, 2012. http://www.ahrq.gov/research/findings/nhqrdr/nhqrdr10/qrdr10.html. Accessed April 1st, 2013.

14. Centers of Disease Control and Prevention. Differences in prevalence of obesity among black, white, and Hispanic adults—United States, 2006-2008. *MMWR.* 2009;58:740-744.

15. Hernandez AF, Fonarow GC, Liang L, et al., GWTG Steering Committee. Sex and racial differences in the use of implantable cardioverter-defibrillators among patients hospitalized with heart failure. *JAMA.* 2007;298:1525-1532.

16. Bonow R, Grant A, Jacobs A. The cardiovascular state of the union: confronting healthcare disparities. *Circulation.* 2005;111:1205-1207.

17. Roger V, Go A, Lloyd-Jones D, et al. Heart disease and stroke statistics—2011 update. A

report from the American Heart Association. *Circulation*. 2011;123:e18-e209.

18. Brown TM, Hernandez AF, Bittner V, et al. Predictors of cardiac rehabilitation referral in coronary artery disease patients: findings from the American Heart Association's Get With the Guidelines program. *J Am Coll Cardiol*. 2009;54:515-521.

19. Spector RE. *Cultural Diversity in Health and Illness*. 4th ed. Stamford, CT: Appleton & Lange, 1999.

20. Cross T, Bazron B, Dennis K, Isaacs M. *Towards a Culturally Competent System of Care, Vol. 1*. Washington, DC: Georgetown University Center for Child and Human Development, CASSP Technical Assistance Center, 1989.

21. Berlin EA, Fowkes W. A teaching framework for cross-cultural health care. *West J Med*. 1983;139:934-938.

22. Levin SJ, Like RC, Gottlieb JE. ETHNIC: a framework for culturally competent clinical practice. *Patient Care*. 2000;34:188-189.

23. Tervalon M, Murray-Garcia J. Cultural humility versus cultural competence: a critical distinction in defining physician training outcomes in multicultural education. *J Health Care Poor Underserved*. 1998;9:117-125.

24. Wenger N. Current status of cardiac rehabilitation. *J Am Coll Cardiol*. 2008;51:1619-1631.

25. Davidson PM, Gholizadeh L, Haghshenas A, et al. A review of the cultural competence view of cardiac rehabilitation. *J Clin Nurs*. 2009;19:1335-1342.

26. Shin HB, Bruno R. Language use and English speaking ability 2000 U.S. Census. http://www.census.gov/prod/2003pubs/c2kbr-29.pdf. Accessed March 29th, 2013. Accessed March 10, 2011.

27. U.S. Department of Health and Human Services, Office of Minority Health. National standards for culturally and linguistically appropriate services in health care (2000). http://minorityhealth.hhs.gov/assets/pdf/checked/executive.pdf. Accessed March 29th, 2013.

28. National Institutes of Health, National Institute on Minority Health and Health Disparities. www.nimhd.nih.gov/default.html. Accessed February 4, 2013.

29. Bild D, Blumke D, Burke G, Detrano R, Diez-Roux A, Folsom A. Multi-ethnic study of atherosclerosis: objectives and design. *Am J Epidemiol*. 2002;156:871-881.

30. Taylor H, Wilson J, Jones D, Sarpong D, Srinivasan A, Garrison R. Toward resolution of cardiovascular health disparities in Africans Americans: design and methods of the Jackson Heart Study. *Ethn Dis*. 2005;15(S6):4-16.

31. Schweigman K, Eichner J, Welty T, Zhang Y. Cardiovascular disease risk factor awareness in American Indian communities: the Strong Heart Study. *Ethn Dis*. 2006;16:647-652.

32. Howard B, Best L, Comuzzie A, et al. C-reactive protein, insulin resistance, and metabolic syndrome in a population with a high burden of subclinical infection: insights from the Genetics of Coronary Artery Disease in Alaska Natives (GOCADAN) study. *Diabetes Care*. 2008;31:2312-2314.

Revascularization and Valve Surgery section

1. Thomas RJ, King M, Lui K, et al. AACVPR/ACC/AHA 2007 performance measures on cardiac rehabilitation for referral to and delivery of cardiac rehabilitation/secondary prevention services. *J Cardiopulm Rehabil Prev*. 2007;27:260-290.

2. Balady GJ, Williams MA, Ades PA, et al. Core components of cardiac rehabilitation/secondary prevention programs: 2007 update. A scientific statement from the American Heart Association and the American Association of Cardiovascular and Pulmonary Rehabilitation. *J Cardiopulm Rehabil Prev*. 2007;27:121-129.

3. Hamm LF, Sanderson BK, Ades PA, et al. Core competencies for cardiac rehabilitation/secondary prevention professionals: 2010 update. Position statement from the American Association of Cardiovascular and Pulmonary Rehabilitation. *J Cardiopulm Rehabil Prev*. 2011;31:2-10.

4. Roger VL, Go AS, Lloyd-Jones DM, et al. Heart disease and stroke statistics – 2012 update. A report from the American Heart Association. *Circulation*. 2012;125:e2-e220. DOI.1161/CIR.0b013e31823ac046.

5. Title 42 Code of Federal Regulations, Section 410.49: Cardiac rehabilitation program and intensive cardiac rehabilitation program: Conditions of coverage. http://edocket.access.gpo.gov/cfr_2010/octqtr/pdf/42cfr410.49.pdf. Accessed September 3, 2011.

6. Hillis LD, Smith PK, Anderson JL, et al. 2011 ACCF/AHA guideline for coronary artery bypass graft surgery. *Circulation*. 2011;124:e652-e735.

7. Thomas RJ, King M, Lui K, et al. AACVPR/ACCF/AHA 2010 update: performance measures on cardiac rehabilitation for referral to cardiac rehabilitation/secondary prevention services. *J Cardiopulm Rehabil Prev.* 2010;30:279-288.

8. Suaya JA, Shepard DS, Normand S-LT, et al. Use of cardiac rehabilitation by Medicare beneficiaries after myocardial infarction or coronary bypass surgery. *Circulation.* 2007;116:1653-1662.

9. American College of Sports Medicine. *ACSM's Guidelines for Exercise Testing and Prescription.* 9th ed. Philadelphia: Lippincott Williams & Wilkins, 2014.

10. Gibbons RJ, Balady GJ, Bricker JT, et al. ACC/AHA 2002 guideline update for exercise testing. A report of the American College of Cardiology/American Heart Association Task Force on Practice Guidelines (Committee on Exercise Testing). 2002;40:1531-40. Erratum in: J Am Coll Cardiol. 2006;48:173.1

11. King III SB, Smith SC, Hirshfield JW, et al. 2007 focused update of the ACC/AHA/SCAI 2005 guideline update for percutaneous coronary intervention. *Circulation.* 2008;117:261-295.

12. Aragam KG, Moscucci M, Smith DE, et al. Trends and disparities in referral to cardiac rehabilitation after percutaneous coronary intervention. *Am Heart J.* 2011;161:544-551.e2.

13. Goel K, Lennon RJ, Tilbury RT, et al. Impact of cardiac rehabilitation on mortality and cardiovascular events after percutaneous coronary intervention in the community. *Circulation.* 2011;123:2344-2352.

14. Miller FA, Rajamannan N, Grogan M, Murphy JG. Prosthetic heart valves. In: JD Murphy, ed. *Mayo Clinic Cardiology Review.* Philadelphia: Lippincott Williams & Wilkins, 2000:337-352.

15. Smith CR, Leon MB, Mack MJ, et al. Transcatheter versus surgical aortic-valve replacement in high-risk patients. *NEJM.* 2011;364:2187-2198.

16. Kodali SK, Williams MR, Smith CR, et al. Two-year outcomes after transcatheter or surgical aortic-valve replacement. *NEJM.* 2012;366:1686-1995.

17. Feldman T, Foster E, Glower DG, et al. Percutaneous repair or surgery for mitral regurgitation. *NEJM.* 2011;364:1395-1406.

18. Williams MA, Haskell WL, Ades PA, et al. Resistance exercise in individuals with and without cardiovascular disease: 2007 update. A scientific statement from the American Heart Association Council on Clinical Cardiology and Council on Nutrition, Physical Activity, and Metabolism. *Circulation.* 2007;116:572-584.

Dysrhythmias section

1. Allen BJ, Casey TP, Brodsky MA, Luckett CR, Henry WL. Exercise testing in patients with life-threatening ventricular tachyarrhythmias: results and correlation with clinical and arrhythmia factors. *Am Heart J.* 1988;116:997-1002.

2. Ryan M, Lown B, Horn H. Comparison of ventricular ectopic activity during 24-hour monitoring and exercise testing in patients with coronary heart disease. *NEJM.* 1975;292:224-229.

3. Sami M, Chaitman B, Fisher L, Holmes D, Fray D, Alderman E. Significance of exercise-induced ventricular arrhythmia in stable coronary artery disease: a coronary artery surgery study project. *Am J Cardiol.* 1984;54:1182-1188.

4. Beckerman J, Mathur A, Stahr S, Myers J, Chun S, Froelicher V. Exercise-induced ventricular arrhythmias and cardiovascular death. *Ann Noninvas Electro.* 2005;10:47-52.

5. Mozaffarian D, Furberg CD, Psaty BM, Siscovick D. Physical activity and incidence of atrial fibrillation in older adults: the cardiovascular health study. *Circulation.* 2008;118:800-807.

6. Abdulla J, Nielsen JR. Is the risk of atrial fibrillation higher in athletes than in the general population? A systematic review and meta-analysis. *Europace.* 2009;11:1156-1159.

7. Mont L, Elosua R, Brugada J. Endurance sport practice as a risk factor for atrial fibrillation and atrial flutter. *Europace.* 2009;11:11-17.

8. Plisiene J, Blumberg A, Haager G, et al. Moderate physical exercise: a simplified approach for ventricular rate control in older patients with atrial fibrillation. *Clin Res Cardiol.* 2008;97:820-826.

9. Mertens DJ, Kavanagh T. Exercise training for patients with chronic atrial fibrillation. *J Cardiopulm Rehabil.* 1996;16:193-196.

10. Leung SK, Lau CP, Tang MO, Leung Z, Yakimow K. An integrated dual sensor system automatically optimized by target rate histogram. *Pacing Clin Electrophysiol.* 1998;21:1559-1566.

11. Shukla HH, Flaker GC, Hellkamp AS, et al. Clinical and quality of life comparison of accelerometer, piezoelectric crystal, and blended sensors in DDDR-paced patients with sinus node dysfunction in the mode selection trial (MOST). *Pacing Clin Electrophysiol.* 2005;28:762-770.

12. Sharp CT, Busse EF, Burgess JJ, Haennel RG. Exercise prescription for patients with pacemakers. *J Cardiopulm Rehabil.* 1998;18:421-431.

13. Fan S, Lyon CE, Savage PD, Ozonoff A, Ades PA, Balady GJ. Outcomes and adverse events among patients with implantable cardiac defibrillators in cardiac rehabilitation: a case-controlled study. *J Cardiopulm Rehabil Prev.* 2009;29:40-43.

14. Vanhees L, Schepers D, Heidbuchel H, Defoor J, Fagard R. Exercise performance and training in patients with implantable cardioverter-defibrillators and coronary heart disease. *Am J Cardiol.* 2001;87:712-715.

15. Vanhees L, Kornaat M, Defoor J, et al. Effect of exercise training in patients with an implantable cardioverter defibrillator. *Eur Heart J.* 2004;25:1120-1126.

16. Kamke W, Dovifat C, Schranz M, Behrens S, Moesenthin J, Voller H. Cardiac rehabilitation in patients with implantable defibrillators. Feasibility and complications. *Z Kardiol.* 2003;92:869-875.

17. Davids JS, McPherson CA, Earley C, Batsford WP, Lampert R. Benefits of cardiac rehabilitation in patients with implantable cardioverter-defibrillators: a patient survey. *Arch Phys Med Rehabil.* 2005;86:1924-1928.

18. Zipes DP, Garson A Jr. 26th Bethesda conference: recommendations for determining eligibility for competition in athletes with cardiovascular abnormalities. Task Force 6: arrhythmias. *J Am Coll Cardiol.* 1994;24:892-899.

19. Philippon F. Cardiac resynchronization therapy: device-based medicine for heart failure. *J Card Surg.* 2004;19:270-274.

20. Schlosshan D, Barker D, Pepper C, Williams G, Morley C, Tan LB. CRT improves the exercise capacity and functional reserve of the failing heart through enhancing the cardiac flow- and pressure-generating capacity. *Eur J Heart Fail.* 2006;8:515-521.

21. De Marco T, Wolfel E, Feldman AM, et al. Impact of cardiac resynchronization therapy on exercise performance, functional capacity, and quality of life in systolic heart failure with QRS prolongation: COMPANION trial sub-study. *J Card Fail.* 2008;14:9-18.

22. Hoth KF, Nash J, Poppas A, Ellison KE, Paul RH, Cohen RA. Effects of cardiac resynchronization therapy on health-related quality of life in older adults with heart failure. *Clin Interv Aging.* 2008;3:553-60.

23. Medtronics. *For Healthcare Professional.* 2013. http://www.medtronic.com/for-healthcare-professionals/products-therapies/cardiac-rhythm/index.htm.

24. Seidl K, Rameken M, Vater M, Senges J. Cardiac resynchronization therapy in patients with chronic heart failure: pathophysiology and current experience. *Am J Cardiovasc Drugs.* 2002;2:219-226.

25. Seifert M, Schlegl M, Hoersch W, et al. Functional capacity and changes in the neurohormonal and cytokine status after long-term CRT in heart failure patients. *Int J Cardiol.* 2007;121:68-73.

26. Steendijk P, Tulner SA, Bax JJ, et al. Hemodynamic effects of long-term cardiac resynchronization therapy: analysis by pressure-volume loops. *Circulation.* 2006;113:1295-1304.

27. Patwala AY, Woods PR, Sharp L, Goldspink DF, Tan LB, Wright DJ. Maximizing patient benefit from cardiac resynchronization therapy with the addition of structured exercise training: a randomized controlled study. *J Am Coll Cardiol.* 2009;53:2332-2339.

28. Conraads VM, Vanderheyden M, Paelinck B, et al. The effect of endurance training on exercise capacity following cardiac resynchronization therapy in chronic heart failure patients: a pilot trial. *Eur J Cardiovasc Prev Rehabil.* 2007;14:99-106.

29. Kelly TM. Exercise testing and training of patients with malignant ventricular arrhythmias. *Med Sci Sports Exerc.* 1996;28:53-61.

30. Pashkow FJ, Schweikert RA, Wilkoff BL. Exercise testing and training in patients with malignant arrhythmias. *Exerc Sport Sci Rev.* 1997;25:235-269.

31. Maron BJ, Zipes DP. Introduction: eligibility recommendations for competitive athletes with cardiovascular abnormalities-general considerations. *J Am Coll Cardiol.* 2005;45:1318-1321.

32. Van Gelder IC, Groenveld HF, Crijns HJ, for the RACE II investigators. Lenient versus strict rate control in patients with atrial fibrillation. *NEJM.* 2010;362:1363-1373.

Heart Failure and Left Ventricular Assist Devices section

1. Roger VL, Go AS, Lloyd D, et al. Heart disease and stroke statistics—2011 update: a report from the American Heart Association. *Circulation.* 2011;123:e18-e209.

2. Lloyd-Jones D, Adams RJ, Brown T, et al. Heart disease and stroke statistics—2010 update: a report from the American Heart Association. *Circulation*. 2010;121:1-170.

3. Jessup M, Abraham WT, Casey DE, et al. Focused update: ACCF/AHA guidelines for the diagnosis and management of heart failure in adults. *Circulation*. 2009;119:1977-2016.

4. Cahalin LP. Heart failure. *Phys Ther*. 1996;76: 516-533.

5. Rector TS, Kubo SH, Cohn JN. Patients' self-assessment of their congestive heart failure. part 2: content, reliability and validity of a new measure, The Minnesota Living with Heart Failure Questionnaire. *Heart Fail*. 1987;3:198-209.

6. Green CP, Porter CB, Bresnahan DR, Spertus JA. Development and evaluation of the Kansas City Cardiomyopathy Questionnaire: a new health status measure for heart failure. *J Am Coll Cardiol*. 2000;35:1245-1255.

7. Ware JE, Sherbourne CD. The MOS 36-item short-form health survey (SF-36): conceptual framework and item selection. *Med Care*. 1992;30:42-49.

8. Keteyian SJ, Pina IL, Hibner BA, Fleg JL. Clinical role of exercise training in the management of patients with heart failure. *J Cardiopulm Rehabil Prev*. 2010;30:67-76.

9. Davies EJ, Moxham T, Rees K, et al. Exercise based rehabilitation for heart failure. *Cochrane Database Syst Rev*. 2010;4:CD003331.

10. Keteyian SJ, Marks CRC, Brawner CA, et al. Responses to arm exercise in patients with compensated heart failure. *J Cardiopulm Rehabil*. 1996;16:366-371.

11. Kitzman DW, Little WC, Brubaker PH, et al. Pathophysiological characterization of isolated diastolic heart failure in comparison to systolic heart failure. *JAMA*. 2002;288:2144-2150.

12. Wilson JR, Martin JL, Schwartz D, et al. Exercise intolerance in patients with chronic heart failure: role of impaired nutritive flow to skeletal muscle. *Circulation*. 1984;69:1079-1087.

13. Mancini D, Walter G, Reicheck N, et al. Contribution of skeletal muscle atrophy to exercise intolerance and altered muscle metabolism in heart failure. *Circulation*. 1992;85:1364-1373.

14. Adams V, Jiang H, Yu J, et al. Apoptosis in skeletal muscle myocytes of patients with chronic heart failure is associated with exercise intolerance. *J Am Coll Cardiol*. 1999;33:959-965.

15. Duscha DB, Kraus WE, Keteyian SJ, et al. Capillary density of skeletal muscle: a contributing mechanism for exercise intolerance in class II-III chronic heart failure independent of other peripheral alterations. *J Am Coll Cardiol*. 1999;33:1956-1963.

16. Duscha DB, Annex BH, Green HJ, et al. Deconditioning fails to explain peripheral skeletal muscle alterations in men with chronic heart failure. *J Am Coll Cardiol*. 2002;39:1170-1174.

17. Piepoli M, Kaczmerik A, Francis D, et al. Reduced peripheral skeletal muscle mass and abnormal reflex physiology in chronic heart failure. *Circulation*. 2006;114:126-134.

18. Olson TP, Snyder EM, Johnson BD. Exercise-disordered breathing in chronic heart failure. *Exerc Sport Sci Rev*. 2006;34:194-201.

19. Keteyian SJL, Brawner CA, Pina IL. Role and benefits of exercise in the management of patients with heart failure. *Heart Fail Rev*. 2010;15:523-530.

20. Keteyian SJ. Exercise training in congestive heart failure: risks and benefits. *Prog Cardiovasc Dis*. 2011;53:419-428.

21. O'Connor CM, Whellan DJ, Lee KL, et al. Efficacy and safety of exercise training in patients with chronic heart failure. *JAMA*. 2009;301:1439-1450.

22. Wisloff U, Stoylen A, Loennechen JP, et al. Superior cardiovascular effect of aerobic interval training versus moderate continuous training in heart failure patients: a randomized study. *Circulation*. 2007;115:3086-3094.

23. Tabet JY, Meurin P, Beauvais F, et al. Absence of exercise capacity improvement after exercise training program a strong prognostic factor in patients with chronic heart failure. *Circ Heart Fail*. 2008;1:220-226.

24. Smart N, Marwick TH. Exercise training for patients with heart failure: a systematic review of factors that improve mortality and morbidity. *Am J Med*. 2004;116:693-706.

25. Hammill BG, Curtis LH, Schulman KA, et al. Relationship between cardiac rehabilitation and long-term risks of death and myocardial infarction among elderly Medicare beneficiaries. *Circulation*. 2010;121:63-70.

26. Van Tol BAF, Huijsmans RJ, Kroon DW, et al. Effects of exercise training on cardiac performance, exercise capacity and quality of life in patients with heart failure: a meta analysis. *Eur J Heart Fail*. 2006;8:841-850.

27. Flynn KE, Pina IL, Whellan DJ, et al. Effects of exercise training on health status in patients with chronic heart failure. *JAMA*. 2009;301:1451-1459.

28. *ACSM's Guidelines for Exercise Testing and Prescription*. 9th ed. Philadelphia: Lippincott Williams & Wilkins, 2014.

29. Keteyian SJ, Issac D, Thadani U, et al. Safety of symptom-limited cardiopulmonary exercise testing in patients with chronic heart failure due to left ventricular systolic dysfunction. *Am Heart J*. 2009;158:S72-S77.

30. Arnold JMO, Liu P, Demers C, et al. Canadian Cardiovascular Society consensus conference recommendations on heart failure. *Can J Cardiol*. 2006;22:23-45.

31. Pina IL, Apstein CS, Balady GJ, et al. Exercise in heart failure: a statement from the American Heart Association Committee on Exercise, Rehabilitation, and Prevention. *Circulation*. 2003;107:1210-1225.

32. Mckelvie RS, McCarthy N, Tomlinson C, et al. Comparision of hemodynamic responses to cycling and resistance exercise in congestive heart faiure secondary to ischemic cardiomyopathy. *Am J Cardiol*. 1995;76:977-979.

33. Feiereisen P, Delagardelle C, Vaillant M, et al. Is strength training the more efficient training modality in chronic heart failure? *Med Sci Sports Exerc*. 2007;39:1910-1917.

34. Pu C, Johnson MT, Forman DE, et al. Randomized trial of progressive resistance training to counteract the myopathy of chronic heart failure. *J Appl Physiol*. 2001;90:2341-2350.

35. Palevo G, Keteyian SJ, Kang M, et al. Resistance exercise training improves heart function and physical fitness in stable patients with heart failure. *J Cardiopulm Rehabil*. 2009;29:294-298.

36. Braith RW, Beck DT. Resistance exercise: training adaptations and developing a safe exercise prescription. *Heart Fail Rev*. 2008;13:69-79.

37. Delagardelle C, Feiereisen P, Autier P, et al. Strength/endurance training versus endurance training in congestive heart failure. *Med Sci Sports Exerc*. 2002;34:1868-1872.

38. Williams MA, Haskell WL, Ades PA, et al. Resistance exercise in individuals with and without cardiovascular disease. *Circulation*. 2007;116:572-584.

39. Bernardi L, Spadacini G, Bellwon J, et al. Effect of breathing rate on oxygen saturation and exercise performance in chronic heart failure. *Lancet*. 1998;351:1308-1311.

40. Johnson PH, Cowley AJ, Kinnear WJM. A randomized controlled trial of inspiratory muscle training in stable chronic heart failure. *Eur Heart J*. 1998;19:1249-1253.

41. Mancini D, Henson D, LaManca J, et al. Benefit of selective respiratory muscle training on exercise capacity in patients with congestive heart failure. *Circulation*. 1995;91:320-329.

42. Weiner P, Waizman J, Magadle R, et al. The effect of specific inspiratory muscle training on the sensation of dyspnea and exercise tolerance in patients with congestive heart failure. *Clin Cardiol*. 1999;22:727.

43. Keteyian SJ. General interview and examination skills. In: JE Ehrman, SJ Keteyian, PM Gordon, PS Visich, eds. *Clinical Exercise Physiology*. 2nd ed. Champaign, IL: Human Kinetics, 2009:61-76.

44. Keteyian SJ, Brawner CA, Schairer JR, et al. Effects of exercise training on chronotropic incompetence in patients with heart failure. *Am Heart J*. 1999;138:233-240.

45. Meyer K, Samek L, Schwaibold M, et al. Interval training in patients with severe chronic heart failure. *Med Sci Sports Exerc*. 1997;29:306-312.

46. Rose EA, Gelijns AC, Moskowitz AJ, et al. Long-term use of a left ventricular assist device for end-stage heart failure. *NEJM*. 2001;345:1435-1443.

47. Mitter N, Sheinberg R. Update on ventricular assist devices. *Curr Opin Anesthesiol*. 2010;23:57-66.

48. McCarthy PM, Smedira NO, Vargo RL, et al. One hundred patients with the HeartMate left ventricular assist device: evolving concepts and technology. *J Thorac Cardiovasc Surg*. 1998;115:904-912.

49. Griffith BP, Kormos RL, Borovetz HS, et al. HeartMate II left ventricular assist system: from concept to first clinical use. *Ann Thorac Surg*. 2001;71:S116-120.

50. Jaski BE, Kim J, Maly RS, et al. Effects of exercise during long-term support with a left ventricular assist device: results of the experience with left ventricular assist device with exercise (EVADE) pilot trial. *Circulation*. 1997;95:2401-2406.

51. de Jonge N, Kirkels H, Lahpor JR, et al. Exercise performance in patients with end-stage heart failure after implantation of a left ventricular

assist device and after heart transplantation. *J Am Coll Cardiol.* 2011;37:1794-1799.

52. Jaski BE, Lingle RJ, Kim J, et al. Comparison of functional capacity in patients with end-stage heart failure following implantation of a left ventricular assist device versus heart transplantation: results of the experience with left ventricular assist device with exercise trial. *J Heart Lung Transplant.* 1999;18:1031-1040.

53. Jakovljevic DG, George RS, Nunan D, et al. The impact of acute reduction of continuous-flow left ventricular assist device support on cardiac and exercise performance. *Heart.* 2010;96:1390-1395.

54. Kennedy MD, Haykowsky M, Humphrey R. Function, eligibility, outcomes, and exercise capacity associated with left ventricular assist devices: exercise rehabilitation and training for patients with ventricular assist devices. *J Cardiopulm Rehabil.* 2003;23:208-217.

55. Nicholson C, Paz JC. Total artificial heart and physical therapy management. *Cardiopulm Phys Ther J.* 2010;21:13-21.

56. Mettauer B, Geny B, Lonsdorfer-Wolf E, et al. Exercise training with a heart device: a hemodynamic, metabolic, and hormonal study. *Med Sci Sports Exerc.* 2001;33:2-8.

57. Rogers JG, Aaronson KD, Boyle AJ, et al. Continuous flow left ventricular assist device improves functional capacity and quality of life of advanced heart failure patients. *J Am Coll Cardiol.* 2010;55:1826-1834.

58. Mancini D, Goldsmith R, Levin H, et al. Comparison of exercise performance in patients with chronic severe heart failure versus left ventricular assist devices. *Circulation.* 1998;98:1178-1183.

59. Pagani FD, Miller LW, Russell SD, et al. Extended mechanical circulatory support with a continuous-flow rotary left ventricular assist device. *J Am Coll Cardiol.* 2009;54:312-321.

60. Allen JG, Weiss ES, Schaffer JM, et al. Quality of life and functional status in patients surviving 12 months after left ventricular assist device implantation. *J Heart Lung Transplant.* 2010;29:278-285.

61. Miller LW, Pagani FD, Russell SD, et al. Use of a continuous-flow device in patients awaiting heart transplantation. *NEJM.* 2007;357:885-896.

62. Slaughter MS, Pagani FD, Rogers JG, et al. Clinical management of continuous-flow left ventricular assist devices in advanced heart fail-ure. *J Heart Lung Transplant.* 2010;29(4, suppl 1):S1-S39.

Cardiac Transplantation section

1. Barnard CN. The operation: a human cardiac transplant: an interim report of a successful operation performed at Groote Schuur Hospital, Cape Town. *S Afr Med J.* 1967;41:1271-1274.

2. Rodeheffer RJ, McGregor CGA. The development of cardiac transplantation. *Mayo Clin Proc.* 1992;67:480-484.

3. Stehlik J, Edwards LB, Kucheryavaya AY, et al. The Registry of the International Society for Heart and Lung Transplantation: twenty-seventh official adult transplant report–2010. *J Heart Lung Transplant.* 2009;29:1089-1103.

4. Raichlin E, Chandrasekaran K, Kremers WK, et al. Sirolimus as primary immunosuppressant reduces left ventricular mass and improves diastolic function of the cardiac allograft. *Transplantation.* 2008;86:1395-1400.

5. Hunt SA, Haddad F. The changing face of heart transplantation. *J Am Coll Cardiol.* 2008;52:587-598.

6. Hummel M, Michauk I, Hetzer R, Fuhrman B. Quality of life after heart and heart-lung transplantation. *Transplant Proc.* 2001;33:3546-3548.

7. Kuhn WF, Davis MH, Lippmann SB. Emotional adjustments to cardiac transplantation. *Gen Hosp Psychiatry.* 1988;10:108-113.

8. Sherry DC, Simmons B, Wung SF, et al. Noncompliance in heart transplantation: a role for the advanced practice nurse. *Prog Cardiovasc Nurs.* 2003;18:141-146.

9. Squires RW. Cardiac rehabilitation issues for heart transplantation patients. *J Cardiopulm Rehabil.* 1990;10:159-168.

10. Niset G, Preumont N. Determinants of peak aerobic capacity after heart transplantation. *Eur Heart J.* 1997;18:1692-1693.

11. Marconi C, Marzorati M. Exercise after heart transplantation. *Eur J Appl Physiol.* 2003;90:250-259.

12. Buendia-Fuentes F, Almenar L, Ruiz C, et al. Sympathetic reinnervation 1 year after heart transplantation, assessed using iodine-123 metaiodobenzylguanidine imaging. *Transplant Proc.* 2011;43:2247-2248.

13. Sanchez H, Bigard X, Veksler V, et al. Immunosuppressive treatment affects cardiac and

skeletal muscle mitochondria by the toxic effect of vehicle. *J Mol Cell Cardiol.* 2000;32:323-331.

14. Squires RW. Transplant. In: FJ Pashkow, WA Dafoe, eds. *Clinical Cardiac Rehabilitation: A Cardiologist's Guide.* 2nd ed. Baltimore: Williams & Wilkins, 1999:175-191.

15. Buendía Fuentes F, Martínez-Dolz L, Almenar Bonet L, et al. Normalization of the heart rate response to exercise 6 months after cardiac transplantation. *Transplant Proc.* 2010;42:3186-3188.

16. Keteyian SJ, Brawner C. Cardiac transplant. In: *ACSM's Exercise Management for Persons with Chronic Diseases and Disabilities.* Champaign, IL: Human Kinetics, 1997:54-58.

17. Kao AC, Van Trigt P, Shaeffer-McCall GS, et al. Central and peripheral limitations to upright exercise in untrained cardiac transplant recipients. *Circulation.* 1994;89:2605-2615.

18. Pope SE, Stinson EB, Daughters GT, et al. Exercise response of the denervated heart in long-term cardiac transplant recipients. *Am J Cardiol.* 1980;46:213-218.

19. Stratton JR, Kemp GJ, Daly RC, et al. Effects of cardiac transplantation on bioenergetic abnormalities of skeletal muscle in congestive heart failure. *Circulation.* 1994;89:1624-1631.

20. Lampert E, Mettauer B, Hoppeler H, et al. Structure of skeletal muscle in heart transplant recipients. *J Am Coll Cardiol.* 1996;28:980-984.

21. Hanson P, Slane PR, Lillis DL, et al. Limited oxygen uptake post heart transplant is associated with impairment of calf vasodilatory capacity. *Med Sci Sports Exerc.* 1995;27:S49.

22. Carter R, Al-Rawas OA, Stevenson A, Mcdonagh T, Stevenson RD. Exercise responses following heart transplantation: 5 year follow-up. *Scott Med J.* 2006;51:6-14.

23. Brubaker PH, Brozena SC, Morley DL, et al. Exercise-induced ventilatory abnormalities in orthotopic heart transplant patients. *J Heart Lung Transplant.* 1997;16:1011-1017.

24. Squires RW, Hoffman CJ, James GA, et al. Arterial oxygen saturation during graded exercise testing after cardiac transplantation. *J Cardiopulm Rehabil.* 1998;18:348.

25. Braith RW, Limacher MC, Mills RM, et al. Exercise-induced hypoxemia in heart transplant recipients. *J Am Coll Cardiol.* 1993;22:768-776.

26. Mettauer B, Zhao QM, Epailly E, et al. VO_2 kinetics reveal a central limitation at the onset of subthreshold exercise in heart transplant recipients. *J Appl Physiol.* 2000;88:1228-1238.

27. Squires RW, Leung TC, Cyr NS, et al. Partial normalization of the heart rate response to exercise after cardiac transplantation: frequency and relationship to exercise capacity. *Mayo Clin Proc.* 2002;77:1295-1300.

28. Richard R, Verdier JC, Duvallet A, et al. Chronotropic competence in endurance trained heart transplant recipients: heart rate is not a limiting factor for exercise capacity. *J Am Coll Cardiol.* 1999;33:192-197.

29. Pokan R, Von Duvillard SP, Ludwig J, et al. Effect of high-volume and -intensity endurance training in heart transplant recipients. *Med Sci Sports Exerc.* 2004;36:2011-2016.

30. Golding LA, Mangus BC. Competing in varsity athletics after cardiac transplant. *J Cardiopulm Rehabil.* 1989;9:486-491.

31. Kapp C. Heart transplant recipient climbs the Matterhorn. *Lancet.* 2003;362:880-881.

32. Haykowsky MJ, Riess K, Burton I, et al. Heart transplant recipient completes ironman triathlon 22 years after surgery. *J Heart Lung Transplant.* 2009;28:415.

33. Kavanagh T. Physical training in heart transplant recipients. *J Cardiovasc Risk.* 1996;3:154-159.

34. Kaye DM, Esler M, Kingwell B, et al. Functional and neurochemical evidence for partial cardiac sympathetic reinnervation after cardiac transplantation in humans. *Circulation.* 1993;88:1110-1118.

35. Scott CD, Dark JH, McComb JM. Evolution of the chronotropic response to exercise after cardiac transplantation. *Am J Cardiol.* 1995;76:1292-1296.

36. Marconi C, Marzorati M, Fiocchi R, et al. Age-related heart rate response to exercise in heart transplant recipients. Functional significance. *Pflugers Arch.* 2002;443:698-706.

37. Schwaiblmair M, von Scheidt W, Uberfuhr P, et al. Functional significance of cardiac reinnervation in heart transplant recipients. *J Heart Lung Transplant.* 1999;18:838-845.

38. Squires RW, Arthur PA, Gau GT, et al. Exercise after cardiac transplantation: a report of two cases. *J Cardiopulm Rehabil.* 1983;3:570-574.

39. Degre S, Niset G, Desmet JM, et al. Effets de l'entrainement physique sur le coeur humain denerve apres transplantation cardiaque ortho-

topique. *Ann Cardiol Angeol (Paris)*. 1986;35:147-149.

40. Niset G, Cousty-Degre C, Degre S. Psychological and physical rehabilitation after heart transplantation: 1 year follow-up. *Cardiology*. 1988;75:311-317.

41. Sieurat P, Roquebrune JP, Grinneiser D, et al. Surveillance et readaptation des transplantes cardiaques heterotopiques a la periode de convalescence. *Arch Mal Coeur*. 1986;79:210-216.

42. Kavanagh T, Yacoub MH, Mertens DJ, et al. Cardiorespiratory responses to exercise training after orthotopic cardiac transplantation. *Circulation*. 1988;77:162-171.

43. Kavanagh T, Yacoub MH, Mertens DJ, et al. Exercise rehabilitation after heterotopic cardiac transplantation. *J Cardiopulm Rehabil*. 1989;9:303-310.

44. Keteyian S, Shepard R, Ehrman J, et al. Cardiovascular responses of heart transplant patients to exercise training. *J Appl Physiol*. 1991;70:2627-2631.

45. Kobashigawa JA, Leaf DA, Lee N, et al. A controlled trial of exercise rehabilitation after heart transplantation. *NEJM*. 1999;340:272-277.

46. Lampert E, Mettauer B, Hoppeler H, et al. Skeletal muscle response to short endurance training in heart transplantation recipients. *J Am Coll Cardiol*. 1998;32:420-426.

47. Horber FF, Scheidegger JR, Grunig BF, et al. Evidence that prednisone-induced myopathy is reversed by physical training. *J Clin Endocrinol Metab*. 1985;61:83-88.

48. Braith RW, Mills RM, Welsch MA, et al. Resistance exercise training restores bone mineral density in heart transplant recipients. *J Am Coll Cardiol*. 1996;28:1471-1477.

49. Zhao QM, Mettauer B, Epailly E, et al. Effect of exercise training on leukocyte subpopulations and clinical course in cardiac transplant patients. *Transplant Proc*. 1998;30:172-175.

50. Balady GJ, Arena R, Sietsema K, et al. Clinician's guide to cardiopulmonary exercise testing in adults: a scientific statement from the American Heart Association. *Circulation*. 2010;122:191-225.

51. Ehrman JK, Keteyian SJ, Levine AB, et al. Exercise stress tests after cardiac transplantation. *Am J Cardiol*. 1993;71:1372-1373.

52. Keteyian SJ, Brawner C. Cardiac transplant. In: *ACSM's Exercise Management for Persons with Chronic Diseases and Disabilities*. 2nd ed. Champaign, IL: Human Kinetics, 2003:70-75.

53. Gibbons RJ, Balady GJ, Beasley JW, et al. ACC/AHA guidelines for exercise testing: a report of the American College of Cardiology/American Heart Association on Practice Guidelines (Committee on Exercise Testing). *J Am Coll Cardiol*. 1997;30:260-315.

54. McGregor CGA. Cardiac transplantation: surgical considerations and early postoperative management. *Mayo Clin Proc*. 1992;67:577-585.

55. Centers for Medicare and Medicaid Services. www.cms.gov.

Peripheral Arterial Disease section

1. Hiatt WR, Hirsch AT, Regensteiner JG, Brass EP. Clinical trials for claudication. Assessment of exercise performance, functional status, and clinical end points. Vascular Clinical Trialists. *Circulation*. 1995;92:614-621.

2. Criqui MH, Langer RD, Fronek A, et al. Mortality over a period of 10 years in patients with peripheral arterial disease. *NEJM*. 1992;326:381-386.

3. Selvin E, Erlinger TP. Prevalence of and risk factors for peripheral arterial disease in the United States: Results from the National Health and Nutrition Examination Survey, 1999-2000. *Circulation*. 2004;110:738-743

4. Gardner AW, Skinner JS, Cantwell BW, Smith LK. Progressive vs single-stage treadmill tests for evaluation of claudication. *Med Sci Sports Exerc*. 1991;23:402-408.

5. Hiatt WR, Nawaz D, Regensteiner JG, Hosack KF. The evaluation of exercise performance in patients with peripheral vascular disease. *J Cardiopulm Rehabil*. 1988;12:525-532.

6. Hirsch AT, Haskal ZJ, Hertzer NR, et al. ACC/AHA 2005 practice guidelines for the management of patients with peripheral arterial disease (lower extremity, renal, mesenteric, and abdominal aortic): a collaborative report from the American Association for Vascular Surgery/Society for Vascular Surgery, Society for Cardiovascular Angiography and Interventions, Society for Vascular Medicine and Biology, and Society of Interventional Radiology. *Circulation*. 2006;47:1239-1312.

7. Gardner AW. The effect of cigarette smoking on exercise capacity in patients with intermittent claudication. *Vasc Med*. 1996;1:181-186.

8. Olin JW, Allie DE, Belkin M, et al. ACCF/AHA/ACR/SCAI/SIR/SVM/SVN/SVS 2010 performance measures for adults with peripheral artery disease. *J Am Coll Cardiol.* 2010;56:2147-2181.

9. Langbein WE, Collins EG, Orebaugh C, et al. Increasing exercise tolerance of persons limited by claudication pain using polestriding. *J Vasc Surg.* 2002;35:887-893.

10. Mika P, Spodaryk K, Cencora A, Unnithan VB, Mika A. Experimental model of pain-free treadmill training in patients with claudication. *Am J Phys Med Rehabil.* 2005;84:756-762.

11. McDermott MM, Ades P, Guralnik JM, et al. Treadmill exercise and resistance training in patients with peripheral arterial disease with and without intermittent claudication: a randomized controlled trial. *JAMA.* 2009;301:165-174.

12. Walker RD, Nawaz S, Wilkinson CH, Saxton JM, Pockley AG, Wood RF. Influence of upper- and lower-limb exercise training on cardiovascular function and walking distances in patients with intermittent claudication. *J Vasc Surg.* 2000;31:662-669.

13. Zwierska I, Walker RD, Choksy SA, Male JS, Pockley AG, Saxton JM. Upper- vs lower-limb aerobic exercise rehabilitation in patients with symptomatic peripheral arterial disease: a randomized controlled trial. *J Vasc Surg.* 2005;42:1122-1130.

14. Zwierska I, Walker RD, Choksy SA, Male JS, Pockley AG, Saxton JM. Relative tolerance to upper- and lower-limb aerobic exercise in patients with peripheral arterial disease. *Eur J Vasc Endovasc Surg.* 2006;31:157-163.

15. Treat-Jacobson D, Bronas UG, Leon AS. Efficacy of arm-ergometry versus treadmill exercise training to improve walking distance in patients with claudication. *Vasc Med.* 2009;14:203-213.

16. Money SR, Herd JA, Isaacsohn JL, et al. Effect of cilostazol on walking distances in patients with intermittent claudication caused by peripheral vascular disease. J Vasc Surg. 1998;27:267-274; discussion 74-75.

Chronic Lung Disease section

1. Global Initiative for Chronic Obstructive Lung Disease (GOLD). Global strategy for the diagnosis, management and prevention of COPD. 2011. Available from: http://www.goldcopd.org.

2. McGoon M, Gutterman D, Steen V, et al. Screening, early detection and diagnosis of pulmonary arterial hypertension. ACCP evidence-based clinical practice guidelines. *Chest.* 2004;126:14S-34S.

3. Martinez FJ, Taczek AE, Seifer FD, et al. Development and initial validation of a self-scored population screener questionnaire (COPD-PS). *J COPD.* 2008;5:85-95.

4. Yawn BP, Mapel DW, Mannino DM, et al. Development of the lung function questionnaire (LFQ) to identify airflow obstruction. *Int J COPD.* 2010;5:1-10.

5. Ries AL, Bauldoff GS, Carlin BL, et al. Pulmonary rehabilitation: joint ACCP/AACVPR evidence-based clinical practice guidelines. *Chest.* 2007;131(5 suppl):4S-42S.

6. Casaburi R, ZuWallack R. Pulmonary rehabilitation for management of chronic obstructive pulmonary disease. *NEJM.* 2009;360:1329-1335.

Chapter 10

1. Suaya JA, Shepard DS, Normand ST, et al. Use of cardiac rehabilitation by Medicare beneficiaries after myocardial infarction or coronary bypass surgery. *Circulation.* 2007;116:1653-1662.

2. Thomas RJ, King M, Lui K, et al. AACVPR/ACC/AHA 2007 performance measures on cardiac rehabilitation for referral to and delivery of cardiac rehabilitation/secondary prevention services. *J Am Coll Cardiol.* 2007;50:1400-1433.

3. Thomas RJ, King M, Lui K, et al. AACVPR/ACC/AHA 2010 update: performance measures on cardiac rehabilitation for referral to cardiac rehabilitation/secondary prevention services. *J Am Coll Cardiol.* 2010;56:1159-1167.

4. LaBresh KA, Fonarow GC, Smith SC, et al. Improved treatment of hospitalized coronary artery disease patients with the Get With the Guidelines program. *Crit Pathw Cardiol.* 2007;6:98-105.

5. Gurewich D, Prottas J, Bhalotra S, et al. System-level factors and use of cardiac rehabilitation. *J Cardiopulm Rehabil Prev.* 2008;28:380-385.

6. Grace SL, Russell KL, Reid RD, et al. Effect of cardiac rehabilitation referral strategies on utilization rates. *Arch Intern Med.* 2011;171:235-241.

7. Department of Health and Human Services, Centers for Medicare and Medicaid Services. Publication No. 100-06. Change request 6850; Transmittal 170(I)(B). May 21, 2010.

8. Department of Health and Human Services, Centers for Medicare and Medicaid Services. Decision memo for intensive cardiac rehabilita-

tion (ICR) program – Pritikin program (CAG-00418N). August 12, 2010.

9. Hamm LF, Sanderson BK, Ades PA, et al. Core competencies for cardiac rehabilitation/secondary prevention professionals: 2010 update. *J Cardiopulm Rehabil Prev.* 2011;31:2-10.

10. Balady GJ, Williams MA, Ades PA, et al. Core components of cardiac rehabilitation/secondary prevention programs: 2007 update: a scientific statement from the American Heart Association and the American Association of Cardiovascular and Pulmonary Rehabilitation. *Circulation.* 2007;115:2675-2682.

11. Audelin MC, Savage PD, Ades PA. Changing clinical profile of patients entering cardiac rehabilitation/secondary prevention programs: 1996-2006. *J Cardiopulm Rehabil Prev.* 2008;28:299-306.

12. Ades PA, Savage PD, Toth MJ, et al. High-calorie-expenditure exercise. A new approach to cardiac rehabilitation for overweight coronary patients. *Circulation.* 2009;119:2671-2678.

13. Donnelly JE, Blair SN, Jakicic JM, et al. ACSM position stand. Appropriate physical activity intervention strategies for weight loss and prevention of weight regain for adults. *Med Sci Sports Exerc.* 2009;41(2):459-471.

14. Savage PD, Ades PA. Pedometer step counts predict cardiac risk factors at entry to cardiac rehabilitation. *J Cardiopulm Rehabil Prev.* 2008;28:370-377.

15. Ayabe M, Brubaker PH, Dobrosielski D, et al. The physical activity patterns of cardiac rehabilitation program participants. *J Cardiopulm Rehabil Prev.* 2004;24:80-86.

16. Jones NL, Schneider PL, Kaminsky LA, et al. An assessment of the total amount of physical activity of patients participating in a phase III cardiac rehabilitation program. *J Cardiopulm Rehabil Prev.* 2007;27:81-85.

17. Leon AS, Franklin BA, Costa F, et al. Cardiac rehabilitation and secondary prevention of coronary heart disease: an American Heart Association scientific statement in collaboration with the American Association of Cardiovascular and Pulmonary Rehabilitation. *Circulation.* 2005;111:369-376.

18. Kokkinos P, Myers J, Kokkinos JP, et al. Exercise capacity and mortality in black and white men. *Circulation.* 2008;117:614-622.

19. Savage PD, Antkowiak ME, Ades PA. Failure to improve cardiopulmonary fitness in car-diac rehabilitation. *J Cardiopulm Rehabil Prev.* 2009;29:284-291.

20. Department of Health and Human Services, Centers for Medicare and Medicaid Services. Publication No. 100-06. Change request 6850. May 21, 2010.

21. *Federal Register,* Vol. 74, No. 226, Section 410.49. November 25, 2009:62004-62005.

22. Sanderson BK, Shewchuk RM, Bittner V. Cardiac rehabilitation and women: what keeps them away? *J Cardiopulm Rehabil Prev.* 2010;30:12-21.

23. Jolliffe J, Rees K, Taylor R, et al. Exercise-based rehabilitation for coronary heart disease. *Cochrane Database Syst Rev.* 2001;1:CD001800.

24. Taylor R, Brown A, Jolliffe J, et al. Exercise-based rehabilitation for patients with coronary heart disease: systematic review and meta-analysis of randomized controlled trials. *Am J Med.* 2004;116:682-692.

25. Tharrett KJ, McInnis KJ, Peterson JA. Health/fitness facility design and construction. In: *ACSM's Health/Fitness Facility Standards and Guidelines.* 3rd ed. Champaign, IL: Human Kinetics, 2007:31-43.

26. Title 42 Code of Federal Regulations: 42 CFR, Part 482. http://ecfr.gpoaccess.gov/cgi/t/text/text-idx?c=ecfr&tpl=/ecfrbrowse/Title42/42cfr482_main_02.tpl. Accessed April 14, 2013.

27. Federal Register, Vol. 74, No. 226, Wednesday, November 25, 2009, pps:62004-62005.

28. Title 42 Code of Federal Regulations, Section 410.49: Medicare conditions of coverage for cardiac rehabilitation program and intensive cardiac rehabilitation program. http://edocket.access.gpo.gov/cfr_2010/octqtr/pdf/42cfr410.49.pdf. Accessed March 12, 2011.

29. Medicare program; payment policies under the physician fee schedule and other revisions to Part B for CY 2010; final rule; Medicare program; solicitation of independent accrediting organizations to participate in the advanced diagnostic imaging supplier accreditation program. *Federal Register,* Vol. 74, No. 266. November 25, 2009:61877.

30. American College of Sports Medicine. http://certification.acsm.org. Accessed March 12, 2011.

31. American Board of Physical Therapy Specialists (ABPTS) Cardiovascular and Pulmonary Specialist Certification. www.abpts.org/Certification/CardiovascularPulmonary. Accessed April 14, 2013.

32. King ML, Williams MA, Fletcher GF, et al. Medical director responsibilities for outpatient cardiac rehabilitation/secondary prevention programs. *J Cardiopulm Rehabil*. 2005;25:315-320.

Chapter 11

1. Porter ME. What is value in health care? *NEJM*. 2010;363:2477-2481.

2. American College of Sports Medicine. *Guidelines for Exercise Testing and Prescription*. 7th ed. Philadelphia: Lippincott Williams & Wilkins, 2006.

3. American Association of Cardiovascular and Pulmonary Rehabilitation (AACVPR) Outcomes Committee. Outcome Tools Resource Guide, 2002. Available to AACVPR members only at www.aacvpr.org/Publications.

4. Pashkow P, Ades PA, Emery CF, et al. Outcome measurement in cardiac and pulmonary rehabilitation by the AACVPR Outcomes Committee. *J Cardiopulm Rehabil*. 1995;15:304-405.

5. Encyclopedia of Public Health. Precede-Proceed Model. http://www.enotes.com/precede-proceed-model-reference/precede-proceed-model.

6. Balady GJ, Williams MA, Ades PA, et al. Core components of cardiac rehabilitation/secondary prevention programs: 2007 update. *J Cardiopulm Rehabil*. 2007;27:121-129.

7. Oldridge NB. Outcome assessment in cardiac rehabilitation: health-related quality of life and economic evaluation. *J Cardiopulm Rehabil*. 1997;17:179-194.

8. American Thoracic Society statement: guidelines for the six minute walk test. *Am J Respir Crit Care Med*. 2002;166:111-117.

9. Podsiadlo D, Richardson S. The timed "up and go" test: a test of basic functional mobility for frail elderly persons. *J Am Geriatr Soc*. 1991;39:142-148.

10. Hlatky MA, Boineau RE, Higginbotham MB, et al. A brief self-administered questionnaire to determine functional capacity (the Duke Activity Status Index). *Am J Cardiol*. 1989;64:651-654.

11. Radloff LS. The CES-D Scale: a self-report depression scale for research in the general population. *Appl Psychol Meas*. 1977;1:385-401.

12. Zigmond AS, Snaith RP. The hospital anxiety and depression scale. *Acta Psychiatr Scand*. 1983;67:361-370.

13. Spitzer R, Kroenke K, Williams J. Validation and utility of a self-report version of PRIME-MD: the PHQ Primary Care Study. *JAMA*. 1999;282:1737-1744.

14. Eichenauer K, Feltz G, Wilson J, Brookings J. Measuring psychosocial risk factors in cardiac rehabilitation. Validation of the Psychosocial Risk Factor Survey. *J Cardiopulm Rehabil Prev*. 2010;30:309-318.

15. Verrill D, Graham H, Vitcenda M, Peno-Green L, Kramer V, Corbisiero T. Measuring behavioral outcomes in cardiopulmonary rehabilitation. *J Cardiopulm Rehabil Prev*. 2009;29:193-203.

16. Connor SL, Gustafson JR, Sexton G, et al. The Diet Habit Survey: a new method of dietary assessment that relates to plasma cholesterol changes. *J Am Diet Assoc*. 1992;92:41-47.

17. Resnick B, Jenkins L. Testing the reliability and validity of the Self-Efficacy for Exercise Scale. *Nurs Res*. 2000;49:154-159.

18. Hallal PC, Victora CG. Reliability and validity of the International Physical Activity Questionnaire (IPAQ). *Med Sci Sports Exerc*. 2004;36:556.

19. Kane RL. *Understanding Health Care Outcome Research*. Gaithersburg, MD: Aspen, 1997.

20. Wicklund I. The Nottingham health profile a measure of health related quality of life. *Scand J Prim Health Care*. 1990(suppl);1:15-18.

21. Thomas RJ, King M, Lui K, et al. AACVPR/ACCF/AHA 2007 performance measures on cardiac rehabilitation for referral to and delivery of cardiac rehabilitation/secondary prevention services. *J Cardiopulm Rehabil Prev*. 2007;27:260-290.

22. Bonow RO, Masoudi FA, Rumsfeld JS, et al. ACC/AHA classification of care metrics: performance measures and quality metrics. *Circulation*. 2008;118:2662-2666.

23. Thomas RJ, King M, Lui K, et al. AACVPR/ACCF/AHA 2010 update: performance measures on cardiac rehabilitation for referral to cardiac rehabilitation/secondary prevention services. *J Cardiopulm Rehabil Prev*. 2010;30:279-288.

24. Spertus JA, Eagle KA, Krumholz HM, et al. American College of Cardiology and American Heart Association methodology for the selection and creation of performance measures for quantifying the quality of cardiovascular care. *J Am Coll Cardiol*. 2005;45:1147-1156.

25. Brøgger J, Bakke P, Eide GE, et al. Comparison of telephone and postal survey modes on respiratory symptoms and risk factors. *Am J Epidemiol.* 2002;155;572-576.

26. Institute for Healthcare Improvement. How to improve. www.ihi.org/knowledge/Pages/Howto-Improve. Accessed July 11, 2012.

27. Donabedian A. The quality of care. *JAMA.* 1988;260:1742-1748.

28. Berwick DM. A primer on leading the improvement of systems. *BMJ.* 1996;312:619-622.

29. The Deming Cycle: or PDSA and PDCA. www.quality-improvement-matters.com/deming-cycle.html. Accessed July 9, 2012.

Index

Note: The italicized *f* and *t* following page numbers refer to figures and tables, respectively.

A

AACVPR. *See* American Association of Cardiovascular and Pulmonary Rehabilitation
ABI (ankle–brachial index) 186
ACC. *See* American College of Cardiology
accelerometers 111, 113*f*, 114*f*, 120
accreditation of facilities 202-203, 226
ACE inhibitors 109
ACLS (advanced cardiac life support) course 62, 229, 231-232, 233
ACSM. *See* American College of Sports Medicine
ACSM's Guidelines for Exercise Testing and Prescription 164
action stage 25
activities of daily living (ADLs)
   as admission criteria 53*f*
   assessment of 44-47, 63, 146
   chronic lung disease and 191
   claudication and 186
   flexibility training and 121
   in older patients 146, 147
   rehabilitation and 147
acute coronary syndrome 6
ADA (Americans with Disabilities Act) 201
adenosine 69
adherence 87-88, 134
adjustment to life change 131-133
advanced cardiac life support (ACLS) course 62, 229, 231-232, 233
advance directives 226
adverse event forms 229. *See also* documentation
AED (automatic external defibrillator) 231, 233
aerobic exercise training 182. *See also* cardiorespiratory endurance training
African Americans
   cardiovascular risk burden in 157*t*
   health care disparities in 156, 158
   hypertension in 108
   population of 156
   women 151
AHA. *See* American Heart Association
alcohol use
   assessment of 134
   hypertension and 107, 108*t*
   smoking cessation and 92

Algorithm for Assessment of Patient Willingness to Quit Smoking 254
allograft vasculopathy 179, 181, 183
alveolar gas diffusion impairment 181
American Association of Cardiovascular and Pulmonary Rehabilitation (AACVPR)
   Cardiac Rehabilitation Outcomes Matrix 212-214, 212*t*-213*t*
   on continuum of care 7
   core competencies 50-51, 51*f*, 194-199, 195*t*-198*t*
   facilities and equipment 200
   PAD Exercise Training Toolkit 188
   performance measures for referral 14-17, 14*t*-17*t*, 47-48, 194, 219
   program certification 17, 194, 210, 219-220
   program core components 8*t*-12*t*, 212-214, 212*t*-213*t*
   race of staff and patients 156
   registry of outcome data 223
American College of Cardiology (ACC)
   on heart failure stages 173*t*
   performance measures of 14, 15*t*
   on peripheral arterial disease exercise 188
   on smoking and tobacco 72*t*
American College of Sports Medicine (ACSM)
   ACSM's Guidelines for Exercise Testing and Prescription 164
   certification for exercise testing supervision 62
   on hypertension 74*t*
   on physical activity 74*t*
   on weight loss and body composition 75*t*
American Dietetic Association 74*t*, 75*t*
American Heart Association (AHA)
   on added sugars 35
   on AEDs 231
   on cholesterol intake 37
   on CPR and ECC 230
   on documenting emergencies 229
   on dyslipidemia and nutrition 73*t*
   on exercise testing supervision 62
   Get With the Guidelines 229
   on heart failure stages 173*t*
   performance measures of 14, 15*t*
   on peripheral arterial disease exercise 188

   on physical activity 75*t*
   recommendations of 37
   on secondary prevention 57
   on smoking and tobacco 72*t*
   Therapeutic Lifestyle Changes Diet 37, 37*t*
   translation of materials by 22-23
American Indians and American Natives (AI/AN) 157*t*
American Lung Association 72*t*
Americans with Disabilities Act (ADA) 201
anger, evaluation of 132
angina
   after heart transplant 181
   rating scale 66, 67, 257
   standing orders for chest pain 257-258
   during supervised exercise 226-227
   typical *versus* atypical 68
ankle–brachial index (ABI) 186
anti-inflammatory diet 35-36
antioxidants 35
anxiety 132, 134
aortic stenosis 163, 166
arhythmias. *See* dysrhythmias
arterial blood gases 190
arterial oxygenation, after transplantation 181
arthritis, claudication *versus* 186
Asian Americans 156, 157*t*
assessment, patient
   of activities of daily living 44, 63, 146
   baseline 42-47, 45, 169-170
   changes in patient conditions 226-228
   core competencies in 195*t*
   core components of 8*t*
   daily 45
   inpatient 42-47
   parameters for inpatient activity program 44
   of patient goals for rehabilitation 43
   preexercise, in patients with diabetes 123-124
   of tobacco use 90-92
asthma 190
atherosclerotic disease. *See also* peripheral arterial disease
   homocysteine and 141
   after revascularization 164-165
   secondary prevention of 79*t*
atherothrombosis 141-142

ATP III classifications 96-97, 100-102, 101*t*
atrial fibrillation 167, 170*t*. *See also* dysrhythmias
atrioventricular (AV) pacing 168
atropine 69
attendance, calculation of 219
audits, program 221
automatic external defibrillator (AED) 231, 233

B

behavior change theory 20, 198-199
behavior modification 19-29. *See also* tobacco cessation
  behavioral outcomes domain 212*t*-213*t*, 214-216, 217
  behavior change theory 20, 198-199
  individualization of 20-21
  outpatient services and 137
  positive cues in 28
  program guidelines for 21
  progress reports in 27
  rewards in 27-28
  role of knowledge in 21-23
  sample diagnosis and plan development 22
  self-efficacy and 23-24
  self-esteem and 23
  self-monitoring skills in 27
  S.M.A.R.T. goals in 26
  stages of change in 20, 24-26
  in weight loss 139, 139*t*
benchmarking program outcomes 222, 229
best practices, promotion of 3
beta-blockers 109
beverages, sweetened 35, 38
bile acid sequestrants 104-105
biventricular pacing 169
blood glucose monitoring 125-126, 127*t*, 128*t*, 129*t*, 130*t*
blood pressure management. *See also* hypertension
  core competencies in 196*t*
  core components of 9*t*
  goals in 79*t*, 109
  after heart transplantation 180
body composition 75*t*
body mass index (BMI) 138, 138*t*
bradycardia 259
breathing exercises 175, 191
bronchodilators 190
Bruce Protocol for treadmill testing 64, 64*t*, 65
buddy system 28
buprorion SR 94

C

CABG. *See* coronary artery bypass graft
CAD. *See* coronary artery disease
CAGE Questionnaire 92, 134, 253
carbohydrates 33-34, 38
cardiac arrest 228, 229, 256-257

Cardiac Arrest Registry to Enhance Survival 229
cardiac dysrhythmias. *See* dysrhythmias
cardiac output, in transplantation 180-181
Cardiac Rehabilitation Outcomes Matrix 212-214, 212*t*-213*t*
cardiac rehabilitation/secondary prevention programs. *See also* inpatient cardiac rehabilitation; outpatient cardiac rehabilitation/ secondary prevention
  benefits of 2, 17
  in continuum of care 6-8, 6*f*, 13-14, 17
  core components of 2-3, 8*t*-12*t*
  guidelines for secondary prevention in 3, 4
  home-based 154, 199, 232-233, 247-248
  Medicare provision for 2-3, 204-206, 221
  nontraditional 232-234
cardiac resynchronization therapy (CRT) 169
cardiac transplantation 179-185
  exercise testing and training after 183-185, 185*t*
  immunosuppression in 179, 180, 182
  inpatient exercise training after 184
  interventions after 182-183
  overview of 179-180
  psychological factors in 180
  responses to exercise after 180-182
cardiographic technician certification 62
cardiopulmonary exercise testing (CPX) 66-67, 190, 191. *See also* exercise testing
cardiopulmonary resuscitation (CPR)
  emergency standing orders for 256-257
  GWTG-R Code Sheet for 263-265
  LVAD patients and 179
  training in 230-231
cardiorespiratory endurance training (CRE). *See also* exercise training
  components of 115, 116*t*, 118-119
  dose–response relationship with outcomes 118
  in heart transplant patients 182
  for patients without a recent exercise test 116*t*, 119
  physical activity outside of rehabilitation and 119-120
  weight loss and 118-119
cardiorespiratory fitness (CRF) 109-111
cardiovascular disease risk
  assessment of 78, 79*t*
  diabetes and 123
  physical inactivity and 109-110
  racial and cultural diversity and 156-158, 157*t*
  risk factors in 43, 96-97, 141-142

supplements and 36
  in women 151
case management 77
Centers for Disease Control and Prevention (CDC) 74*t*
Centers for Medicare and Medicaid Services (CMS) 202, 204-205. *See also* Medicare
certification. *See also* accreditation
  cardiographic technician 62
  for exercise testing supervision (ACSM) 62
  program (AACVPR) 17, 194, 210, 219-220
chart review 42, 45
CHD. *See* coronary heart disease
chest pain, standing orders for 257-258
CHF (congestive heart failure) 45, 80. *See also* heart failure
cholesterol. *See also* lipid management; low-density lipoprotein cholesterol
  absorption inhibitors 105
  classification of lipoproteins 95, 96
  coronary heart disease and 95
  dietary intake of 37
  high-density lipoprotein 95, 97, 101*t*, 138*t*
  measurement of 95-96
  recommended levels of 97, 99*f*
  smoking and 90
chronic lung disease 189-191
chronic obstructive pulmonary disease (COPD) 189-191
chronic venous insufficiency 186
cilostazol 189
CLAS (National Standards for Culturally and Linguistically Appropriate Services) 159-160
claudication. *See also* peripheral arterial disease
  evaluation of 185-186
  intermittent 228
  pharmacologic treatment in 189
  rating scale 66, 67
clinical pathways 49-50, 49*t*, 51*t*
clinical review entries 235
CMS (Centers for Medicare and Medicaid Services) 202, 204-205
coaching approach 77
communication
  documentation of 205, 207
  in emergency planning 232-234
  reading ability and 22-23
community-site programs 233-234
completion rate 219
computer software 88
Conditions for Coverage (CfC) 202
Conditions of Participation (CoP) 202
confidentiality 238, 245
congestive heart failure (CHF) 45, 80. *See also* heart failure
consciousness raising 27
contemplation stage 24
Continuous Quality Improvement (CQI) 199

continuum of care 5-18
  core components in 8*t*-12*t*
  importance of 5
  organizational culture and 17-18
  program administration and 210
  reducing gaps in 13-17, 14*t*-17*t*
  role of cardiac rehabilitation in 17
  steps in 6-8, 6*f*
  in transitional care 54, 56
contracts, in behavior modification 28, 78
COPD (chronic obstructive pulmonary disease) 189-191
Core Competencies (AACVPR) 50-51, 51*f*, 194-200, 195*t*-198*t*
corneal arcus 96
coronary artery bypass graft (CABG)
  cardiac rehabilitation participation after 145*t*
  practice considerations for patients with 162-165
  sternal bone healing after 60
  in women 150
coronary artery disease (CAD) 96, 104-105, 157*t*
coronary heart disease (CHD)
  drug therapy for 105
  dyslipidemia and 95, 100*t*
  hypertension and 109
  insulin resistance and 100-102, 101*t*
  obesity and 137
  risk categories for 80, 98, 99*f*, 100*t*
  risk factors in 96-98
  treatment guidelines 103-105, 104*f*
  triglycerides and 95, 101*t*, 102-103, 102*t*
  in women 150-154, 151*t*, 152*t*, 153*t*
counselors
  home exercise parameters 179
  mental health 133-134, 135
  nutritional 8*t*
  physical activity 11*t*-12*t*, 198*t*
  spiritual needs 133
  substance abuse 135
  vocational rehabilitation 210
CPR. *See* cardiopulmonary resuscitation
CRE. *See* cardiorespiratory endurance training
C-reactive protein (CRP) 142
critical limb ischemia 186
CR/SP. *See* cardiac rehabilitation/secondary prevention programs
CR specialists 50, 51*f*, 51*t*
CR/SP Entry Clinical Review 235
cues, in behavior modification 28
cultural competency 158-160
cultural diversity. *See* racial and cultural diversity
cultural humility 159
cycle ergometers 63, 65, 65*t*, 186
cyclosporine 179

D

Daily Emergency Cart Checklist 266-267

Daily Exercise Record, Outpatient 245
Daily Exercise Session Report 244
DASH (Dietary Approaches to Stop Hypertension) diet 32, 108
data collection and management 220-221
defibrillators 231
denial 131
depression
  measurement of 92
  medications for 134
  in older patients 149
  risk stratification and 81, 228
  signs and symptoms of 132
  smoking cessation and 92
  in women 152, 153
diabetes and diabetes management 122-126. *See also* insulin resistance; Type 2 diabetes
  blood glucose monitoring in 124-126, 127*t*, 128*t*, 129*t*
  cardiovascular disease risk and 43*f*
  complications in 123
  core competencies in 197*t*
  core components of 10*t*
  exercise benefits and risks in 121-123
  exercise prescription in 124
  foot care in 124, 125-126
  hypoglycemia or hyperglycemia with exercise 227-228
  in minorities 157*t*
  nutrition and 33-34, 37
  in older patients 147*t*, 148
  in outcomes matrix 213*t*
  peripheral arterial disease and 185
  precautions for patients in 124-125
  preexercise assessment and testing in 123-124
  statements on 74*t*
  statistics on 122
  therapeutic goals in 79*t*
  Type 1 diabetes 122-123, 128*t*
Diabetes Prevention Program (DPP) 33
Dietary Guidelines for Americans (USDA) 35, 37-39, 107-108. *See also* nutrition
dietary supplements 36
digitalis therapy 82
dipyridamole 69
discharge planning 47-49, 47*f*, 55, 136
disease-specific approaches. *See* special populations
diuretics 109
dobutamine stress echocardiography (DSE) 69, 186-187
documentation
  CAGE questionnaire 92, 134, 253
  CR/SP Entry Clinical Review 235
  Daily Emergency Cart Checklist 266-267
  Daily Exercise Session Report 244
  Education Flow Sheet 246
  of emergencies 229, 261-265, 272
  Emergency Equipment Maintenance Log 271

Emergency Standing Orders 256-260
  Get With the Guidelines-Resuscitation Code Sheet 263-265
  Home Exercise Program 247-248
  individualized treatment plans 205, 206, 221
  informed consent for exercise rehabilitation 242-243
  informed consent for exercise testing 237-238
  Inpatient Rehabilitation Services Record 236
  intervention summaries 228-229
  Long-Term Outpatient Program Daily Exercise Record 245
  Mock Code and Emergency In-Service Log 272
  Monthly Emergency Cart Checklist 268-270
  of new symptoms during exercise 227-228
  for outcome analysis 221-222
  Physician Notification 261-262
  Quick Look Patient Record 241
  requirements for 205, 207, 221
  of resuscitation events 263-265
  screening before each session 227-228, 235
  Smoking History Questionnaire 249-252
  Standing Orders to Initiate Outpatient Cardiac Rehabilitation 255
Doppler arterial testing 186
dose–response relationship, of physical activity 110
drug therapy. *See* medications
dyslipidemia 95-105. *See also* lipid management
  causes of 96
  insulin resistance and metabolic syndrome in 100-102, 101*t*
  lipid classification 95-96, 97
  long-term follow-up 105
  in minorities 157*t*
  nutrition and 73*t*-74*t*, 98, 100
  in older patients 147*t*, 148
  risk factors in 96-98, 99*f*
  statistics on 95
  therapeutic lifestyle changes for 98-103, 100*t*, 104*f*
  treatment guidelines in 79*t*, 103-105, 104*f*
  triglycerides and 95, 101*t*, 102-103, 102*t*
dyspnea
  in chronic lung disease 189, 190
  emergency standing order for 259-260
  with exercise 45, 228, 259-260
  in heart failure 172, 173, 175, 176
  after heart transplantation 182
  in medical history and assessment 59, 228
  in mitral stenosis 166

dyspnea *(continued)*
  in outcomes analysis 220
  rating scale 66, 67, 202
  in revascularization patients 164
  in younger and older women 151*t*
dysrhythmias 166-170
  atrial fibrillation 167, 170*t*
  cardiac resynchronization therapy
    and 169
  emergency standing orders for 167,
    170*t*, 259
  factors associated with 167, 168*f*
  implantable cardioverter-defibrilla-
    tors and 168-169
  pacemakers and 167-168
  practice considerations in 169-170,
    170*t*-171*t*
  during supervised exercise 164, 166-
    167, 227

E
ECGs. *See* electrocardiograms
echocardiography 69, 186-187
ED (erectile dysfunction) 133
education. *See also* behavior modifi-
    cation
  of cardiac rehabilitation staff 207-208
  for clinical supervision during exer-
    cise 62, 82
  continuing, for health professionals
    51, 210
  Education Flow Sheet 246
  for emergencies 230-234
  for heart transplant patients 183
  inpatient 44*f*, 45-47, 55
  learning assessment tools 46-47
  for LVAD patients 178-179
  in maintenance programs 87
  for older adults 147
  outpatient 82, 83, 85-87, 134-135
  principles for patient 20-28, 83
  on psychosocial issues 134-135
  safety-related information 47
Education Flow Sheet 246
egg consumption 37
electrocardiograms (ECGs)
  in exercise testing 68-69
  in initial exams 59
  monitoring during exercise 80, 83, 85
  remote monitoring 232
  risk stratification and 82
emergency cardiac care (ECC) 230-231
emergency code forms 229
Emergency Equipment Maintenance
    Log 271
emergency planning
  advance directives 226
  for at-home services 232-233
  for community-site facilities 233-234
  Daily Emergency Cart Checklist
    266-267
  documentation of emergencies 229,
    261-265, 272
  Emergency Equipment Mainte-
    nance Log 271
  emergency plans 62, 83, 200, 201, 232

Emergency Standing Orders 256-260
  equipment and maintenance 230
  intervention summaries 228-229
  Mock Code and Emergency In-
    Service Log 272
  Monthly Emergency Cart Checklist
    268-270
  physician notification 261-364
  potential risks in programs 226-228
  site preparation 232
  staff training 230-232
  transportation of patients to hospi-
    tals 232, 260
emergency standing orders 256-260
  cardiopulmonary arrest/code 99
    256-257
  chest pain 257-258
  dyspnea 259-260
  dysrhythmias 167, 170*t*, 259
  hyperglycemia 258
  hypertension 258-259
  hypoglycemia 258
  hypotension 258
  intravenous line placement 260
  patient transportation 260
emotions 20, 131. *See also* psychosocial
    management
emphysema 190-191
energy balance–weight loss equation 139
enrollment, calculation of 219
equipment
  educational 52
  for emergencies 230, 268-270, 271
  general considerations for 201
  for inpatient rehabilitation 200
  maintenance of 230, 266-271
  for outpatient rehabilitation 201-202
erectile dysfunction (ED) 133
ethnic diversity. *See* racial and cultural
    diversity
ETHNIC model 158-159
European Atherosclerosis Society 73*t*
European Society of Cardiology 73*t*, 76
exercise. *See also* exercise testing; exer-
    cise training; physical activity
  adverse responses to 45, 228
  cardiac transplantation and 180-181
  clinical supervision during 82, 83, 85
  contraindications for 61, 62
  hypertension and 107
  physical activity *versus* 109
  readiness to change model and 26
  recommendations for 115
  risk stratification for 62, 69, 80-82,
    115, 228
  in smoking cessation 94
  in weight loss 140-141
exercise capacity 66-68
exercise intolerance 228
exercise physiologists 209
exercise specialists 208-209
exercise testing
  cardiopulmonary 66-67, 190, 191
  contraindications to 61-62
  controlled job simulation 70
  diabetes and 123-124

dysrhythmias and 170
facilities and equipment for 202
heart failure and 176
heart transplantation and 183-184
with imaging modalities 68-69
informed consent in 62, 237-238
interpretation of 67-68
interviews and questionnaires and 70
medications and 62
modality and protocols for 62-66,
    64*t*, 65*t*, 66*f*
in older adults 146
in outcomes matrix 212*t*
pharmacologic stress testing 69, 82,
    186-187
revascularization and 164, 165
safety in 62
6-minute walk test 58, 70, 239-240
symptom rating scales for 66-67
termination of 63
uses of 61-62
valve replacement and 166
exercise training. *See also* cardiore-
    spiratory endurance training;
    resistance training
cardiorespiratory endurance train-
    ing 115-120, 116*t*
chronic lung disease and 191
contraindications for 60-61
core components of 12*t*, 115, 116*t*,
    117*t*, 118-119
dose–response relationship with
    outcomes 118
dysrhythmias and 167-169
evaluation of 198*t*
flexibility training 117*t*, 121
heart failure and 173-175, 175*t*,
    177-178
heart transplantation and 182-183,
    184-185, 185*t*
in home settings 232-233, 247-248
informed consent in 242-243
LVAD and 177-178
for older adults 146-147, 146*t*
in outcomes matrix 212*t*
for patients without an exercise
    tolerance test 116*t*, 119
peripheral arterial disease and 188-
    189
physical activity outside of rehabili-
    tation and 119-120
progression of activity in 44-45, 45*t*
revascularization and 164, 165
valve replacement and 166
eye exams 96, 107

F
facilities and equipment 52-53, 53*f*,
    200-202
fats, dietary 33-34, 37*t*
fiber, dietary 38
fibrates 105
fibrinogen 142
fiscal accountability 3, 199-200
5 Rs of intervention 91
flexibility training 117*t*, 121

foot care 124, 125-126, 187
Functional Independence Measure 53

G

Gardner-Skinner protocol 187
genetic effects 33, 96
Geriatric Depression Questionnaire 149
Get With the Guidelines (AHA) 229,
    263-265
Get With the Guidelines-Resusci-
    tation (GWTG-R) Code Sheet
    263-265
GISSI study 36
glucose monitoring 125-126, 127t, 128t,
    129t, 130t
goals 26, 78, 79t
group means 221
group therapy 139

H

HDL-C. *See* high-density lipoprotein
    cholesterol
health and health care disparities
    155-162
    cardiovascular disease and 156,
        157t, 158
    cultural competency 158-159, 160
    definition of health disparities 155
    eliminating 159, 161
    ethnicity and 155-156
    resources on raising awareness 161
    studies on 156
Health Belief Model 20
Healthcare Provider BLS 231, 234
health educators 209
health insurance companies 204
health-related quality of life (HRQL)
    216-217
Healthy People 156
heart failure (HF)
    clinical manifestations of 172
    disability evaluation 173
    exercise training 173-175, 175t,
        177-178
    left ventricular assist devices 176-
        179, 177f
    in minorities 157t
    pathophysiology of 171-172, 172t
    practice considerations in 175-176,
        176t
    secondary prevention after 170-171
    during supervised exercise 227
HeartMate left ventricular assist
    devices 177f
heart rate (HR)
    in cardiac transplantation 180, 181,
        184
    daily assessment of 44, 45, 84, 227
    diabetes and 125, 130t
    ECG monitoring of 85
    heart transplantation and 180
    pacemakers and 168
    risk stratification and 81, 82
    target 247, 255
    tobacco use and 90
heart rate reserve 115, 119, 181

heart transplantation. *See* cardiac
    transplantation
heat shock protein 142
HF. *See* heart failure
HF-ACTION study 62, 174
Hiatt protocol 187
high-density lipoprotein cholesterol
    (HDL-C)
    measurement of 95
    in metabolic syndrome 101t, 138t
    recommended levels of 97
high-fructose corn syrup (HFCS) 34
high-sensitivity C-reactive protein
    (hs-CRP) 142
Hispanics 151, 155-156, 157t
HMG Co-A reductase inhibitors
    (statins) 96, 103-104, 104f
home-based secondary prevention
    154, 199, 232-233, 247-248
home health care 53-54, 53f, 232-233
homocysteine 96, 141
hostility, evaluation of 132
HRQL (health-related quality of life)
    216-217
hs-CRP (high-sensitivity C-reactive
    protein) 142
hyperglycemia
    blood glucose monitoring guidelines
        125-126
    care in 128t, 129t, 130t
    emergency standing orders for 258
    during supervised exercise 227-228
hypertension 106-109
    cardiovascular disease and 97
    drug therapy for 106t, 108-109
    emergency standing orders for 258-259
    guidelines on 74t, 79t
    lifestyle modifications in 107-108, 108t
    measurement and classification of
        106-107, 106t, 109
    in minorities 157t
    in older patients 147t, 148
    in outcomes matrix 213t
    pre- or postexercise 228
    pulmonary 190
    statistics on 106
hypoglycemia
    blood glucose monitoring guidelines
        125-126
    care in 127t, 128t
    emergency standing orders for 258
    signs and symptoms 130t
    during supervised exercise 227-228
hypotension, postexercise 227, 228, 258
hypoxemia 190

I

ICR (Intensive Cardiac Rehabilita-
    tion) 82-85, 194, 204-205
imaging, in exercise testing 68-69
immunosuppression, in transplanta-
    tion 179, 180, 182
implantable cardioverter-defibrillators
    (ICD) 168-169
incident reports 229. *See also* docu-
    mentation

individualized treatment plans (ITP)
    205, 206, 221
inflammation 35-36, 142
information management 203
informed consent
    in exercise rehabilitation 242-243
    in exercise testing 62, 237-238
initial patient assessment 42, 45, 169-170
inpatient cardiac rehabilitation
    (IPCR) 41-47. *See also* cardiac
    rehabilitation/secondary preven-
    tion programs
    admission criteria for 53, 53f
    adverse responses to 45
    clinical pathways 49-50, 49t, 51t
    components of 42, 67
    decreasing length of stay and 41
    discharge planning in 47-49, 47f, 55
    education program in 44, 45-47, 55
    facilities and equipment for 52-53,
        53f, 200
    heart transplantation and 184
    initial patient assessment in 42-47
    progression of activities in 44-45, 45t
    staffing in 50-51, 51t, 67-68
    transitional programming in 52-54,
        53f
inpatient rehabilitation facilities (IRF)
    52-53, 53f, 200
Inpatient Rehabilitation Services
    Record 236
Institute of Medicine (IOM)
    on dyslipidemia and nutrition 74t
    on racial and ethnic disparities 156,
        159
insulin resistance. *See also* diabetes
    coronary heart disease and 100-102,
        101t
    measurement of 33
    metabolic syndrome and 100-102, 101t
    nutrition and 33-34
    in older patients 147t, 148
    therapeutic goals on 79t
    treatment of 102
insurance and reimbursement 203-205
Intensive Cardiac Rehabilitation
    (ICR) 82-85, 194, 204-205
interleukin-6 142
intermittent claudication (IC). *See*
    claudication
International Physical Activity Ques-
    tionnaire (IPAQ) 111-113, 112f
Internet sites 120
interstitial fibrosis 190
interventions
    clinical problems requiring 227
    in heart transplant recipients 182-183
    intervention summaries 228-229
    in outpatient services 137
    for revascularization or valve
        patients 163
    risk factor guidelines 79t, 80
    for smoking cessation 46, 92-94,
        134-135
    for weight management 137-138
interviews 70, 91

intravenous line placement 260
intubation 231-232
IPAQ (International Physical Activity Questionnaire) 111-113, 112f
IPCR. See inpatient cardiac rehabilitation
ischemia
    as contraindication to exercise training 59, 60, 62
    critical limb 186, 228
    dysrhythmias and 169-170
    exercise testing and 58, 61, 67-68, 124
    heart transplantation and 181, 183
    imaging modalities and 69-70
    in outcomes analysis 198
    revascularization and 164-165
    risk stratification and 81, 226-227
    during supervised exercise 45, 226-227
    termination of exercise testing and 63
ITP (individualized treatment plans) 205, 206, 221

J

Jackson Heart Study 161
job simulation, controlled 70
Joint Commission (TJC) 202-203, 226

L

lapse and relapse stage 25
LDL-C. See low-density lipoprotein cholesterol
learning assessment tools 46-47
LEARN Model 158
left ventricular assist devices (LVAD) 176-179, 177f
left ventricular function, in transplantation 180
length of stay (LOS) 41
lipid management. See also dyslipidemia
    clinical evaluation 96
    core competencies in 196t
    core components of 9t-10t
    dietary guidelines for 73t-74t, 98, 100
    estimate of 10-year risk 99f
    insulin resistance and metabolic syndrome 100-102, 101t
    long-term follow-up in 105
    in minorities 157t
    in older patients 147t, 148
    in outcomes matrix 213t
    therapeutic lifestyle changes for 98-103, 100t, 104f
    treatment guidelines in 79t, 103-105, 104f
lipoprotein(a) (Lp(a)) 141-142
lipoproteins. See also low-density lipoprotein cholesterol
    classification of 95, 96
    high-density lipoprotein cholesterol 95, 97, 101t, 138t
    measurement of 95-96
    smoking and 90
LOS (length of stay) 41
low-carbohydrate diets 33-34
low-density lipoprotein cholesterol (LDL-C)

dietary supplements and 36
    measurement of 95
    in older patients 148
    recommended levels of 97, 100t, 148
    saturated fats and 34
    treatment of 103
low-fat diets 33-34
LVAD (left ventricular assist devices) 176-179, 177f

M

MACs (Medicare Administrative Contractors) 204
maintenance stage 25, 85-88
Making Health Communication Programs Work (NCI) 23
maximal oxygen uptake 66-67
medical director 62, 84, 207, 208
medical evaluation 58-60
medical history
    for hypertension 106-107
    for inpatient rehabilitation 58-59
    for outpatient rehabilitation 78
    smoking history 91-92, 249-252
Medicare
    on cardiac rehabilitation 2-3, 204-206
    coverage by 204
    documentation for 205, 221
    on health care providers 202, 208
    on heart transplant patients 184
    on Intensive Cardiac Rehabilitation 82-85, 194, 204-205
    on transitional care 54
Medicare Administrative Contractors (MACs) 204
medications
    in chronic lung disease 190
    exercise testing and 62
    in hypertension 106t, 108-109
    in lipid management 103-105, 104f
    in peripheral arterial disease 189
    psychotropic 134
    in smoking cessation 93, 94-95
Mediterranean diet 32, 35
men 145t, 149
mental health professionals 133-134, 135, 137, 209
metabolic equivalents (METs) 111, 118-119
metabolic syndrome
    diagnosis of 100-102, 101t, 138-139, 138t
    insulin resistance in 33, 100, 102
    in older patients 148
    treatment of 102, 137
MI (myocardial infarction) 145t, 150
MI FREEE trial 2
minimally invasive coronary bypass (MID-CAB) 162-165
Minnesota Living with Heart Failure Questionnaire 174
minorities. See racial and cultural diversity
Missing Persons: Minorities in the Health Profession 156

Mock Code and Emergency In-Service Log 272
Monthly Emergency Cart Checklist 268-270
motivational interviews 91
Multi-Ethnic Study of Atherosclerosis (MESA) 161
muscle structure, after transplantation 181
muscular strength 120-121
myocardial infarction (MI) 145t, 150
MyPlate 37, 38-39

N

National Cholesterol Education Program (NCEP)
    on egg consumption 37
    on low-density lipoprotein-cholesterol 96-97
    older patients and 148
    risk estimates 99f
    treatment guidelines 100t, 103-105, 104f
National Health and Nutrition Examination Survey (NHANES) 34
National Institutes of Health (NIH) 159, 161
National Registry of Cardiopulmonary Resuscitation 229
National Standards for Culturally and Linguistically Appropriate Services (CLAS) 159-160
Native Americans 157t
NCEP. See National Cholesterol Education Program
negative predictive value 68
neuropathy, peripheral 124-126
New York Heart Association (NYHA) function classes 172
niacin 105
nicotine 90. See also tobacco use
nicotine replacement therapy 94
NIH (National Institutes of Health) 159, 161
nuclear imaging, in exercise testing 69
nuclear perfusion imaging 69
nuclear scintigraphy 69, 186-187
nurses 208
Nurses' Health Study 37
nutrient density 34
nutrition 31-39
    AHA recommendations 35, 37
    dietary patterns 32
    dietary supplements 36
    diets, specific 32, 35-36, 37, 37t
    for dyslipidemia 98, 100
    egg consumption 37
    fat *versus* sugar intake 34-35
    hypertension and 107-108, 108t
    low carbohydrate *versus* low fat diets 33-34
    nutritional counseling 8t, 195t
    in obesity and weight control 32-34, 140
    for older patients 148

statements on 73t-74t
U.S. Dietary Guidelines 35, 37-39, 73t

O

obesity
  classification of 138-139, 138t
  energy balance–weight loss equation 139
  health effects of 137-138
  in minorities 156, 157t
  nutrition guidelines in 33-34
  in older patients 147t, 148
  rising rates of 32-33, 156
  sugar and fructose consumption and 34
  therapeutic goals for 79t
  in women 151, 151t
occupational therapists 209
Office of the Surgeon General 72t
older patients 144-149
  baseline evaluation of 145-146
  diabetes in 147t, 148
  dyslipidemia in 147t, 148
  education of 147
  exercise training by 146-147, 146t
  health disparities in 158
  hypertension in 108, 147t, 148
  obesity in 147t, 148
  participation rate of 144-145, 145t
  physical activity by 147t, 148-149
  psychosocial dysfunction in 147t, 149
  after revascularization 164
  secondary prevention in 147-149, 147t
  smoking cessation by 147t, 149
omega 3-acid ethyl esters 105
omega-3 fats 34, 35, 36, 37
one-repetition maximum (1RM) 121
organizational policies and procedures 202-203. See also program administration
outcomes 211-223
  behavioral outcomes domain 212t-213t, 214-216, 217
  benchmarking 222
  Cardiac Rehabilitation Outcomes Matrix 212-214, 212t-213t
  clinical outcomes domain 212t-213t, 214, 215
  data analysis 221-222
  data collection and management 220-221
  documentation and reporting of 221-222
  health outcomes domain 212t-213t, 216-217
  national registries 221, 222-223
  performance measures versus 218
  purposes for measuring 218-220
  Quality Improvement and 222-223
  service outcomes domain 212t, 218
outcomes-based programming 194
outpatient cardiac rehabilitation/ secondary prevention 71-88.
  See also cardiac rehabilitation/ secondary prevention programs

clinical supervision during exercise 82, 83, 85, 86
coaching and case management 77
core components of 76, 212-214, 212t-213t
daily risk assessment 84
early outpatient exercise program 82
ECG monitoring in 85, 86
facilities and equipment for 201-202
implementation of 88
innovation in 85
intensive cardiac rehabilitation in 82-85, 194, 204-205
maintenance phase 25, 85-88
physician roles in 84
practice guideline documents for 72-76, 72t-75t
publication requirement for programs 84-85
reducing complications during exercise 83
risk factor assessment and management 77-78, 79t
risk stratification for cardiac events in exercise 80-82, 86, 115, 226
secondary prevention program structure in 76-77
statistics on 75-76
outpatient education 82, 83, 85, 86, 87
outpatient services 137
overweight 138-139, 138t. See also obesity
oxygen extraction, after transplantation 181
oxygen therapy 190-191
oxygen uptake, after transplantation 181, 182

P

pacemakers 167-168
Pacific Islanders 157t
PAD. See peripheral arterial disease
PAD Exercise Training Toolkit: A Guide for Health Care Professionals 188
PAD Physical Activity Recall Questionnaire 186
Patient Health Questionnaire 149, 152
patient records 200, 203, 241
PDSA (Plan-Do-Study-Act) model 222-223
peak oxygen uptake, after transplantation 181
pedometers 120
pentoxifylline 189
percentage change calculations 221
percutaneous transluminal coronary angioplasty (PCI) 162, 163, 165
performance measures
  applying 194
  development of 14, 17
  in discharge planning 47-48
  examples of calculations 218, 219
  outcomes versus 14, 218
  referral from inpatient setting 14t-15t
  referral from outpatient setting 16t-17t
  service outcomes domain 212t, 218

performance review, of staff 210
pericardial effusions 164
peripheral arterial disease (PAD) 185-189
  claudication evaluation 185-186
  diagnosing 186
  exercise prescription 188-189
  patient assessments 186-187
  pharmacologic treatment 189
  practice considerations 187-188, 189
  risk factors in 187
personnel 207-210
  in cardiac rehabilitation and secondary prevention 84
  at community-site facilities 233-234
  emergency training of 230-232
  exercise physiologists 209
  exercise specialists 208-209
  in exercise testing supervision 62
  health educators 209
  knowledge and technical skills of 207-208
  medical director 62, 84, 207, 208
  mental health professionals 133-134, 135, 137, 209
  need for minority 156
  occupation therapists 210
  physical therapists 209
  program director 208
  registered dietitians 209
  registered nurses 208
  respiratory therapists 209
  staff education and performance review 210
  vocational rehabilitation counselors 210
pharmacologic stress testing 69, 82, 186-187
pharmacologic therapy. See medications
physical activity. See also exercise
  assessment of 111-114, 112f, 113f, 114f
  counseling 11t-12t, 198t
  dose–response relationship with health 118
  exercise versus 109
  hypertension and 108t
  inactivity as risk factor 109-111
  lifestyle activity 141
  by older patients 147t, 148-149
  outside of cardiac rehabilitation 119-120
  recommendations for 110, 111, 115
  statements on 74t-75t
  statistics on 109
  therapeutic goals for 79t
  after valve repair or replacement 166
  in weight loss 140-141
Physical Activity Guidelines for Americans, 2008 111
physical examination 59-60
physical therapists 209, 232-233
physician notification of untoward event 261-262
physicians 84, 261-262
Physicians' Health Study 37

Plan-Do-Study-Act (PDSA) model 222-223
plant-based diet 32. *See also* nutrition
pleural effusions 164
policies and procedures, organizational 202-203. *See also* program administration
positive predictive value 68
posttraumatic stress disorder (PTSD) 132
PRECEDE Model 214
precontemplation stage 24
prednisone 180, 182
premature ventricular complexes (PVCs) 167, 171t, 259
preparation stage 25
processes *versus* systems 218
program administration 193-210. *See also* performance measures
  alternative rehabilitation delivery models 195, 198-199
  Continuous Quality Improvement 199
  continuum of care and services 210
  core competencies 195t-198t
  documentation 205, 207
  facilities and equipment 200-202
  fiscal accountability 3, 199-200
  information management 203
  insurance and reimbursement 203-205
  maximizing program utilization 194
  organizational policies and procedures 202-203
  outcomes-based programming 194
  personnel 207-210
  program comprehensiveness 194
  program priorities 194-200, 195t-198t
  staff education and performance review 210
program director 208
program utilization, maximizing 194
progress reports, in behavior modification 27
prompts, in behavior modification 28
Protection Motivation Theory 20
prudent diet 32, 35. *See also* nutrition
psychosocial management. *See also* counselors; education; interventions
  adherence and 87-88, 134
  assessments in 130-131
  in cardiac transplantation 180
  core competencies in 197t
  core components of 11t
  discharge planning 47-49, 47f, 55, 136
  evaluation of 131-133
  after heart transplantation 183
  medications in 134
  in older patients 147t, 149
  in outcomes matrix 213t
  relaxation training in 133, 135
  social support in 28, 133, 135, 154
  specialized consultation in 134
  spiritual needs and counseling in 133
  stress management in 108, 132, 133, 135, 137

tobacco and alcohol in 134
in women 152, 152t
PTSD (posttraumatic stress disorder) 132
pulmonary ventilation, after transplantation 181
PVCs (premature ventricular complexes) 167, 171t, 259

Q
Quality Improvement (QI) 222-223
quality of life 216-217
questionnaires
  outcome data from 220, 223
  physical activity assessment by 111, 112f
  on smoking history 249-252
Quick Look Patient Record 241
quit lines, in smoking cessation 94

R
racial and cultural diversity 154-162
  cardiac rehabilitation participation and 145t
  cardiovascular risk burden and 156-158, 157t
  culturally competent care and 158-160
  eliminating health care disparities 159, 161
  health disparities and 155, 156, 159, 161
  historical perspective on disparities 156
  resources in raising awareness 161
  statistics on 155-156, 155f
rate-responsive pacing 168
rating scales
  angina 66, 67, 257
  claudication 66, 67
  dyspnea 66, 67
ratings of perceived exertion (RPE) 115, 120, 146, 178
readiness to change 24-26
reading ability 22-23
record keeping 200
referrals. *See* performance measures
registered dietitians 209
registered nurses 208
registries, participation in 221
relapse 25, 93-94
relative risk 110
relaxation training 133, 135
religious needs and counseling 133
REMATCH 176
remote ECG monitoring 232
resistance training
  benefits of 120
  components of 117t
  in heart failure patients 175, 178
  in heart transplant recipients 182, 184
  in LVAD patients 178
  in older adults 146, 146t
  in outcomes matrix 213t
  in peripheral arterial disease 188-189
  after revascularization 164, 165
  strength assessment in 121

respiratory arrest 228
respiratory therapists 209
resting electrocardiogram 59
revascularization
  in coronary artery bypass graft 162-165
  in percutaneous transluminal coronary angioplasty 163, 165
  in peripheral arterial disease 189
  statistics on 162
rewards, in behavior change 27-28
risk factors 89-143. *See also* diabetes; dyslipidemia; hypertension; interventions; obesity; tobacco use
  assessment and management of 77-78, 79t
  in cardiovascular disease 43, 96-97, 141-142
  in coronary heart disease 96-98
  C-reactive protein as 142
  in dyslipidemia 96-98, 99f
  homocysteine as 96, 141
  inactivity as 109-111
  intervention guidelines and 79t, 80
  lipoprotein(a) as 141-142
  in peripheral arterial disease (PAD) 187
  psychosocial 130-133
risk reduction. *See* behavior modification
risk stratification
  in cardiac or respiratory arrest 228
  in exercise planning 81, 115, 226
  in exercise testing 62, 69
  model of 80-82
  for therapeutic lifestyle changes 98-100, 100t
role models 28
RPE (ratings of perceived exertion) 115, 120, 146, 178

S
safety. *See also* emergency planning
  clinical supervision during exercise 82, 83, 85
  in exercise planning 115
  in exercise testing 62
  facilities and equipment and 200-201
  in heart failure patients 176t
  in heart transplant patients 184
  inpatient education on 47
  intervention summaries 228-229
  in LVAD patients 178-179
  potential risks in programs 226-228
  statistics on 226
saturated fats 34
secondary prevention. *See also* outpatient cardiac rehabilitation/secondary prevention
  atherosclerotic disease and 79t, 164-165
  in home settings 232-233, 247-248
  hypertension and 107
  implementation of 88
  importance of 2, 3, 4
  initiation of 6

in older cardiac patients 147-149, 147*t*
outpatient services 137
smoking and 72*t*
structure of 76-77
"Secondary Prevention and Risk Reduction Therapy for Patients with Coronary and Other Atherosclerotic Vascular Disease" 3-4
selective serotonin reuptake inhibitors (SSRIs) 134
self-efficacy 23-24, 212*t*
self-esteem 23
self-monitoring skills 27
sensitivity, in exercise testing 68
service outcomes domain 212*t*, 218
sexual dysfunction and adjustment 133, 137
SF-36 Healthy Survey 152
sICAM-1 (soluble intercellular adhesion molecule type 1) 142
sitting time 109-110, 149
6-minute walk test (6MWT) 58, 70, 239-240
skilled nursing facilities (SNFs) 53, 53*f*
skin assessment, in peripheral artery disease 187
S.M.A.R.T. goals 26
smoking. *See* tobacco use
smoking cessation. *See* tobacco cessation
smoking history 91-92, 249-252
social economic status (SES), health disparities and 158
socialization, for older adults 147
social networks 28
social support
    in behavior modification 28
    in cardiac rehabilitation/secondary prevention programs 133, 135
    for women 154
sodium reduction 107-108, 108*t*
soluble intercellular adhesion molecule type 1 (sICAM-1) 142
space requirements 200
special populations 143-191
    cardiac transplantation 179-185, 185*t*
    chronic lung disease 189-191
    dysrhythmias 166-170, 168*f*, 170*t*-171*t*
    guidelines for 144
    heart failure and left ventricular assist devices 170-179, 172*t*, 173*t*, 175*t*, 176*t*, 177*f*
    older patients 144-149, 145*t*, 146*t*, 147*t*
    peripheral arterial disease 185-189
    racial and cultural diversity 145*t*, 154-162, 155*f*, 157*t*
    revascularization and valve surgery 162-166
    women 145*t*, 150-154, 152*t*, 153*t*, 154*t*, 158
    younger patients 149
specificity, in exercise testing 68
spiritual needs and counseling 133
SSRIs (selective serotonin reuptake inhibitors) 134
stages of change 20, 24-26

standing orders. *See* emergency standing orders
Standing Orders to Initiate Outpatient Cardiac Rehabilitation 255
stanol esters 36
strength training. *See* resistance training
stress management
    general strategies in 137
    hypertension and 108
    lapse and relapse and 25
    posttraumatic stress disorder 132
    relaxation training in 133, 135
stress testing. *See* exercise testing
Strong Heart Study 161
sugar intake 34-35, 38
supervising physicians 84
survival skills 48
symptom rating scales 66-67
syncope or near-syncope 228
systems *versus* processes 218

T
tachycardia 259
telemedicine 204
theophylline 190
Theory of Reasoned Action/Planned Behavior 20
Therapeutic Lifestyle Changes (TLC) 37*t*, 98-103, 104*f*. *See also* lipid management
thromboembolic disease 189
TJC (Joint Commission) 202-203, 226
tobacco cessation
    action stage of 25
    alcohol use and 92
    algorithm for assessment of willingness 254
    core competencies in 197*t*
    core components of 11*t*
    education in 135-136
    health benefits of 90
    intervention for inpatients 46
    intervention for outpatients 92-94
    motivational interviews in 91
    by older patients 147*t*, 149
    in outcomes matrix 213*t*
    pharmacologic therapy 93, 94-95
tobacco use 90-95. *See also* tobacco cessation
    assessment of 90-92, 134
    health effects of 90
    history of 91-92, 249-252
    in minorities 157*t*
    statements on 72*t*
    therapeutic goals on 79*t*
trans fats 34
transitional planning 47-49, 47*f*, 52-54, 53*f*
transplantation. *See* cardiac transplantation
transportation of patients to hospitals 232, 260
Transtheoretical Model (TTM) 20
treadmill ergometers 63-66, 64*t*, 187
trend graphs 27
triglycerides 95, 101*t*, 102-103, 102*t*

Type 1 diabetes 122-123, 128*t*. *See also* diabetes and diabetes management
Type 2 diabetes. *See also* diabetes and diabetes management
    exercise benefits in 122
    health effects of 122
    hyperglycemia care in 129*t*
    monitoring during exercise 227-228
    in older patients 147*t*, 148
type D personality pattern 132

U
Unequal Treatment: Confronting Racial and Ethnic Disparities in Health Care 156
United States Department of Agriculture (USDA)
    Dietary Guidelines for Americans 35, 37-39
    on dyslipidemia and nutrition 73*t*
    MyPlate 37, 38-39
unsaturated fats 34
"usual care" 76
Utstein guidelines 229

V
valvular heart disease (VHD) 163, 165-166
varenicline 94
vocational rehabilitation counselors 210

W
waist circumference measurements 138, 138*t*
Walking Impairment Questionnaire 186
weekly logs 120
weight management
    behavioral modification in 139, 139*t*
    core competencies in 196*t*
    core components of 9*t*
    in CR/SP programs 137-138
    dietary guidelines for 32-34, 140
    energy balance–weight loss equation 139
    exercise and physical activity in 118-119, 140-141
    hypertension and 108*t*
    identifying overweight patients 138-139, 138*t*
    individual factors in 33
    insulin resistance and 33-34
    in outcomes matrix 213*t*
    statements on 75*t*
whites, cardiovascular risk burden in 157*t*
whole grains 38
women 150-154
    health care disparities in 158
    program participation by 145*t*, 152-153, 153*t*
    program tailoring for 153-154, 154*t*
    psychosocial considerations for 152, 152*t*
    younger 149

Y
younger patients 149

About the AACVPR

The **American Association of Cardiovascular and Pulmonary Rehabilitation (AACVPR)** is the worldwide leader in promoting the value and practice of cardiovascular and pulmonary rehabilitation. AACVPR's mission is improving the quality of life for patients and their families by reducing morbidity, mortality, and disability from cardiovascular and pulmonary diseases through education, prevention, rehabilitation, research, and aggressive disease management.

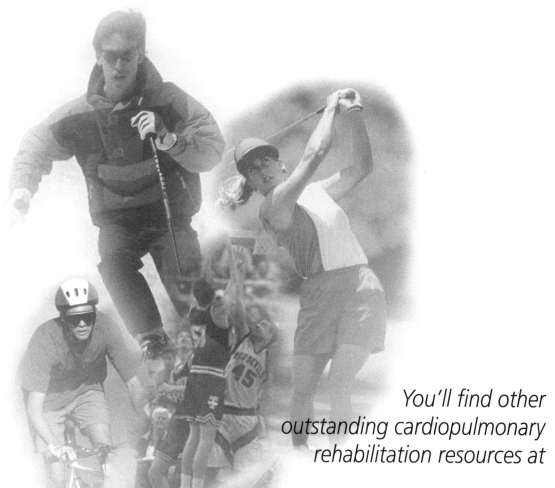

You'll find other outstanding cardiopulmonary rehabilitation resources at

www.HumanKinetics.com

In the U.S. call

1-800-747-4457

Australia	08 8372 0999
Canada	1-800-465-7301
Europe	+44 (0) 113 255 5665
New Zealand	0800 222 062

HUMAN KINETICS
The Information Leader in Physical Activity & Health
P.O. Box 5076 • Champaign, IL 61825-5076 USA